Praise for *Women's Health For Dummies*

"*Women's Health For Dummies* is one smart book. It's brimming with up-to-date information that all women can use to take better charge of their own health. Best of all, the book isn't patronizing or frightening. It reads instead like an invitation to better health, which is a lot harder to turn down!"

> — Madge Kaplan, Health Desk Editor for public radio's night business show *Marketplace*

"*Women's Health For Dummies* helps the reader to understand — and conquer — whatever ails her. A useful guide to everything from depression to nutrition and pregnancy to breast cancer, this book helps the reader take charge of her health and her health care."

> — Lori Andrews, Professor of Health Law at Chicago-Kent College of Law and Author of *The Clone Age: Adventures in the New World of Reproduction Technologies*

Praise for *Men's Health For Dummies*

"No matter how take-charge they think they are, most men don't take much charge of their health. Now, thanks to Charles Inlander's *Men's Health For Dummies,* every man can take charge of his body, mind, and health. A must-read if you care at all about feeling well and staying well."

> — Ted David, CNBC Network Anchor

"A smart read! Translating the newest medical discoveries into plain and fun-to-read English, Inlander tells men how to *get* healthy and how to *stay* healthy. If you want to reach your maximum potential physically and mentally, this is the resource you need."

> — Sydney Walker III, M.D., Director, Southern California Neuropsychiatric Institute

"We men worry a lot about 'fitness,' but far less about what it takes for real health. Charles Inlander has boiled down tons of information to give us simple, easy to read rules that can make us fitter and healthier."

> — Victor Cohn, former Science Editor *The Washington Post* and Author of *News & Numbers: A Guide to Reporting Scientific Claims and Controversies in Health and Other Fields*

"Charlie cuts right to the chase. You will get the essential health information you need clearly and concisely."

— Joe Graedon, Pharmacologist, Author of the bestselling *People's Pharmacy* books

"With baby boomers aging and health costs rising, one of the most important tasks we face as a society is to persuade people to live healthier lives. This book gives men straightforward, basic advice on how to do that. I recommend it to men of all ages who want to be active and healthy well into their senior years."

— Steven Findlay, Health Policy Analyst, National Coalition of Health Care

"This book is an excellent and direct approach to achieving and maintaining positive health status and possibly an excellent way to improving one's quality of life."

— J. Lyle Bootman, Ph.D. Dean and Professor, University of Arizona Health Sciences Center and Executive Director, Health Outcomes & Pharmacoeconomics Center (HOPE)

Praise for Family Health For Dummies

"Once or twice in a century, the paths of medical science, common sense, and clarity intersect. *Family Health For Dummies* has captured all three. A lightning strike of useful and healthy information."

— Dr. Philip P. Gerbino, President, University of the Sciences in Philadelphia

"In my lectures as President of the UCLA Center on Aging, I often say 'you can't turn the clock back — but you *can* rewind it!' That's what my friend Charles Inlander is all about in this practical guide to living *better*, longer."

— Art Linkletter, Author, Entertainer, TV Star, and President of the UCLA Center on Aging

"This book is priceless! It covers the ABCs of almost every family health question. Next to living in perfect health yourself comes the wonderful knowledge of what to do and not to do in any emergency. Read it before you need it!"

— Bonnie Prudden, Bonnie Prudden School and Pain Erasure Clinic

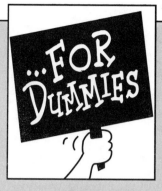 ™

References for the Rest of Us!™

BESTSELLING BOOK SERIES

Do you find that traditional reference books are overloaded with technical details and advice you'll never use? Do you postpone important life decisions because you just don't want to deal with them? Then our *...For Dummies*® business and general reference book series is for you.

...For Dummies business and general reference books are written for those frustrated and hard-working souls who know they aren't dumb, but find that the myriad of personal and business issues and the accompanying horror stories make them feel helpless. *...For Dummies* books use a lighthearted approach, a down-to-earth style, and even cartoons and humorous icons to dispel fears and build confidence. Lighthearted but not lightweight, these books are perfect survival guides to solve your everyday personal and business problems.

> *"More than a publishing phenomenon, 'Dummies' is a sign of the times."*
>
> — The New York Times

> *"A world of detailed and authoritative information is packed into them..."*
>
> — U.S. News and World Report

> *"...you won't go wrong buying them."*
>
> — Walter Mossberg, Wall Street Journal, on IDG Books' ...For Dummies books

Already, millions of satisfied readers agree. They have made *...For Dummies* the #1 introductory level computer book series and a best-selling business book series. They have written asking for more. So, if you're looking for the best and easiest way to learn about business and other general reference topics, look to *...For Dummies* to give you a helping hand.

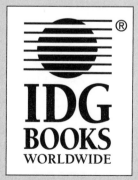

1/99

WOMEN'S
HEALTH
FOR
DUMMIES®

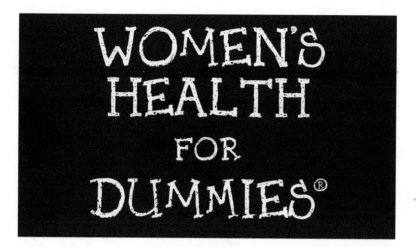

WOMEN'S HEALTH FOR DUMMIES®

by Pamela Maraldo and The People's Medical Society

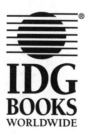

IDG Books Worldwide, Inc.
An International Data Group Company

Foster City, CA ♦ Chicago, IL ♦ Indianapolis, IN ♦ New York, NY

Women's Health For Dummies®

Published by
IDG Books Worldwide, Inc.
An International Data Group Company
919 E. Hillsdale Blvd.
Suite 400
Foster City, CA 94404
www.idgbooks.com (IDG Books Worldwide Web site)
www.dummies.com (Dummies Press Web site)

Library of Congress Catalog Card No.: 99-61118

ISBN: 0-7645-5119-1

Printed in the United States of America

10 9 8 7 6 5 4 3 2 1

1B/RS/QT/ZZ/IN

Distributed in the United States by IDG Books Worldwide, Inc.

Distributed by CDG Books Canada Inc. for Canada; by Transworld Publishers Limited in the United Kingdom; by IDG Norge Books for Norway; by IDG Sweden Books for Sweden; by Woodslane Pty. Ltd. for Australia; by Woodslane (NZ) Ltd. for New Zealand; by TransQuest Publishers Pte Ltd. for Singapore, Malaysia, Thailand, Indonesia, and Hong Kong; by ICG Muse, Inc. for Japan; by Norma Comunicaciones S.A. for Colombia; by Intersoft for South Africa; by Le Monde en Tique for France; by International Thomson Publishing for Germany, Austria and Switzerland; by Distribuidora Cuspide for Argentina; by Livraria Cultura for Brazil; by Ediciones ZETA S.C.R. Ltda. for Peru; by WS Computer Publishing Corporation, Inc., for the Philippines; by Contemporanea de Ediciones for Venezuela; by Express Computer Distributors for the Caribbean and West Indies; by Micronesia Media Distributor, Inc. for Micronesia; by Grupo Editorial Norma S.A. for Guatemala; by Chips Computadoras S.A. de C.V. for Mexico; by Editorial Norma de Panama S.A. for Panama; by American Bookshops for Finland. Authorized Sales Agent: Anthony Rudkin Associates for the Middle East and North Africa.

For general information on IDG Books Worldwide's books in the U.S., please call our Consumer Customer Service department at 800-762-2974. For reseller information, including discounts and premium sales, please call our Reseller Customer Service department at 800-434-3422.

For information on where to purchase IDG Books Worldwide's books outside the U.S., please contact our International Sales department at 317-596-5530 or fax 317-596-5692.

For consumer information on foreign language translations, please contact our Customer Service department at 1-800-434-3422, fax 317-596-5692, or e-mail rights@idgbooks.com.

For information on licensing foreign or domestic rights, please phone +1-650-655-3109.

For sales inquiries and special prices for bulk quantities, please contact our Sales department at 650-655-3200 or write to the address above.

For information on using IDG Books Worldwide's books in the classroom or for ordering examination copies, please contact our Educational Sales department at 800-434-2086 or fax 317-596-5499.

For press review copies, author interviews, or other publicity information, please contact our Public Relations department at 650-655-3000 or fax 650-655-3299.

For authorization to photocopy items for corporate, personal, or educational use, please contact Copyright Clearance Center, 222 Rosewood Drive, Danvers, MA 01923, or fax 978-750-4470.

About the Author

Pamela Maraldo, Ph.D., R.N., chairperson of the board of the People's Medical Society, is one of the nation's foremost women's health advocates. She is a professor of nursing at the Columbia School of Nursing and has appeared on numerous radio and television programs, including *Talk of the Nation* and the *McLaughlin Special Report*.

The People's Medical Society is the nation's largest nonprofit consumer health organization. Its mission is to provide consumers with up-to-date health information from health care professionals and the latest medical research. Its health care experts have published more than 70 health titles and are frequently seen on such television programs as *Oprah, Today,* and *Good Morning America*.

ABOUT IDG BOOKS WORLDWIDE

Welcome to the world of IDG Books Worldwide.

IDG Books Worldwide, Inc., is a subsidiary of International Data Group, the world's largest publisher of computer-related information and the leading global provider of information services on information technology. IDG was founded more than 30 years ago by Patrick J. McGovern and now employs more than 9,000 people worldwide. IDG publishes more than 290 computer publications in over 75 countries. More than 90 million people read one or more IDG publications each month.

Launched in 1990, IDG Books Worldwide is today the #1 publisher of best-selling computer books in the United States. We are proud to have received eight awards from the Computer Press Association in recognition of editorial excellence and three from Computer Currents' First Annual Readers' Choice Awards. Our best-selling ...For Dummies® series has more than 50 million copies in print with translations in 31 languages. IDG Books Worldwide, through a joint venture with IDG's Hi-Tech Beijing, became the first U.S. publisher to publish a computer book in the People's Republic of China. In record time, IDG Books Worldwide has become the first choice for millions of readers around the world who want to learn how to better manage their businesses.

Our mission is simple: Every one of our books is designed to bring extra value and skill-building instructions to the reader. Our books are written by experts who understand and care about our readers. The knowledge base of our editorial staff comes from years of experience in publishing, education, and journalism — experience we use to produce books to carry us into the new millennium. In short, we care about books, so we attract the best people. We devote special attention to details such as audience, interior design, use of icons, and illustrations. And because we use an efficient process of authoring, editing, and desktop publishing our books electronically, we can spend more time ensuring superior content and less time on the technicalities of making books.

You can count on our commitment to deliver high-quality books at competitive prices on topics you want to read about. At IDG Books Worldwide, we continue in the IDG tradition of delivering quality for more than 30 years. You'll find no better book on a subject than one from IDG Books Worldwide.

IDG BOOKS WORLDWIDE

John Kilcullen
Chairman and CEO
IDG Books Worldwide, Inc.

Steven Berkowitz
President and Publisher
IDG Books Worldwide, Inc.

*Eighth Annual
Computer Press
Awards ➤1992*

*Ninth Annual
Computer Press
Awards ➤1993*

*Tenth Annual
Computer Press
Awards ➤1994*

*Eleventh Annual
Computer Press
Awards ➤1995*

IDG is the world's leading IT media, research and exposition company. Founded in 1964, IDG had 1997 revenues of $2.05 billion and has more than 9,000 employees worldwide. IDG offers the widest range of media options that reach IT buyers in 75 countries representing 95% of worldwide IT spending. IDG's diverse product and services portfolio spans six key areas including print publishing, online publishing, expositions and conferences, market research, education and training, and global marketing services. More than 90 million people read one or more of IDG's 290 magazines and newspapers, including IDG's leading global brands — Computerworld, PC World, Network World, Macworld and the Channel World family of publications. IDG Books Worldwide is one of the fastest-growing computer book publishers in the world, with more than 700 titles in 36 languages. The "...For Dummies®" series alone has more than 50 million copies in print. IDG offers online users the largest network of technology-specific Web sites around the world through IDG.net (http://www.idg.net), which comprises more than 225 targeted Web sites in 55 countries worldwide. International Data Corporation (IDC) is the world's largest provider of information technology data, analysis and consulting, with research centers in over 41 countries and more than 400 research analysts worldwide. IDG World Expo is a leading producer of more than 168 globally branded conferences and expositions in 35 countries including E3 (Electronic Entertainment Expo), Macworld Expo, ComNet, Windows World Expo, ICE (Internet Commerce Expo), Agenda, DEMO, and Spotlight. IDG's training subsidiary, ExecuTrain, is the world's largest computer training company, with more than 230 locations worldwide and 785 training courses. IDG Marketing Services helps industry-leading IT companies build international brand recognition by developing global integrated marketing programs via IDG's print, online and exposition products worldwide. Further information about the company can be found at www.idg.com. 1/24/99

Author's Acknowledgments

Books of this magnitude are never written alone. And this book was no exception. Many talented people have helped craft and create this volume. Each of them has my utmost respect and gratitude.

My list of thank yous begins with Jennifer Hay, who served as the editorial project manager for the People's Medical Society. Jen oversaw every aspect of this book, from contributing text to editing it. She did a whale of a job keeping everything on track and in focus. There would be no book without her.

And she was not alone at the People's Medical Society. Special thanks to Director of Projects Michael Donio, Vice President for Editorial Services Karla Morales, Editorial Project Manager Annette Doran, and President Charles B. Inlander. Each played a major role in making this book possible.

Our literary agent Gail Ross deserves our sincere thanks for helping to make this collaboration between the folks at IDG Books and the People's Medical Society possible.

Many gifted and talented writers contributed to this book. Special thanks to: Janet Benton, Marcy Caplin, Kristin Casler, Angela Cerf, Martha Capwell Fox, Christine Kuehn Kelly, Luci Patalano, Miranda Barrett Potter, Bernadette Sukley, and Patricia Webb.

We have had a wonderful working relationship with IDG Books. Much of that is due to Tammerly Booth, executive editor, who conceived the idea for this book and wanted to work with us. It's been a wonderful working relationship. Kelly Ewing and Colleen Esterline were our IDG project editors. Their guidance and insight were invaluable in making this a relevant, readable, and informative work. Tammy Castleman served as the copy editor, Kathryn Born as illustrator, and Dr. Ramona Slupik and Dr. Barb Robinson as technical editors. Obviously, without their considerable talents this book would still be in the idea stage.

Publisher's Acknowledgments

We're proud of this book; please register your comments through our IDG Books Worldwide Online Registration Form located at http://my2cents.dummies.com.

Some of the people who helped bring this book to market include the following:

Acquisitions and Editorial

Project Editor: Colleen Esterline

Executive Editor: Tammerly Booth

Editorial Coordinator: Maureen F. Kelly

Copy Editor: Tamara Castleman

Aquistions Coordinator: Karen Young

Technical Editors: Dr. Ramona Slupik, Dr. Barb Robinson

Associate Permissions Editor: Carmen Krikorian

Editorial Managers: Leah P. Cameron, Mary C. Corder

Media Development Manager: Heather Heath Dismore

Production

Project Coordinator: E. Shawn Aylsworth

Layout and Graphics: Linda M. Boyer, Angela F. Hunckler, Jane E. Martin, Brent Savage, Jacque Schneider, Janet Seib, Kate Snell, Michael A. Sullivan, Brian Torwelle

Proofreaders: Christine Berman, Mary Lea Ginn, Jennifer Mahern, Nancy Price, Ethel M. Winslow, Janet M. Withers

Illustrator: Kathryn Born

Indexer: Joan Griffitts

Special Help

Suzanne Thomas

General and Administrative

IDG Books Worldwide, Inc.: John Kilcullen, CEO; Steven Berkowitz, President and Publisher

IDG Books Technology Publishing: Brenda McLaughlin, Senior Vice President and Group Publisher

Dummies Technology Press and Dummies Editorial: Diane Graves Steele, Vice President and Associate Publisher; Mary Bednarek, Director of Acquisitions and Product Development; Kristin A. Cocks, Editorial Director

Dummies Trade Press: Kathleen A. Welton, Vice President and Publisher; Kevin Thornton, Acquisitions Manager

IDG Books Production for Dummies Press: Michael R. Britton, Vice President of Production and Creative Services; Cindy L. Phipps, Manager of Project Coordination, Production Proofreading, and Indexing; Kathie S. Schutte, Supervisor of Page Layout; Shelley Lea, Supervisor of Graphics and Design; Debbie J. Gates, Production Systems Specialist; Robert Springer, Supervisor of Proofreading; Debbie Stailey, Special Projects Coordinator; Tony Augsburger, Supervisor of Reprints and Bluelines

Dummies Packaging and Book Design: Patty Page, Manager, Promotions Marketing

♦

The publisher would like to give special thanks to Patrick J. McGovern, without whom this book would not have been possible.

♦

Contents at a Glance

Cartoons at a Glance

By Rich Tennant

The 5th Wave — By Rich Tennant

"Well, nothing shows up on the tests. I think your headaches are probably just stress related."

page 107

The 5th Wave — By Rich Tennant

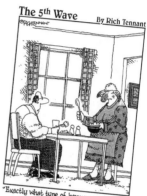

"Sandy says she's going to work on her cat-cow. Sounds more like a science experiment than a yoga posture to me."

page 373

The 5th Wave — By Rich Tennant

"Exactly what type of hormone replacement therapy are you taking?"

page 231

The 5th Wave — By Rich Tennant

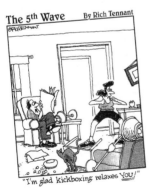

"I'm glad kickboxing relaxes YOU!"

page 5

The 5th Wave — By Rich Tennant

"I'd like you to welcome Grinda to our group. Grinda has issues with potion abuse, poison apples, and a history of negative relationships with men and toads."

page 65

The 5th Wave — By Rich Tennant

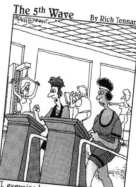

"I exercised so much during my first pregnancy that the baby was born with athlete's foot."

page 331

Fax: 978-546-7747 • E-mail: the5wave@tiac.net

Table of Contents

Part VI: The Part of Tens 373

Chapter 27: Ten Questions to Ask a Prospective Childbirth Practitioner 375

Chapter 28: Ten Ways to Make a Gynecologic Exam More Comfortable 379

Chapter 29: Ten Best Medical Web Sites to Visit 383

Introduction

. . . .

Oh, no! Not another book on women's health! Aren't there more than enough handbooks, guidebooks, manuals, and encyclopedias aimed specifically at women? Could there possibly be a need for still one more?

As surprising as it may sound, there really is a need for another book on women's health. Impossible, you say? After all, in this era of information overload, health information for women is everywhere. But despite this glut of information, most women are still confused. One day you read that only women over 50 should get an annual mammogram. The next day someone says you should start getting them at age 40. HMOs say our primary care doctor can handle most of our routine gynecological needs; ob-gyns tell us otherwise.

We're overwhelmed with conflicting and confusing information. For example, what does it mean when some expert says you have a one in eight chance of developing breast cancer? Most of us think the risk is constant throughout our adult life. In reality, the one in eight risk applies to women above the age of 80! We're told there are too many cesarean sections being performed on us, but we're not being told how to avoid one.

I'm convinced that to some extent the women's health information explosion has caused a credibility implosion. Women have heard so many conflicting and confusing facts, they do not know what to believe. And many of us have thrown up our hands and ignored it all (or at least much of it).

But that does not diminish the need for useful and credible information. In fact, it only underscores it. And that's why the People's Medical Society and I wanted to write this book. Our goal is to give you the information you need to make better and more informed health care decisions.

About This Book

All right — we've posed the challenge. What makes this book so different? Well, for starters, this is a book based on real medical studies. This isn't a book of opinions. That's one difference. And it's a major one. Plus, we've gone to only the most credible sources.

Even more important, we've made sure the information in this book is what you want to know. Too often, health books for women are little more than an advertisement for the physician author or the medical institution whose name appears on the cover. That's not the case here. Because the People's Medical Society is a consumer health organization, we're continually hearing from consumers — and, believe me, they tell us the information they want to know.

For example, we don't just tell you about living wills, we tell you about many of your other medical rights — things such as having the medical power of attorney for a loved one. And, of course, we talk about conditions — not just a few — but most of the major ones that might affect you.

In other words, this is a complete women's health book. It's not just about one health problem or one age range. We think of it as a woman's health insurance policy — because we cover all the health issues and conditions most of us confront in our lives.

Foolish Assumptions

Obviously, you're now convinced you own the perfect book. Just about everything you need to know to maintain your health and get through the health care system will be found in the following pages. And that's pretty much the case. But remember: This book cannot do certain things. For example, an accurate diagnosis cannot be made from a book. Nor can the correct dosage of a medication be prescribed. This book is a guide to be used in conjunction with a medical professional. Don't make the foolish assumption that you can do it all alone.

How This Book Is Organized

How do you use this book? Well, the first thing to know is how we've organized it. Actually, it's pretty logical. We've divided the book into six sections. Each section stands alone — meaning you can just about open it to any page and still find what you need. So here are the different sections and an overview of what you'll find in each.

Part I: Smart Health Care for Women

Knowing how to take care of yourself and how to use the health care system to your advantage is crucial to living a long, healthy life. In this section we discuss diet and exercise — key ingredients in the recipe for a healthy body — along with screening information and other maintenance techniques. We also offer pointers for negotiating your way through the U.S. health care system, from choosing a doctor to choosing an insurer.

Part II: Righting the Wrongs

Self-care involves more than prevention. It also means addressing and confronting any problems that may confront you. This section provides the information you need to right common wrongs, including overweight, eating disorders, addictions, and violence. It also provides tips on dealing with more acute conditions, such as bruises or splinters.

Part III: All That Ails You

Despite your best efforts, you may still fall victim to illness. This section addresses many conditions common to women, from minor conditions such as colds to life-threatening diseases such as cancer. We provide an overview of each condition to help you recognize when there's a problem, what that problem might be, and what can be done about it.

Part IV: Your Reproductive Health

Your reproductive system distinguishes your body from that of a man — and gives you health concerns unique to you, a woman. This section offers you the information to keep your system — and your sex life — healthy. We provide information on conditions that may affect your reproductive organs and your reproductive health — from endometriosis and breast lumps to infertility and menopause. We also offer a frank discussion of your reproductive options, how to avoid sexually transmitted diseases, and what to do when things don't go well between the sheets.

Part V: Pregnancy

Pregnancy and childbirth change your life — and present you, at least temporarily, with different health needs and problems. This section walks you through the whole pregnancy scene — from choosing who will deliver your child and where, to what to expect during your pregnancy and delivery.

Part VI: The Part of Tens

A traditional element of ...*For Dummies* books, the Part of Tens offers short chapters packed with tips and useful information. In this book, we include a list of ten questions you should ask a prospective childbirth practitioner, ten ways to make a gynecologic exam more comfortable, and ten medical Web sites that will keep you on top of women's health.

Icons Used in the Book

To help you efficiently find information you need, we've included icons in the margins to point to various types of information. The following are the icons we've used and what they mean.

Tips point out information that can help you take better care of yourself.

Warnings let you know that you need to exercise extra caution.

Myth Busters dispel commonly held beliefs, letting you know the difference between fact and fiction.

When you see this icon, you know that the information that follows deals with care you must receive from your doctor.

This icon tells you that the information that follows is self-care information.

Health information changes rapidly. This icon keys you in to the very latest information.

Part I
Smart Health Care for Women

The 5th Wave   By Rich Tennant

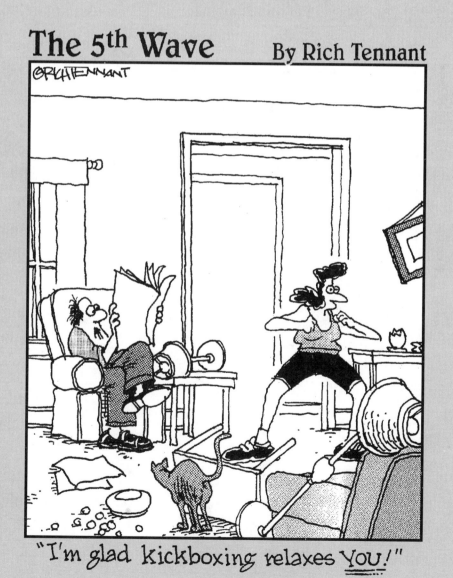

"I'm glad kickboxing relaxes YOU!"

In this part . . .

Think of your body as a machine. For it to operate efficiently, you need to give it the proper fuel (a well-balanced diet), run it periodically (exercise), and make sure it gets the routine maintenance it needs (periodic checkups and physical exams). You also need to establish a good working relation with the mechanics (health care professionals and insurance representatives) that keep it running. This section briefs you on how to maintain your unique, feminine machine.

Chapter 1
Recipe for a Healthy Body

. . . .

In This Chapter

▶ Getting the lowdown on nutrition

▶ Eating a balanced diet

▶ Understanding the importance of vitamins and minerals

▶ Incorporating exercise into your life

▶ Understanding how stress affects the body

▶ Relaxing for your health

. . . .

*L*ife, as you know, comes without guarantees. Although all women want to lead healthy lives, their family histories, their attitudes, and even being at the wrong place at the wrong time can wreak havoc on their health. Nevertheless, if women take care of their bodies, they increase their chances of staying healthy, reduce their risk of becoming ill, and feel good to boot. The recipe is simple: eat a balanced diet, get adequate amounts of necessary vitamins and minerals, exercise to maintain physical fitness, and effectively counter the stress faced on a day-to-day basis. This chapter takes a close look at each of these essential ingredients.

Diet and Nutrition

Eat a balanced, varied diet: You've heard this message before. But when you look further, eating right begins to seem like a full-time job. Do you really have to memorize serving sizes for dozens of foods, and then count how many servings of each food group you have each day?

Learning to read your body's signals may help you reach your goal more comfortably. You may have already noticed that what you eat can influence how you feel. Paying more attention to the news your own body supplies, coupled with some basic nutritional information, can lead you to a better diet. After you notice over and over that certain foods give you indigestion or a headache or that breakfast improves your concentration in the morning, you'll probably want to repeat the choices that make you feel best. You may even start placing grains, fruits, and vegetables at the center of your diet — not because medical experts tell you to do so, but because these foods help you feel well and attain or maintain a healthy weight.

Boosting energy levels with food

The three basic components of food are carbohydrates, proteins, and fats. Most foods are dominated by one or two of these components, or *macronutrients,* but foods often contain at least a tiny bit of all three. Understanding a few things about these components can help you eat wisely.

Carbohydrates: A simple or complex group

Carbohydrates include starches, sugars, and two forms of fiber — soluble and insoluble. Starches and sugars supply you with most of your energy and do so most quickly because you digest them faster than you digest proteins or fats. *Soluble fiber,* such as that found in oatmeal, dissolves in water and passes slowly through the digestive system, helping you to keep feeling full. It reduces cholesterol levels, helps stabilize blood sugar, and much more. You can't digest *insoluble fiber,* which is what makes it a great aid in moving food through your intestines and colon. Eating a diet high in insoluble fiber, such as that found in wheat products and cruciferous vegetables, has even been linked to lower rates of colon and rectal cancers, possibly for this reason.

All vegetables, fruits, grain products, beans, and sugars contain carbohydrates. But not all carbohydrates offer the same nutritional value. The nutrient content of fruits and vegetables, for example, varies according to the individual fruit or vegetable, its age, and how it has been prepared. Fruits and vegetables are generally most nutritious when they are eaten raw or lightly cooked because some of the vitamins they contain are lost during processing.

Carbohydrates from grain sources (such as pastas and flours) vary in what nutrients they have to give, depending on whether they are *complex* or *refined.* Whole grains and whole-grain products, such as brown rice and whole-wheat bread, give you all or most of the nutrients a whole grain has to offer, including complex carbohydrates, or starches. (*Whole* means no edible parts have been removed.) These complex carbohydrates are digested more slowly, so they supply your blood with a lower but more steady level of *glucose* (blood sugar) for a longer time. They also contain plenty of fiber: a slice of whole-grain bread supplies about 15 percent of the recommended daily amount of fiber.

Refined carbohydrates such as white rice and white flour are made from grains whose outer layers (including the bran and the germ) have been removed. Many of the grain's vitamins and minerals — and much of its fiber — are removed with those outer layers, and other nutrients are destroyed during the refining process, which can include bleaching. Some refined products are labeled enriched, which means that some of the missing vitamins have been added back. Keep in mind that even these enriched, refined-grain products often contain little or no fiber and generally provide fewer vitamins and minerals than whole grains.

Proteins: The powerful bodybuilders

Proteins are your body's basic building blocks. They provide raw materials to build and renew your cells, muscles, and tissues, aid your immune system, and keep you strong in general. Only water makes up more of your body weight than protein.

The problem with protein intake in an average American diet is that many protein sources such as red meat and eggs also have a high level of cholesterol. Your best protein sources on a daily basis would be those with low cholesterol, such as chicken, fish, or legumes. Incorporate lean red meat and eggs only on an occasional basis. According to the National Academy of Sciences' Food and Nutrition Board, which sets recommended intakes for many nutrients, girls and women ages 11 to 24 need about 45 grams of protein each day. Women 25 and older should aim for 50 grams.

Even vegetarians who eat no eggs or milk products can meet that protein goal by eating more beans and legumes. The recommended serving of 2 to 3 ounces of protein is about the size of a deck of cards.

Fats: Get the skinny

Dietary fats supply fatty acids that your body can't produce (the ones known as *essential fatty acids*), and they help your body absorb the fat-soluble vitamins A, D, E, and K. They also supply you with energy. Fats take the longest to digest, so they keep you feeling full longer. Whether in plant or animal foods, fats supply more than twice as many calories (units of energy) per gram as proteins or carbohydrates — nine calories compared to four. That means that burning off the same quantity of fat takes longer.

High-fat diets have been linked to high cholesterol, heart disease, some cancers, and obesity and its related illnesses. So when you talk about fats, you have to address how much is safe to eat. National health organizations, including the U.S. Departments of Agriculture and Health and Human Services and the American Heart Association (AHA), recommend that healthy people get no more than 30 percent of their calories from fats. The AHA also sets a bottom limit, endorsing the World Health Organization's recommendation that fat intake be no lower than 15 percent. If you have heart disease or high cholesterol or are at risk for these conditions, ask your doctor for guidelines most appropriate for you.

How about cholesterol?

Your body is able to manufacture all the cholesterol it needs, so cholesterol is not considered an essential nutrient. Consuming excess cholesterol in foods can result in higher levels of low-density lipoprotein (LDL) cholesterol in your blood and a higher risk of coronary heart disease. Because the American Heart Association reports that half of each year's deaths in this country are related to coronary heart disease, many women would benefit by cutting their cholesterol intake as low as they can. Meats, poultry, egg yolks, shrimp, and high-fat dairy products, such as butter, are among the foods to eat in small amounts because they are high in cholesterol.

Remember: The AHA's guidelines don't refer to your daily intake, but to your average daily intake over the course of a week, which gives some flexibility to those women with healthy hearts. If you eat a hamburger and french fries one night, for example, you can counteract that by eating low-fat foods the next day. But keep in mind that this approach is definitely not recommended for those at high coronary risk — a recent study indicates that a fatty meal can increase the risk of heart attack by limiting the arteries' ability to dilate.

When it comes to fats, you also have to address what kind you should eat most often. Certain fats — including the much maligned saturated fats — have important things to contribute to the body. Yet substantial research concludes that the healthiest diet consists of mostly unsaturated fats, which means polyunsaturates and monounsaturates. You find these in vegetable and fish oils, nuts, and in some grains and beans. You may already know that it's considered best to eat so-called monounsaturated oils such as olive oil. Study after study has shown that eating olive oil can lower blood levels of low-density lipoprotein (LDL), the so-called bad cholesterol, and reduce heart disease risk.

But calling an oil "monounsaturated" or "polyunsaturated" is not entirely correct because each vegetable oil actually contains several kinds of fat in unique proportions. Oils containing mostly polyunsaturates are what we call polyunsaturated oils. These oils include safflower and sunflower. The AHA and many other groups recommend getting some of your polyunsaturated fats from fish, especially cold-water fish, which contains essential fatty acids that are thought to have beneficial effects.

Look on the jars of the oils you use to see what their fat proportions are. Choose a balance of oils, using most often those with the most monounsaturated fat, such as olive or canola, or ones with nearly equal amounts of polyunsaturates and monounsaturates, such as sesame and peanut.

Calculating your recommended fat intake

What does "30 percent of calories from fat" mean for you? Here's how you can find out. Estimate your average daily caloric intake, multiply that number by .3 (for 30 percent), and divide the result by 9 (the number of calories in a gram of fat). For example, if you eat about 2,000 calories a day, figure out your recommended fat intake as follows:

2,000 calories X .3 = 600 calories from fat

600 calories divided by .9 = 67 grams of fat

What about saturated fat? The AHA and other groups recommend eating less than 10 percent of your total calories — less than a third of the 30 percent maximum fat intake they recommend — as saturated fat. This fat is most prevalent in the type of oil that hardens at room temperature, such as bacon grease and coconut oil. High intake of saturated fat increases blood levels of LDL cholesterol and the risk of heart disease. Saturated fat is found in meats, poultry, milk, milk products, and certain vegetable oils. These oils include palm kernel oil and coconut oil, which are often used in stored bakery products and candies because they are inexpensive. Read labels to avoid these hidden saturates.

Climbing the pyramid to good nutrition

The safest and smartest way to meet your nutritional needs is to eat a varied, balanced diet. Eating well can have wonderful fringe benefits. The cancer risk for Americans who eat five servings of fruits and vegetables every day may actually be 50 to 70 percent lower than for those who eat lower amounts of fruits and vegetables. And fruits and vegetables also help guard against cardiovascular disease. Fruits and vegetables get some of their power from the fiber they provide and the antioxidant vitamins they contain.

But what do "varied" and "balanced" mean? We'll start with basics. Did you grow up seeing a chart in the school nurse's office that pictured "the four food groups"? If you have children, they're now looking at a poster that depicts a pyramid made up of six food groups (see Figure 1-1). What has changed is not the actual foods mentioned, but the *amounts* of each. Recommendations for protein intake have decreased, especially protein obtained from animal foods. Consequently, the central place that meat used to occupy on the plate has been given to carbohydrates, such as fruits, vegetables, grains and grain products, and beans. Next should be lean and low-fat foods from the meat group and the milk group. The smallest place on your plate should be given to high-fat, high-sugar foods.

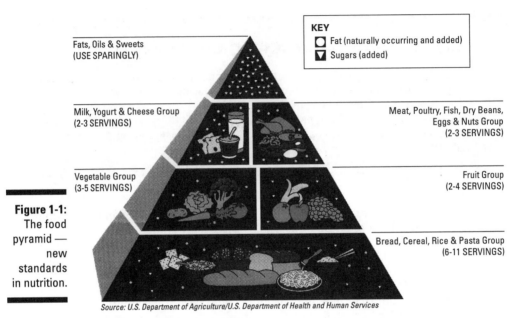

KEY
- ⬭ Fat (naturally occurring and added)
- ▼ Sugars (added)

Fats, Oils & Sweets
(USE SPARINGLY)

Milk, Yogurt & Cheese Group
(2-3 SERVINGS)

Meat, Poultry, Fish, Dry Beans,
Eggs & Nuts Group
(2-3 SERVINGS)

Vegetable Group
(3-5 SERVINGS)

Fruit Group
(2-4 SERVINGS)

Bread, Cereal, Rice & Pasta Group
(6-11 SERVINGS)

Figure 1-1:
The food
pyramid —
new
standards
in nutrition.

Source: U.S. Department of Agriculture/U.S. Department of Health and Human Services

As shown in Figure 1-1, the pyramid recommends certain numbers of servings of each food group. A serving usually means one of something, as in one egg, one slice of bread, or one piece of fruit. Or it may mean a ¹/₂ cup of vegetables, fruits, or cooked cereal, rice, or pasta. A serving from the meat and beans group means 2 to 3 ounces of lean cooked meat, poultry, or fish, or a ¹/₂ cup of cooked beans. (For more details on the food pyramid, call 719-948-4000 and ask for pamphlet 321D, *Dietary Guidelines for Americans,* from the U.S. Department of Health and Human Services and the U.S. Department of Agriculture. Or visit www.pueblo.gsa.gov on the World Wide Web. Many of these agencies' booklets are available, either free or at very low cost.) If you don't want to get hung up on counting servings, think of the recommended numbers of servings as a measure of what your plate should look like — heavy on the complex carbohydrates, lighter on proteins, and very light on fats and sugars.

And what about "variety"? Consider this: Every fruit, vegetable, grain, bean, meat, poultry, fish, nut, and oil contains a unique combination of nutrients, and some highly beneficial nutrients exist in only a few foods. So eating an orange every morning, or lettuce and tomato every night, is not enough. A varied diet provides you with the widest range of nutrients. So broaden your palate with vegetables, fruits, grains, beans, nuts, oils, lean meats, poultry, fish, and low-fat dairy products such as buttermilk. Your pleasures may increase along with your energy.

On liquids: How much should you drink?

You can go 60 days without food, but only about 3 without water. Next to the air you breathe, water is the most important substance to your body. It makes up a huge amount of your blood and parts of everything else, from bone to brain. Water helps clear out wastes, among many other things. The standard recommendation of health professionals is to drink 2 quarts (8 cups) of water per day.

As for other liquids, keep in mind that many of them contain calories. There is no harm in drinking low to moderate amounts of caffeine-containing beverages. However, a high caffeine consumption may result in jitteriness, irritability, or insomnia. And the typical soda offers little other than 3 tablespoons of sugar or lots of artificial sweetener. Keep in mind that caffeine and alcohol are diuretics — they cause your body to lose water — so don't count them as fluid replacement. Most fruit juices don't provide the fiber that whole fruits do, so try to get some of your fruit servings from whole fruits.

Vitamins and Minerals

Vitamins are *nutrients* — food components obtained from your diet — that have been found to be essential in small quantities for human life. If even one vitamin is missing from your diet, your body doesn't function normally. Vitamins perform numerous functions in your body: They promote growth, help the body utilize other essential nutrients, help maintain mental alertness, help maintain the health of various body tissues, and help the body resist infection, among other things. These compounds, which are found in most foods, are organic, which means that they contain the chemical element carbon and come from living materials.

Minerals are nonorganic nutrients — they come from nonliving materials — but they, too, are essential for the proper functioning of our bodies: They play roles in numerous biochemical and physiological processes necessary for good health, including regulation of blood pressure, heartbeat, body temperature, and metabolism.

With all that vitamins and minerals do, you may have trouble believing that scientists did not begin to isolate these nutrients from foods until the early 1900s. By now, 52 of several thousand nutrients in foods have been isolated. Some have been reproduced in laboratories and made available in pill form as nutritional supplements.

Vitamins and minerals are vital to health: You couldn't live without them. But experts disagree over the best ways to get those nutrients — whether from food alone or from both food and pills.

Deciding whether to supplement

Here's the strongest case in favor of food. Whole foods contain thousands of chemicals — many more than the 52 scientists have isolated and studied. The many untested and even unknown chemicals in foods are likely to be at least as important as the ones you know a fair bit about. In fact, the *combinations* of chemicals existing naturally in foods may be what makes them so effective. Singling some out in pills, this argument says, is not a good idea.

But you can't get therapeutic doses (doses that may help prevent or lessen disease) of some vitamins and minerals through food. For instance, many studies indicate that vitamin E boosts health and prevents disease, including heart disease, in amounts ranging from 100 to 1,000 international units (I.U.) per day. To get just 100 I.U. of vitamin E from your diet, you'd have to eat more than 13 cups of wheat-germ oil or 50 avocados. Even if you could fit these into your stomach, your fat intake would hit the roof. So if you want to get the therapeutic dose of vitamin E, this argument says, you need to take a pill.

Supplementation is not without risks. Taking a large amount of certain vitamins or minerals can be toxic or can lead to deficiencies of other nutrients. Nutrients known to be harmful in excessive doses include the minerals zinc and selenium and the vitamins A, D, and B_6.

Getting the right amounts

The American Heart Association and the National Cancer Institute suggest that Americans should rely on a balanced, varied diet with at least five servings of fruits and vegetables a day. Some experts suggest adding a multivitamin-mineral supplement when your dietary intake is limited for any reason, such as pregnancy, dieting, or illness. But many other experts recommend routine use of supplements so that people can reach therapeutic doses. Here are some of the nutrients you should attempt to get plenty of, whether through foods or foods and supplements. Recommended Dietary Allowances (RDAs) for these nutrients and others appear in Table 1-1. (If you're pregnant, see Chapter 25 for RDAs.) Keep in mind that the RDAs are the amounts believed to prevent the symptoms of deficiency, not the amounts believed to lead to optimal health (see the sidebar, "The RDA is almost passe").

✔ **Vitamins C, E, and A:** These vitamins are *antioxidants* — compounds that prevent *free radicals* from damaging your cells. Free radicals are unstable, often harmful chemicals that your body makes, both during normal processes and in response to outside toxins such as cigarette smoke and air pollutants. Free radicals can cause cell mutations, which can lead to cancer. By neutralizing free radicals, antioxidants are thought to help prevent cancer. Some studies associate high amounts of antioxidants in the blood with lowered rates of many disorders that accompany aging. And adequate blood levels of vitamins A and E have been linked to lower rates of heart disease.

Foods rich in vitamin C include citrus fruits, bell peppers, guava, kiwi fruits, broccoli, brussels sprouts, and many other fruits and vegetables. Vitamin C is known to assist wound healing, strengthen bones, cartilage, and skin, among other things.

Foods with ample vitamin E include nuts, oils made from nuts and seeds (such as sunflower and sesame), whole wheat, wheat germ, eggs, and whole-grain cereals. Vitamin E shows great promise in preventing heart disease, probably by reducing the risk of *atherosclerosis* (clogged arteries).

Very high doses of vitamin A can have unpredictable, even unsafe effects for some people. So unless your doctor has determined otherwise or until more research has been done, it may be wise to get most or all of your vitamin A and its precursors from foods, where they are plentiful. About 30 substances known as carotenoids are *precursors* of vitamin A, which means that your body can turn them into vitamin A. Because your body converts those carotenoids (including beta carotene) to vitamin A only in the amounts you need, you can't overdose. Carotenoids are found abundantly in red, orange, and yellow fruits and vegetables and in green vegetables. You can obtain vitamin A itself in safe levels in foods such as whole milk, butter, beef liver, egg yolks, fish oil, and oysters.

✔ **Calcium:** Building up your bones with calcium before you turn 30 decreases your risk of osteoporosis. If your bones are well fortified before age 30, your postmenopausal loss of bone mass can be reduced by more than 40 percent. And if you are elderly, taking calcium and vitamin D supplements (1,200 milligrams and 800 I.U., respectively) may reduce your bone fracture rate by 20 percent. The National Institutes of Health recommends these daily calcium intakes: 1,000 milligrams for premenopausal women as well as for postmenopausal women taking estrogen, and 1,500 for postmenopausal women not taking estrogen and all women over 65. Calcium is abundant in dairy products; canned salmon and sardines; leafy greens such as kale and turnip tops; whole grains such as buckwheat, brown rice, and quinoa; and many beans, including soybeans and soy products such as tofu.

✔ **Iron:** Because premenopausal women lose about 15 to 20 milligrams of iron each month during menstruation, they need more iron than men. However, women's bodies store extra iron whenever they consume more than they need. So most women do have enough iron, and excessive iron consumption can pose serious risks. But if you feel tired or look pale, ask your doctor for a blood test for anemia (iron deficiency), which is easily remedied with modest supplementation. Eat foods rich in iron such as leafy greens, liver, shellfish, red meat, and soy products. Some grains also contain iron, including buckwheat, rye, and quinoa.

✓ **Folic acid and vitamins B6 and B12:** Among other things, a deficiency of these B vitamins has been linked to higher blood levels of the amino acid *homocysteine*. Recent studies suggest that having a high blood level of homocysteine is even worse than high cholesterol and smoking in promoting heart disease and stroke. For folic acid, look to beans (including black turtle, garbanzo, kidney, lima, navy, and pinto — one-half cup of cooked pinto beans contains 73 percent of the RDA of folic acid), peas, leafy greens, oranges, bananas, seeds, and liver. Good sources of vitamin B6 include poultry, fish, pork, whole grains, dried beans and peas, bananas,Ï and avocados. Vitamin B12 is found in meats, dairy products, eggs, liver, and fish. (Vegetarians who eat no eggs or dairy products may wish to consider a low-dose supplement.)

Table 1-1	RDAs for Adult Women
Vitamins	*Recommended Dietary Allowance*
Vitamin A	800 Retinol Equivalents (RE) (4,000 I.U.)
Thiamin (B1)	1.1 milligrams
Riboflavin (B2)	1.1 milligrams
Niacin (B3)	14 milligrams
Vitamin B6	1.3 milligrams (1.5 milligrams for women 51 and over)
Folic acid	400 micrograms
Vitamin B12	2.4 micrograms
Vitamin C	60 milligrams (100 milligrams for smokers)
Vitamin D	5 micrograms (200 I.U.) (10 micrograms [400 I.U.] for women 51-70 and 15 micrograms [600 I.U.] for women over 70)
Vitamin E	8 milligrams (12 I.U.)
Vitamin K	65 micrograms (60 micrograms for women 19-24)

The RDA is almost passe

Change is happening at the National Academy of Sciences' Food and Nutrition Board, the government advisory group that sets national standards for nutrient intake. The RDAs they set represent the amount of each nutrient a person needs to prevent a deficiency. But now the group is working its way through the nutrients to provide another useful measure, the DRIs — Dietary Reference Intakes. These will let you know what amount the board finds essential for good health. This shift from preventing deficiencies to promoting health is just one result of the huge amount of research taking place around the world on disease prevention and nutrition. For listings of the DRIs already set and more, look at the National Academy of Sciences' Web site at www.nas.edu/new.

Minerals	Recommended Dietary Allowance
Calcium	1,000 milligrams (1,200 milligrams for women 51 and over)
Phosphorus	700 milligrams
Magnesium	320 milligrams (310 milligrams for women 19-30)
Iron	15 milligrams (10 milligrams for women 51 and over)
Zinc	12 milligrams
Iodine	150 micrograms
Selenium	55 micrograms

Physical Fitness

What does physical fitness mean to you? The American College of Sports Medicine defines it as "being able to do medium to difficult activities, such as raking leaves, shoveling snow, and cleaning windows, without becoming fatigued, and being able to maintain that ability throughout life." What this definition tells you is that physical fitness doesn't mean being able to run a marathon. It means getting through your days, whatever your age, with energy and without strain. It means welcoming the chance to stretch your physical abilities and not getting hurt or exhausted in the process.

Benefiting from exercise

In a study that tracked almost 16,000 healthy men and women for an average of 19 years, just six, brisk, half-hour walks or jogs per month were found to cut the risk of death by 44 percent. This study, reported in 1998, was the first to separate the effects of heredity and exercise on life span by comparing twins. The study also accounted for various factors such as smoking habits and chronic diseases.

Physical benefits

Exercise is just plain good for the body. Its benefits include the following:

- **Improved cardiovascular health:** Regular aerobic exercise lowers cholesterol levels, increases blood and, thus, oxygen supply to the heart, strengthens the heart muscle, reduces blood pressure, and reduces the tendency to be overweight.

- **Immune system boost:** Numerous studies suggest that a moderate workout results in increased immunity for up to a few hours and that regular, moderate exercise leads to more lasting increases.

- **Increased strength and flexibility:** With regular exercise, many tasks are easier, such as opening a jar or lifting a load of laundry. Weight-bearing exercise is an effective way to strengthen muscles and bones. As an added bonus, you may notice an increase in your range of movement. This benefit is even more pronounced if you include stretching or yoga in your routine.

- **Reduced cancer risk:** Because exercise boosts the immune system, it may help the body locate and kill cancer cells before they have the chance to multiply and become tumors. Several large studies support this theory. One study took into account the nutritional and other health-influencing habits of participants and still found that the moderately active women had a 23 percent lower chance of getting cancer.

Mental benefits

Whether the cause is increased *endorphins* (natural opiates in the body), increased levels of *neurotransmitters* (brain chemicals) that control mood, more oxygen-rich blood flow to the brain, or just distraction from other concerns, exercise can make you feel better mentally. It can energize your body and relax your mind at the same time. Among its best-known mental benefits are

- **Less depression:** Several studies have found that exercise, whether vigorous or mild, makes a positive impact on mild to moderate depression, even for the chronically ill.

✔ **Less anxiety:** A review of more than 150 studies on exercise and anxiety revealed that exercise reduces anxiety as much as meditation and other relaxation techniques. And its benefits can linger well past the after-glow of a workout, especially for those suffering from chronic anxiety. The longer you continue to exercise, the greater the results.

✔ **More self-esteem and confidence:** Exercise can increase self-esteem and the feeling of being able to face challenges. This ability may result in part from an increased stamina and improved physical appearance.

✔ **Increased mental sharpness:** Evaluating the findings of more than 100 studies on physical activity and mental function, researchers found that exercise improves at least three measures of an energetic mind: reaction time, the ability to perceive patterns, and math skills. Some experts think that the decreasing mental function that people associate with aging results partly from decreased blood flow to the brain. Because exercise increases that blood flow, it helps elderly people improve their thinking skills, too. A few studies also link exercise to increased creative thinking.

Determining the right amount for you

There's no doubt that exercise is beneficial, but how often do you need to exercise to reap those benefits? The National Institutes of Health (NIH) recommends 30 minutes of moderate exercise per day, which can be divided into three 10-minute spurts. What qualifies as moderate? The good news is that you don't have to put on fancy clothes, use odd machines, or work out until you're dripping with sweat. A lively walk qualifies, as do bicycling, swimming, yard work, and a host of other enjoyable activities. (Despite the simplicity and flexibility of these guidelines, recent NIH statistics reveal that less than half of adult Americans get any exercise at all.)

Be still my beating heart

Exercise intensity is measured by heart rate. To determine yours, place your index and middle fingers on your opposite wrist or the side of your neck to feel your pulse. Looking at a watch, clock, or the timekeeper on an exercise machine, count the number of beats that occur in 10 seconds. Multiply that number by six. That's your heart rate per minute at that moment. It may or may not be within the target zone experts recommend that you stay within.

Here's one way to figure out your target zone: Subtract your age from 220; that's your maximum heart rate. Multiply that number first by .6, then by .9. Those are the bottom and top limits your heart rate should stay within for at least 20 minutes. Slow down if you're above your range. As your exercise tolerance increases, you'll be able to keep your heart rate within the target zone longer and with less exertion.

If you want to go beyond these minimum recommendations, the traditional prescription is to exercise at least three times a week for 20 minutes or more in your target heart range.

A combination of aerobic and anaerobic exercise gives you the widest range of benefits. *Aerobic exercise* is sustained movement that increases your heart rate. Your body uses oxygen to supply energy during aerobic exercise. Options include walking briskly, jogging, biking, cross-country skiing, swimming, aerobic dance, using exercise machines such as treadmills and stair-steppers, and playing sports, from racquetball to soccer to basketball.

Anaerobic exercise is weight-bearing exercise. It demands so much energy at once that your body has to create energy without oxygen. This kind of exercise is effective at building and strengthening muscle and bones. Activities such as weight training can substantially alter body composition by increasing lean body weight and decreasing fat. Even elderly women can increase their strength and bone mass by lifting weights.

Getting started

If you are coming out of a long period of little exercise, have heart disease, or are at high risk of developing heart disease, be sure to discuss your wish to exercise with your medical practitioner before you start. And if you're recovering from an illness or injury, it is important to begin an exercise program gradually and to seek the advice of a practitioner you trust.

Choose an activity you enjoy that increases your heart rate. Everyone works differently when it comes to setting goals, but here's one approach: Set a long-term goal, such as walking or stretching every day and doing more strenuous exercise three days a week. Then set some short-term goals to get you there. If you've been sedentary for a while, a good first step may be to start stretching or walking for 15 minutes every day. When you have achieved that short-term goal and you're feeling stronger, you may add a stretch-and-tone class twice a week or another activity you enjoy. Even if you're in fairly good shape, build gradually to your ultimate goal. Don't feel bad about taking a step back if you feel you're overdoing it.

This method builds confidence and strength and helps prevent injury. You're likely to start noticing mental improvements soon after you start moving more regularly. It may take a few months before changes in your body match the changes in your mood, but it will happen.

Ouch! Avoiding strains and pains

One of the best ways to help prevent injury is to keep your body strong and flexible, especially your legs, abdomen, and back. This means both stretching and building muscle. Allow time to stretch before and after your workouts to lessen stiffness. Try to warm up a little before you stretch so that your muscles will be less tight. Don't bounce as you stretch, and don't force your body to move beyond mild discomfort.

Bone and muscle grow in response to stress, but this growth takes time. So increase the difficulty of your workouts gradually, allowing time for your body to grow into the task. Take a minimum of one or two days off each week from vigorous exercise to allow your body to recuperate. If you feel sore after exercising, you may find that a sauna or bath helps ease the discomfort. In case of significant pain, consult your doctor.

Breathe In, Breathe Out: Stress and Your Body

Upsetting events often enter your life without an invitation. At other times, you may choose to make major changes, which can also make stress levels skyrocket. This section discusses ways to handle stress and looks into what stress is and what it can do.

Are you stressed out?

Stress is the body's reaction to any kind of upset. Often this upset comes in the form of a change, whether positive or negative. A wedding and a funeral are both events that cause considerable emotional response, and our bodies react as well.

Experts speak of two kinds of stress, *acute* and *chronic*. Acute stress results from a sudden, drastic change — losing your job or winning a million dollars in a lottery, for example. Your body responds to acute stress by giving you a burst of energy, increased immune response, and higher blood pressure — exactly what you need to get through the crisis (unless, of course, this kind of shock happens repeatedly or you are at a high risk for heart attack). If an acute situation becomes long-term (maybe you can't find a new job), or if a daily irritant is driving you nuts or reducing you to tears, the resulting stress is considered chronic.

People respond to chronic stress by living in an ongoing state of agitation. Its primary cause can be external, such as living in a dangerous neighborhood, regularly being asked to do more than you possibly can at work, or taking care of an ailing parent while raising your children. Or it can be something positive, such as planning a wedding, which although exciting, can prove wearing. Chronic stress may even be caused by something few people would find disturbing, but which for you is upsetting. Sources of stress can be internal, too, such as ongoing depression, or anxiety that feels out of control.

Remember: In most cases of chronic stress, the individual does have some choices but may not yet be exercising them. She may be able to change the situation, change her response to the situation, or leave the situation. Reaching out for social support and assistance is also a highly important coping mechanism, one that can make the difference between collapse and recovery.

If something in your life upsets you regularly and you don't seem to be able to get used to it, don't think that ignoring the discomfort that chronic stress produces is a good idea. Ongoing stress is not only emotionally exhausting; it can also have damaging effects on your body. Medical research into the connections between stress and illness began more than 70 years ago and by now has proven a strong link between high stress levels and high rates of illness. But stress can only make you more likely to get sick — it doesn't always result in illness. The crucial component is how you respond to the stress that comes your way.

Stressful events that can affect your life

You may think that only negative events, such as a death in the family, cause stress. But positive events can be equally stressful. Here is a list of stressful life events. If you experience several of these simultaneously and find yourself exhibiting stress-related symptoms such as those listed in the accompanying sidebar, it may be time to take stress-relieving action:

Death of a loved one	Conflicts with family members	Financial difficulties
Change in job or career	Illness of a family member or friend	Change in residence
Loss of job	Retirement	Holidays
Pregnancy	Divorce	Personal illness
Birth of a baby	Vacation	

How does stress affect the human body?

Some of the ways your body can respond are noticeable, including a dry mouth, headaches, insomnia, fatigue, stomachaches, irritability, lack of concentration, hostility, demoralization, decreased sexual desire, painful intercourse, and *amenorrhea* (cessation of menstrual periods). Other changes are invisible until they take their toll. These include a lowering of your resistance to diseases of all kinds, from colds to cancer; excessive release of stress hormones such as cortisol and adrenaline; high blood pressure; the decreased ability of parts of the brain to respond appropriately to stress; and even the deterioration of brain functions that support some aspects of memory.

Relaxation and other coping techniques

Whether you need them now or will need them in the future, here are some excellent ways to relieve the pressure and spare yourself its ill effects:

- **Alternative therapies:** Alternative therapies such as Chinese medicine, homeopathy, and shiatsu (a form of therapeutic massage) may provide relief. A massage or a hot tub can offer short-term relief. And many herbs have a reputation for calming effects. These include chamomile, valerian, ginkgo, linden flower, and passionflower. Hot baths containing a tincture of herbs may provide relief. Some scents, such as lavender, rose, chamomile, marjoram, neroli, and sandalwood, are said to be soothing, whether used in a scent diffuser, in a bath, or on your body. A book on aromatherapy can offer further guidance.

- **Diet:** Providing your body with good nutrition is vital when you're under stress. In contrast, a high-fat diet worsens the negative effects of stress. If you feel that your diet isn't providing adequate support for you, consider seeing a nutritionist for assistance.

- **Exercise:** Whether it's brisk walking or vigorous yard work, exercise gives your body a boost that helps it cope with stress. It does this in part by discharging extra adrenaline and by increasing oxygen flow to your brain. Exercise also provides other benefits, including distraction from what's bothering you and some significantly relaxing aftereffects.

- **Meditation:** Like deep sleep, meditation can take you far from your surroundings and bring mental peace. Although meditation techniques vary, the basic principles are usually to sit comfortably in a quiet place for a predetermined amount of time and pay attention to your breathing. If you'd like to learn more about meditation, look for a book that describes meditation techniques aimed specifically at reducing stress.

✔ **Stress management programs:** If you have a medical condition that is worsened by the stress you're under (such as high blood pressure), consider asking your doctor about a stress reduction and relaxation program at a hospital or clinic in your area. These medically supervised and approved programs can help you learn to identify sources of stress and to handle them better. They do so partly by teaching a simple meditation technique. They may also provide audio or video relaxation tapes, which can help induce a calmer state. Other sources of informational tapes include bookstores and catalogs. If stress keeps you from sleeping well, a tape that aims to improve sleep quality may be worth a try.

✔ **Visualization:** Some people find visualization effective. Try closing your eyes and remembering or inventing a place you find totally relaxing — a sun-drenched beach or a peaceful woodland stream, for example. If it works, you can "go there" whenever you need to calm down.

✔ **Yoga:** Many people find yoga a dependable way to release tension. Yoga is an ancient discipline that offers a system of poses designed to relax and invigorate the entire body, including the spine, internal organs, and muscles. It also includes meditation, as well as other breathing methods that can cause relaxation and increase energy. Classes are a good way to begin your acquaintance with yoga.

Medications

If your symptoms are ongoing or severe, you should see a doctor. The symptoms of stress may mask those of an underlying physical problem or of depression. After ruling out other medical conditions, your doctor may recommend some form of mental health counseling or some type of medication.

Drugs used to treat anxiety and stress include several types of antidepressants. These include benzodiazepines such as Valium, Librium, and Xanax, which are usually prescribed for short-term treatment to make a person less anxious so she can get sleep; tricyclic antidepressants such as Tofranil, Elavil, and Pamelor, which raise levels of calming brain chemicals; selective serotonin reuptake inhibitors such as Prozac and Zoloft, which raise levels of the calming brain chemical serotonin; and monamine oxidase inhibitors such as Marplan, Nardil, or Parnate. Benzodiazepines are addictive and are usually prescribed only for short periods under medical supervision. Monoamine oxidase inhibitors and selective serotonin reuptake inhibitors are approved for long-term use. For more information on antidepressants, see Chapter 14.

Chapter 2
Maintaining the Machine

....

In This Chapter

▶ Choosing a doctor

▶ Looking into complementary medicine

▶ Knowing what to expect from a physical or a gynecologic exam

▶ Getting screenings and other tests

▶ Keeping your medical records

▶ Using medications

▶ Knowing what to expect from surgery

....

*E*ven the most finely tuned machines must be properly maintained in order to run well, and the human body is no exception. In addition to the fuel, rest, and regular operation outlined in Chapter 1, the human "machine" needs periodic checkups, occasional tests, and, at times, adjustments and repairs.

Choosing a Doctor or Gynecologist

The physician is the "mechanic" responsible for maintaining the human machine. But as a quick glance through your Yellow Pages will tell you, choosing a physician is not as simple as looking up the number of the nearest grocery store. You have a mind-boggling choice of different specialists and alternative practitioners from which to choose. And while each has a place in the health care system, it's important to find the physician who is appropriate to your own needs and problems.

Your general mechanic: The primary care physician

If you're in the market for a primary care physician, your choices may include the following:

- ✔ **General practioner:** A generalist doctor with one year of postgraduate training after medical school.

- ✔ **A family practitioner:** A doctor who after medical school has taken a three-year residency that covers certain aspects of internal medicine, gynecology, minor surgery, obstetrics, pediatrics, orthopedics, and preventive medicine.

- ✔ **An internist:** A doctor who after medical school has completed a three-year residency in primary care internal medicine, which involves an understanding of the health care of adults in the areas of disease prevention, wellness, substance abuse, mental health; treatment of common problems of the eyes, ears, skin, nervous system, and reproductive organs; diagnosis and management of problems in such areas as the gastrointestinal system, heart, kidney, liver, and endocrine system; and training in emergency medicine and critical care. These doctors can also take further subspecialist training in specific areas.

Many women receive their primary care from a *gynecologist,* a doctor who specializes in the diagnosis and treatment of problems associated with the female reproductive organs. But gynecologists are actually specialists; in addition to four years of medical school, they complete a four-year residency in obstetrics and gynecology, in which they learn routine gynecologic and obstetrical procedures and surgery. And while gynecologists can provide primary care for most women with common health problems, they may not provide the same kind of specialized care that a primary care doctor would provide. For this reason, many women prefer to see a gynecologist for reproductive care and a primary care doctor for other types of care.

Conducting your search

Regardless of the type of practitioner you are looking for, your selection process will be the same.

Start by asking family members, friends, and neighbors for their recommendations. You may also want to ask a nurse or your present doctor.

Other sources you may want to consider include the following:

- ✔ **Your health insurance company:** If you're in a managed care plan, you will have to contact the plan to find out if the doctors you are considering are plan participants. You may also wish to consult with the plan to get a list of participating physicians from which to begin your search.

  Some managed care plans will allow you to choose a gynecologist as your primary care physician.

✔ **Doctor referral services operated by local medical societies and hospitals:** These services refer only those doctors who are members of the society or who are on the hospital staff. Neither type of service will comment on the ability of physicians, but they do give you a list of names to contact in your search.

✔ **Listings in the telephone directory:** Doctors' names are usually arranged according to their practice or specialty.

Responding to a newspaper advertisement may not be the best way to find a doctor. Although an ad is good way to find out if a doctor is accepting new patients, you have to ask yourself why the doctor is advertising. Is he trying to attract patients because he just finished his internship? Because he's new to the area? Because he's in a highly competitive market? Or has he just moved in from a state where his license was revoked?

Once you come up with a list of possible candidates, you want to find out more about them, starting with their qualifications:

✔ **Check credentials:** Where and when did your prospective doctor obtain her medical degree? Does she hold a doctor of medicine (M.D.) degree or a doctor of osteopathy (D.O.) degree? Did she undergo any postgraduate study? Does she specialize in a certain area of medicine? How long has she been practicing? Is she board certified? Physicians who are board certified have met additional training requirements and passed a rigorous examination administered by a specialty board. To check the board certification status of a physician, call the American Board of Medical Specialties at 800-776-CERT.

✔ **Check history:** Contact your state's medical licensing agency and ask if the doctor has had any actions taken against him. Check with your local courts to see if any malpractice suits have been filed against the doctor in your jurisdiction and learn the disposition of those cases.

✔ **Find out about the practice:** Does the doctor participate in your health maintenance organization or accept your insurance? Does she practice in a group or by herself? Is she affiliated with or does she have admitting privileges at the local hospital of your choice?

✔ **Schedule a get-acquainted visit:** This 10- to 15-minute visit will help you determine whether you and the doctor are right for each other. You can use this time to ask the doctor questions about his credentials, history, and practice as well as about his philosophy of care. Does he emphasize prevention? Does he consider the patient as a partner? Does he favor conservative or aggressive treatment? Pay particular attention to the doctor's manner and attitude when he answers your questions.

The detail expert: The specialist

A specialist is a doctor who concentrates on a specific body system, age group, or disorder, much in the way an internist or family practitioner specializes in primary care medicine. After obtaining a Doctor of Medicine (M.D.) or Doctor of Osteopathy (D.O.) degree, a specialist undergoes two to four years of supervised specialty training called a *residency*. Many specialists also take one or more years of additional training (called a *fellowship*) in a specific area of their specialty (called a *subspecialty*).

Be aware that a doctor can say she specializes in a certain area of medicine without having received any advanced training in that area. If you want to be sure that your doctor is trained in a particular area of medicine, look for one who is board certified in that area.

To become board certified, a specialist must not only complete the advanced training detailed earlier, she must also pass a rigorous test administered by a board of professionals in her field. But in general, board certification is a good sign that the doctor is up-to-date on the procedures, theories, and success-failure rates in her specialty.

You usually encounter a specialist when your primary care physician wants to confirm a diagnosis or wants a second opinion, although you can seek one on your own. Before you schedule an appointment with a specialist, make sure you need one. Going to a specialist should not be a casual next step routinely taken in every medical situation. If your doctor wants you to see a specialist, ask him to explain why. Ask him what he thinks is wrong with you and why he's recommending a particular type of specialist. If your doctor says he wants you to see a specialist for further testing, ask him what he expects the tests to show.

Complementary Medicine

Modern medicine can do wonders, but it doesn't have all the answers. As a result, millions of Americans are turning to complementary, or alternative, therapies.

Complementary medicine encompasses a wide range of healing philosophies and therapies that are generally considered to be outside the scope of mainstream medicine. These treatments and approaches are generally not taught in traditional medical schools or used in hospitals. But these alternatives are being used more and more with traditional medicine in complementary fashion. In fact, many doctors are starting to recommend some complementary therapies to be used along with their own traditional medicine, and some medical schools have begun offering courses in various complementary therapies.

A glossary of medical specialties

The list that follows is what the American Medical Association (AMA) calls "self-designated [medical] specialty classifications." This means that these specialties are the ones that doctors use to describe themselves and their primary and secondary fields of practice.

- *Allergy and immunology* involves the diagnosis and treatment of all forms of allergies and other disorders involving the immune system.

- *Anesthesiology* involves putting a patient to sleep or preventing her from feeling pain during surgery or diagnostic procedures by giving her anesthetic drugs.

- *Cardiology* deals with diseases of the heart and blood vessels.

- *Dermatology* involves the diagnosis and treatment of cancerous and noncancerous disorders of the skin.

- *Endocrinology* is concerned with disorders of the glands. It also deals with disorders such as diabetes and sexual problems.

- *Gastroenterology* is concerned with problems involving the digestive tract, including the gallbladder, liver, stomach, and other related organs.

- *Geriatrics* involves the problems associated with aging and diseases of the elderly.

- *Hematology* specializes in disorders and treatment of the blood and blood-forming parts of the body.

- *Nephrology* is concerned with disorders of the kidney.

- *Oncology* involves the diagnosis and treatment of all types of cancer and other malignant and benign tumors.

- *Ophthalmology* diagnoses, monitors, and provides medical and surgical treatment of vision problems and other disorders of the eyes.

- *Otolaryngology* deals with diseases and disorders of the ear, nose, and throat.

- *Preventive medicine* involves preventing disease through immunization and good health habits, and focuses on occupational and environmental factors.

- *Proctology* diagnoses and treats disorders of the intestinal tract, rectum, and anus.

- *Psychiatry* involves evaluating, treating, and preventing behavioral, emotional, and mental disorders.

- *Pulmonary disease* deals with diseases of the lungs.

- *Rheumatology* specializes in diseases of the tendons, muscles, and joints, including arthritis.

- *Surgery* involves surgical procedures. Some surgeons may be generalists or specialists in a particular specialty such as cardiovascular or reconstructive surgery.

- *Urology* deals with diseases of the urinary system, as well as the reproductive organs in men.

If you're considering using complementary therapies, talk with your doctor. She can let you know if the therapy is appropriate for your health problem or if it may have side effects that may be harmful to you.

Some of the more common complementary therapies are

- **Acupressure:** Acupressure is a form of manipulative therapy that originated in China. Pressure is applied with the fingertips along the meridians of your body — invisible pathways in which the life force (called chi) flows — letting chi flow to various parts of your body, theoretically restoring health.

- **Acupuncture:** Similar to acupressure, this ancient Chinese healing art uses very thin needles that are inserted under the skin and along your meridians to treat disease and restore health.

- **Chiropractic:** Chiropractic is a therapy that manipulates the spinal vertebrae to attempt to restore health. This healing art holds that the spinal column is central to a sense of well-being because it is instrumental in maintaining the health of the nervous system. Manipulating the vertebrae restores or keeps the nervous system healthy.

- **Herbal medicine:** Herbal medicine is a healing art that uses plants to treat and prevent illnesses.

- **Homeopathy:** Homeopathy is a system of medicine founded on the idea that "like cures like." Homeopathy holds that the whole person must be treated, not just the disease. Therefore, symptoms indicate an imbalance of the life force and balance must be restored for a healthy mind, body, and spirit. Homeopathic medications are from natural sources, such as plants, animal material, and natural chemicals.

- **Massage therapy:** Massage therapy relaxes, relieves tension, soothes aches and pains, improves circulation and digestion, and stimulates the body's systems. Massage therapy can also treat stress and fatigue, insomnia, lower back pain, headaches, and muscle fatigue. The philosophy of massage therapy is based upon the balance in the body. When the balance is disturbed, illness occurs.

- **Naturopathy:** This healing art focuses on the body's natural healing force and makes use of massage, herbal therapy, homeopathy, and other complementary therapies to treat a range of conditions.

- **Reflexology:** Related to acupuncture, reflexology uses the hands to stimulate certain areas of the feet that are thought to correspond to various organs and other parts of the body.

Visiting Your Doctor: What to Expect

Okay, you've found a doctor, and you've made an appointment. Perhaps it's for a standard physical. Perhaps you have a specific complaint. Whatever the reason, you need to be prepared — that means that you need to know what you should do and what the doctor will do.

The preliminaries

If you're seeing your doctor for a specific complaint, make a list of the problems you've been experiencing. Be as detailed as possible. If you're experiencing pain, for example, describe it. Is it dull? sharp? throbbing? Explain when the symptom started, how long it lasts, whether it's affected by activities such as sleeping or eating and whether it's relieved by over-the-counter medications. These details give your doctor a better idea of what to look for. Even if you're seeing your doctor for a routine physical, you may have questions about your health or health care. Write these questions down before your appointment so that you'll remember to ask them. Your doctor will likely have questions of her own. Depending on the purpose of your visit and whether you've seen the doctor before, she may ask you about your medical history, family history, lifestyle, work, and any symptoms you are experiencing. She will also want to know the names and dosages of any medications you take. To prepare yourself for these questions, you might want to make a list all of your prescription and nonprescription drugs or bring the medications in their original containers along with you. If your appointment is with a new doctor, you should have your medical records from your previous doctor transferred or collect them before you go.

The exam

Depending on the purpose of your visit, your age, and your medical and family history, your doctor may want you to have certain tests. These tests fall into four categories:

- ✔ **Screening tests:** These tests look for a potential problem in an otherwise healthy woman. Common screening tests for women, depending on their age, include blood pressure monitoring, a weight check, a Pap test and pelvic exam, and a screening mammogram.

- ✔ **Diagnostic tests:** These tests also look for problems. If a screening test is abnormal, your doctor will order a diagnostic test. For example, if a suspicious spot showed up on your mammogram, your doctor may recommend a biopsy (in which a sample of tissue from the suspicious area is removed and examined under a microscope) to determine whether you have breast cancer.

> ✔ **Prognostic, or monitoring, tests:** These tests are performed to give additional information after the doctor has already made a diagnosis. If the doctor has already diagnosed lung cancer, for example, she may order an MRI (magnetic resonance imaging) to see whether the cancer has spread from the lungs to other areas of the body. Monitoring tests can also be used to determine the effects of medical treatment on a disease or condition.

During a standard regular exam, or checkup, you're most likely to only have basic screening tests, along with the exam itself.

A basic physical exam should include your medical and family history along with a head-to-toe examination. Your doctor may check your eyes, ears, and skin; listen to your heart; check the inside of your mouth and throat; measure your height and weight; and check your reflexes. Some of the screening tests mentioned in Table 2-1 may also be performed at this time.

The following general guidelines for medical testing and screening are based on various sources, including groups of medical experts and the U.S. Preventive Services Task Force. Keep in mind that there is no agreement among the medical community on what tests should be performed, how often, or if at all. And your own health and family history may suggest a different timetable. You and your doctor should discuss what's best for you.

Questions to ask about medical tests

If your doctor orders a test, ask her the name of the test and its purpose. If you think you may have had the test recently, tell her. The test may not need to be repeated. Ask your doctor the following questions:

✔ Why do I need this test?

✔ Why this particular test?

✔ How accurate and reliable is the test? Every test carries the risk of resulting in a *false-positive* result (a result that falsely indicates the presence of a disease or condition) or a *false-negative* result (a result that fails to show the presence of an existing disease or condition).

✔ What will be done if the test is positive or negative?

✔ Is the test *invasive* (any test beyond a simple blood sample that pierces or invades the body is invasive and carries a risk of infection or other conditions) or noninvasive? If the test is invasive, what risks are involved? Is there a noninvasive test that can provide similar information?

✔ Does the test require any special preparation, such as fasting for several hours?

✔ How much does it cost?

✔ Will my insurance cover it?

✔ Are there any alternatives if I refuse this test?

Table 2-1	Preventive Screening Recommendations
Test	**Timetable**
Blood pressure check	Periodic blood pressure screening is recommended for all people 21 years and older. Some experts recommend a check every time you visit your doctor.
Cholesterol test	Periodic cholesterol screening is recommended by most groups for women between the ages of 45 and 65. The National Cholesterol Education Program Adult Treatment Panel II recommends testing at least once every five years for all adults 20 years and older.
Colorectal cancer screening tests	Virtually all groups recommend regular screening for all people 50 and over. The American Cancer Society recommends an annual digital rectal exam (DRE) beginning at age 40, an annual fecal occult blood test beginning at age 50, and sigmoidoscopy every three to five years beginning at age 50.
Electrocardiogram (EKG)	Some experts recommend getting a baseline EKG at age 40 to use as a comparison with future EKGs.
Mammogram	The Task Force recommends screening every one to two years with mammography alone or mammography and an annual clinical breast exam for women ages 50 to 69. Most other groups now recommend that mammograms be given every one to two years beginning at age 40.
Pap test	A Pap test is recommended at least once every three years for women who are sexually active or who are 18 or older. The American Cancer Society, National Cancer Institute, American College of Obstetricians and Gynecologists, and American Academy of Family Physicians recommend annual tests but permit testing less frequently at the discretion of the physician after three or more annual smears have been normal.
Visual and glaucoma screening	The American Academy of Ophthalmology recommends periodic comprehensive eye exams, including a glaucoma screen, beginning at age 40.

Another type of routine exam that you may encounter — either as part of your routine physical or during a visit to your gynecologist — is the gynecologic examination.

The gynecologic examination

Regular gynecologic examinations help you maintain your health and fertility and help assure that you have an uncomplicated pregnancy and childbirth. The exams, which are recommended annually for sexually active teens and all women 18 and over, are designed to detect problems with your reproductive system early, when treatment is most successful. These exams usually include a pelvic exam with a Pap test and a breast exam. They often also include weight and blood pressure checks, and, on occasion, blood and urine tests.

You may feel uncomfortable or anxious before a gynecologic exam, especially if you've never had one before or are seeing a new doctor. This is perfectly normal. Knowing what to expect, however, can help relieve the anxiety somewhat (Chapter 28 offers additional tips to put you at ease).

When you're called into the examination room, you're asked to undress and put on a hospital gown. When the doctor arrives, you lie down on the examining table. Your doctor may start with either a pelvic exam or a breast exam. For the pelvic exam, she asks you to bend your knees and put your feet into metal footrests known as *stirrups*. She also asks you to slide your body down toward the end of the examining table. This position gives the doctor the best view of the visible internal reproductive structures.

After donning surgical gloves, your doctor begins the examination with a visual inspection of your external genitals. She gently spreads the folds of skin around your vagina to look for irritation, herpes sores, genital warts, or anything else unusual. Next, she inserts an instrument called a *speculum* into your vagina. This device, which is shaped like a duckbill with a handle, allows the doctor to spread apart the walls of the vagina to view the cervix and to insert and withdraw instruments without touching the sides of your vagina. While the speculum is open, the doctor looks at the vagina and cervix for signs of redness, discharge, and rough spots, which can be precancerous cell changes. She then performs a Pap test.

The Pap test

For this test, which screens for cervical cancer, the doctor uses a small, plastic brush, a wooden spatula (like a Popsicle stick), or a long cotton-tipped swab to gently scrape cells from your cervix, (see Figure 2-1). She places the cells on a slide, which is sent to a laboratory for examination.

The Pap test can detect cell changes long before they progress to cancer. In fact, it's estimated that 90 percent of deaths from cervical cancer could have been prevented if the women had had Pap tests. But what happens if the test indicates an abnormality?

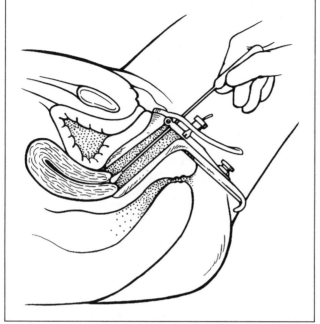

Figure 2-1:
Your doctor
takes a
sample of
cells for
testing
during the
Pap test.

First, take a deep breath. An abnormal Pap test does not usually mean a woman has cancer; instead, it may indicate a precancerous condition or inflammation. Pap tests are not always 100 percent accurate. Sometimes they find suspicious cells when no cancer is present, and sometimes abnormal cells in the cervix were not scraped off during the procedure.

If your test results reveal abnormal but not obviously cancerous cells, ask your doctor to explain the abnormality. It could be caused by a vaginal infection or inflammation.

If your test results reveal mild *dysplasia* (abnormal development of cells) or *cervical intraepithelial neoplasia* (CIN, which indicates a combination of dysplasia and early surface cancer that has not spread), your doctor may recommend regular Pap tests to monitor the condition or a diagnostic procedure such as a cervical biopsy.

If your test results show moderate or severe dysplasia or CIN, it means that cellular abnormalities may be present that could progress to invasive cancer if they are not treated. Your doctor will recommend a biopsy to determine the need for treatment and to select the best type of treatment. For more information on the treatment of cervical cancer, see Chapter 16.

After completing the Pap test, the doctor removes the speculum and performs what is called a bimanual exam. She inserts one or two gloved, lubricated fingers into the vagina until they are against your cervix. She places her other hand on your lower abdomen and applies pressure. This enables her to feel the size and shape of your uterus and check for any masses that might be on the ovaries or fallopian tubes. To complete the pelvic exam, the doctor may insert one finger into your rectum and one finger into your vagina to feel your ovaries.

Breast exam

Many gynecologic exams also include a breast examination. For this test, you lie back on the examining table and stretch your arms above your head as the doctor checks your breasts and armpits for lumps. She asks you if you perform regular breast self-exams. If you don't, she should offer to show you how. (See "How to perform a breast self-examination.")

When the exam is over, your doctor should take a few minutes to discuss any results she's found or to tell you when you'll find out the results of your Pap test. She should also ask if you have any additional questions.

How to perform a breast self-examination

It is estimated that between 50 and 80 percent of breast cancers are first detected by women through breast self-examination. Regular breast self-examination enables you to become familiar with your breasts so that you can learn what is normal for you and become aware of any early subtle changes.

Most experts recommend that you perform the exam monthly — generally two or three days after the end of your menstrual period. If you are postmenopausal, experts recommend that you pick a particular day to perform the exam, then do it at the same time each month.

Here are the basics:

✔ Stand in front of a mirror and look for changes in the size or contour of your breasts, dimpling or puckering of the skin, nipple discharge, or other abnormalities. Do this first with your arms at your sides, then stretch your arms above your head and look again. Finally, stand with your hands on your hips and flex your chest muscles, again looking for any changes or abnormalities.

✔ Lie on your back and place a pillow under the shoulder of the side you are examining. Raise the arm above your head and use the finger pads of the three middle fingers of the opposite hand to feel for lumps or thickening, pressing hard enough to know how the breast feels.

You can choose from three different patterns to perform this part of the exam: an up-and-down line, a wedge, or a starburst pattern, in which you radiate from the nipple out. Do it the same way every time.

After checking the breast for lumps, gently squeeze the nipple and look for any discharge. Repeat the entire process on the other side.

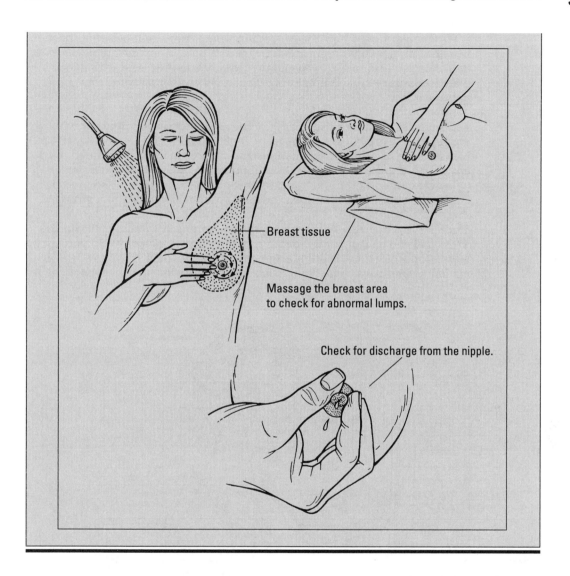

Breast tissue

Massage the breast area
to check for abnormal lumps.

Check for discharge from the nipple.

Mammograms

Mammograms should be a part of your preventive health care, although
they generally don't take place during your gynecologic exam. These breast
x-rays can detect growths that are too small to be felt during breast examinations and, thus, detect cancer at an early stage, when it can be more
easily treated. When performed as part of routine, preventive care,
mammograms are known as *screening mammograms*. When performed to
obtain an image of a suspicious lump, mammograms are known as *diagnostic
mammograms*.

In either case, here's how the procedure works. You stand before a special x-ray machine with your chest bare. One at a time, a technician places each breast onto a plastic platform and then gently compresses it with another plate (see Figure 2-2). The x-ray is taken while your breast is in this compressed state.

A radiologist compares the images of the breast with each other or with images from a previous mammogram, looking for changes in the density of breast tissue as well as calcifications and nipple changes. Mammograms do not always show cancer; they show abnormal or suspicious areas, which help determine whether further tests need to be done. They also provide information about the size, location, and possible spreading of a growth.

Studies show that regular screening mammograms in women between the ages of 50 and 65 can cut the death rate from breast cancer by 30 percent or more. And while there is still disagreement about whether routine mammograms are as beneficial to women in their 40s, most groups now

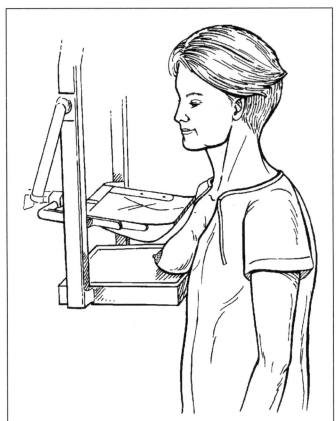

Figure 2-2:
During a mammogram, your breast is compressed while an x-ray is taken of the tissue.

recommend that women should begin routine screening at age 40. You should be aware however, that because breast tissue is denser in younger women, they are more likely to experience false-negative mammogram results (results that indicate an abnormality when none is present).

Maintaining Your Medical Record

Your medical record is a collection of all the charts and notes your doctors have made about your health over the years. This record, which is generally kept in a central location at the hospital you've attended or at your doctor's office, usually includes the following information:

- ✔ Your biographical information
- ✔ Your medical and family history
- ✔ The results of your physical exams
- ✔ Any medical diagnoses that have been made
- ✔ The results of any diagnostic and laboratories tests that have been conducted on you, such as x-rays and blood tests
- ✔ Your medication records
- ✔ Your doctor's orders
- ✔ Progress notes written by doctors, nurses, consultants, and other health care workers
- ✔ Informed consent forms (see the "Informed consent" section later in the chapter)
- ✔ Care plans

This is important information — important to you, your doctor, and any other practitioner from whom you seek health care. But some doctors and hospitals are reluctant to share medical records with you. Ironically, however, other people are able to see your record without a problem — health and life insurance carriers and your employers, for example. And to make matters worse, some medical records contain errors and inaccuracies. For this and other reasons, it is important to know what is in your medical record. Knowing what is in your record can help you correct any misinformation that may be there and be better informed about your health care.

Accessing your medical record

Your right to see your record depends on the law in the state where you live. Some states have laws that specifically permit you direct access to your record; other states have no regulations. This does not mean, however, that you are forbidden access. Access is not illegal in any state.

Here's how to go about it:

- ✔ **Ask for your medical records:** Start by asking your doctor directly. If this fails, call the office or hospital that holds the records and ask what you must do to obtain them.

- ✔ **Put your request in writing:** This documents your efforts and offers proof that you are working through normal channels. Include your name, address, patient identification number, and the specific entry or file you want and indicate that you are willing to pay a reasonable copying fee. If your request is denied, ask for the denial to be put in writing with the reasons listed.

- ✔ **Seek legal action:** If all else fails, contact a lawyer familiar with your state's laws. You may be able to obtain a court order from a magistrate or civil court judge.

- ✔ **Contact the Medical Information Bureau (MIB):** If you've ever completed an insurance company application form that includes health information, that information is on file with the MIB. If the MIB has a file on you, you can obtain a copy for $8 by calling the MIB at 617-426-3660.

Keeping your own medical record

Medical records are sometimes inaccurate or incomplete. The latter is particularly true if you move often or consult numerous doctors and hospitals. It is quite possible that each doctor or hospital holds only a piece of the puzzle. For this reason, it's a good idea for you to maintain your own medical record.

Here's what your record should include

- ✔ **A record of your individual visits:** This is a record of the details of each visit to a doctor or hospital. It should include the date, the doctor, your symptoms or complaints, and the doctor's diagnosis and treatment. Make sure you include all visits to any medical practitioner, including your primary care doctor and specialists.

- ✔ **A record of major hospitalizations:** This record lets you keep track of everything that happens to you during a hospitalization. It includes personal data about each visit, including admission and discharge dates, the name and address of the hospital, the name of the doctor who admitted you, the name of any consulting doctors or surgeons, the reason for your admission, and your diagnosis and treatment. It should also include a record of the daily activities that accompanied your visit. This includes not only a record of visits by various doctors and other practitioners but also a daily log of tests you experienced (and their results) and medications you were given.

✔ **A record of your medications:** This, of course, is a record of the medications you take. It includes all prescription medications you take (especially if you have them filled at different pharmacies). It can also include nonprescription, or over-the-counter, medications. Information you need in this section includes the name of the medication, what it is for, the name of the doctor who prescribed it, the pharmacy where the prescription was filled, the expiration date, and any side effects or adverse reactions you experienced. If you're taking more than one medication, you run the risk of experiencing a drug interaction. By keeping track of the medications you're taking and sharing this information with your doctors, you can help avoid unpleasant side effects.

Using Medications

Medications are an important part of medical care. In some cases, the benefits are the difference between life and death. Yet most people know very little about the medications they take. Studies suggest that almost half of all prescriptions filled are not fully used. Consumers report confusion about side effects, shelf life, and even how to read or interpret the instructions given to them by a doctor or pharmacist or printed on a label.

Whenever you have a question about medications — whether your doctor prescribes them or you purchase them over the counter — don't hesitate to ask your doctor or pharmacist. Taking the wrong medication or taking the right medication incorrectly can be as dangerous (or more so) as failing to take a medication that you need.

Prescription medications

Prescription medications are medications that your doctor must order, or prescribe, for you. Your doctor can either phone the order in to the pharmacy or provide you with a written order form. You should find out the following every time your doctor prescribes a new medication:

✔ The name of the medication

✔ What the medication is designed to do

✔ The dose of the medication

✔ The amount you're supposed to take

✔ How often you're supposed to take the medication

✔ Any particular instructions for taking the medication (whether you should take it with meals, for example)

✔ Any possible side effects

✔ Whether the medication interacts negatively with any other medications you are taking

Your doctor may prescribe a brand name drug, but depending on what she marks on the prescription form and the laws of your state, your pharmacist may give you a drug with a different name — a generic drug. A *generic drug* is a drug whose active ingredients duplicate those of the brand name product. Acetaminophen, for example, is the generic name of the pain-relieving and fever-reducing drug Tylenol.

Generally, generic drugs are cheaper than their brand name counterparts. You may wish to ask your doctor or pharmacist whether a generic form of the drug you are being prescribed exists.

Over-the-counter drugs

Unlike prescription drugs, which must be ordered by a doctor and obtained from a licensed pharmacy, you can purchase over-the-counter (OTC) drugs just about anywhere. But just because these drugs are more readily available doesn't mean that they aren't strictly regulated. Because OTC products can be purchased without a doctor's prescription, the Food and Drug Administration (FDA) requires them to have a higher standard of safety than prescription products. So OTC products generally consist of ingredients that have a long and established safety record at lower dosages. They also must carry labels that contain all the information you need to use the product safely and effectively. This does not mean, however, that these drugs cannot be dangerous if used incorrectly or in combination with other medications.

Here are some things you should consider when buying an OTC medication:

✔ **Shop around:** Competition for OTC drugs is fierce, and prices vary significantly. In any given store, you may find several products with the same active ingredient. Look for the product with the best price.

✔ **Ask your pharmacist for a recommendation:** If you're not sure what type of OTC medication you need or which brand may be best for you, your pharmacist may be able to help you narrow down your decision.

✔ **Look for expiration dates.**

✔ **Check the packaging:** Make sure safety seals are intact. Before making your purchase, check to see if the seals are broken. If you have any question about the integrity of the package, return it immediately or throw it away. Don't use it.

What to Do If Your Doctor Recommends Surgery

So your doctor has just recommended surgery. Don't panic, and don't rush home to pack just yet. Before you make such a major decision, you need a thorough understanding of your problem, the surgical procedure itself, and your other treatment options. Depending on your particular circumstances, it is possible that surgery may not be necessary.

Is it necessary?

Studies show that as many as 10 to 20 percent of all surgeries may be unnecessary. A study published in *The New England Journal of Medicine*, for example, estimated that almost half of the more than 100,000 carotid endarterectomies performed in the United States (carotid endarterectomy is a procedure that cleans out the arteries that supply blood to the brain) were performed on patients without symptoms of carotid disease. Other studies show that between 15 and 40 percent of appendectomies are performed on a normal appendix. And experts are now rethinking the old belief that a woman who gave birth by cesarean section must deliver by c-section in all future deliveries.

With this information in mind, it's important that you determine whether your surgery is necessary before you consent to undergo it. If your doctor recommends surgery, ask her the following questions:

- ✔ Is this surgery really necessary?
- ✔ Are there other alternatives to treat my problem, such as medication, diet, bed rest, or physical therapy?
- ✔ What will happen if I don't have this surgery?
- ✔ Will the problem recur even after surgery is done?
- ✔ What are the risks and potential complications of the surgery?

If you and your doctor have determined that surgery is necessary, find out about the procedure that is being recommended. Ask her the following:

- ✔ Are there less invasive or less risky surgical alternatives?
- ✔ Is it possible to perform the surgery on an outpatient basis?
- ✔ What are the predicted success rates of the surgery?

In addition to asking questions of the doctor who has recommended surgery, consider getting a second opinion. In fact, your doctor might recommend this herself. And your insurance company may insist on it.

Go to a doctor who's not a friend or colleague of your doctor for an unbiased second opinion. And consider the source of that opinion. If you seek the opinion of a surgeon, for example, she may be less likely to recommend a treatment other than surgery than another type of practitioner.

If the second opinion differs from your doctor's recommendation, seek a third or even a fourth opinion, if necessary. And research the issue on your own at the library or on reputable Internet Web sites so that you can make an educated decision. (See Chapter 29 for a list of helpful Web sites.)

Informed consent

Informed consent is simply the idea that you have the right to available information about your condition and about the benefits and risks of any procedures doctors want to perform on you. That way, you can make an informed decision about what is done to your body before you give the go-ahead or refusal. In other words, your doctor must fully explain in simple terms the pros and cons of any proposed procedure, including surgery. She must also tell you why she feels the procedure is needed and what risks accompany it.

How does informed consent affect you when you're contemplating surgery? There are two likely scenarios. You may be asked to sign a blanket consent form and/or a form that gives your consent for a specific procedure.

The blanket consent form

If your surgery involves admittance to a hospital, your admittance paperwork will likely include a consent form. This form may be a blanket consent form. By signing it, you are basically giving the hospital permission to do with you as it sees fit. Some hospitals may also ask you to sign a consent form that includes a release against negligence on the hospital's part or that requires you to surrender your right to sue due to malpractice. These types of forms are not legally binding, however, because they give the hospital an unfair advantage over you.

If you don't sign the consent form, chances are you may not be admitted to the hospital. Here's what you can do if that happens:

- Make changes to the form that you feel are necessary and sign your initials next to the changes.
- Write on the form that you are signing it only because you would not be admitted otherwise and that you have no intention of giving up any of the rights the form is forcing you to give up.
- Ask to speak with a supervisor if the admissions clerk tells you that you cannot alter the form.

Protecting yourself against nosocomial infections

You can increase your chances of remaining infection-free by heeding the following advice:

✔ Request that all hospital personnel who come in direct contact with you wash their hands.

✔ Request to change your room if your roommate develops an infection.

✔ Refuse to be shaved the night before a surgery or a procedure that requires the removal of hair.

✔ If you have a urinary catheter, have the nurse routinely check the drainage to help you maintain cleanliness.

Consent form for a specific procedure

The other type of consent form you may be asked to sign gives your approval for a specific procedure or operation. You should be given a consent form for each procedure done, not a blanket consent form.

Make sure the doctor who is performing the procedure explains it to you clearly. Before you give your consent, be sure your doctor has explained the following:

✔ Your condition and diagnosis

✔ The benefits of the procedure

✔ The risks of the procedure

✔ The survival rates and the effectiveness or success rate of the procedure

✔ Alternative treatments and how feasible they might be

Read the consent form carefully. If you don't agree to any of the items on the form, revise and amend it.

Surviving a hospital stay

Whether you go to a hospital for surgery or some other treatment, you hope that you return feeling better. What you may not know is that you have a good chance of picking up another ailment altogether. This scenario is referred to as *iatrogenesis*.

Iatrogenesis is a condition or illness that is inadvertently introduced by a doctor or by a medical treatment or diagnostic procedure. Among the most common types of iatrogenic illness are *nosocomial infections*. These infections, which can be deadly, are caused by microorganisms that dwell within hospitals. You're at greater risk if you're having surgery because microbes can multiply quickly in an open wound. Nosocomial infections are often spread by hand contact, usually by direct contact with medical staff that has had contact with other seriously ill patients. But organisms can also be spread in food, water, intravenous fluids, and transfused blood.

Nosocomial infections are not the only type of iatrogenic illness that routinely occur in hospitals. Medication errors are also common. Because many workers are involved in giving you medication, numerous chances for mistakes exist. A doctor can write the order for the wrong drug; a nurse may misinterpret a doctor's handwriting; a pharmacist may not properly label a medication; a drug allergy may be overlooked, or the wrong drug may be given to the wrong patient.

Protecting yourself against medication errors

Here are some steps you can take to protect yourself against medication errors:

✔ Keep a record of all prescription and over-the-counter medications you take.

✔ Inform your doctor, nurses, and pharmacists of any drug allergies or sensitivities you have and what medications you are currently taking.

✔ Make sure you know the names of all drugs prescribed and given to you.

✔ Make sure you receive the drug you are supposed to receive.

✔ Examine the drug you are given. Speak out if it looks different from the norm.

✔ Read labels carefully before taking medications.

✔ Take medications as directed.

✔ Report any problems with or adverse reactions to your doctor immediately.

Chapter 3

Insurance for a Healthy Life

In This Chapter
▶ An insurance primer
▶ Managed care versus fee-for-service
▶ Understanding Medicare and Medicaid
▶ Long-term-care insurance

A single hospital stay can cost thousands of dollars. If you or a family member is sick enough to require a long hospital stay, you don't need the added stress that comes with trying to determine how to pay the hospital bill or how to cover your living expenses if the hospital bill wipes out your annual salary. Health insurance can take away some of your worry.

A Health Insurance Primer

Health insurance pays the large expense that can be incurred when you or a family member sees doctors, goes to the hospital, or seeks other costly medical services. If you have some type of health insurance, you can obtain the high-quality medical care you want without severely impacting your wallet. Not that your wallet won't feel at least a pinch. Like health care costs, health insurance premiums have skyrocketed over the past two decades.

Many employers offer some type of health insurance as part of their benefits package. If you do not work for a company that provides any type of health insurance, you should strongly consider purchasing it on your own.

 Don't assume that you will be able to purchase health insurance on your own with little or no difficulty. If your health is poor or you are suddenly diagnosed with a long-term illness, many insurance companies will tell you that your preexisting condition will prohibit you from getting the coverage you probably really need.

The Classic Approach: Indemnity Insurance

When many people think of health insurance, they think of indemnity insurance. For years, this pay-as-you-go type of insurance dominated the industry. Even now, many Americans receive coverage from these plans.

In this type of insurance plan, also known as a *fee-for-service* plan, you or your employer pays a premium for insurance coverage. Then, after you meet your *deductible* (the amount you must pay before your insurance kicks in), the plan pays for services as you receive them. Depending on the type of insurance, you may also have to pay a *co-payment* or *coinsurance*, generally a percentage of the service's cost.

Table 3-1 explains the three major types of indemnity insurance.

Table 3-1	Types of Indemnity Insurance
Type	*Description*
Hospital insurance	This type provides coverage for inpatient and outpatient hospital services. Policies usually specify the number of days of hospitalization and the percentage of costs they will cover in a certain time period or set a dollar limit on the total benefits they will pay.
Medical-surgical insurance	The medical portion pays for doctors' visits to the hospital and may pay for office visits that lead to inpatient or surgical care. It also pays for some drugs, x-rays, anesthesia, and laboratory tests performed outside the hospital. The surgical portion pays the surgeon's and anesthesiologist's fees for surgery performed in the hospital or in an ambulatory surgical center. It may also cover procedures performed in a doctor's office.
Major medical insurance	This type covers the medical and surgical expenses associated with illness. Most plans include a deductible. After you meet the deductible, the plans generally pay a portion of covered expenses. You are responsible for the remaining percentage (the co-payment, or coinsurance). If your health care provider doesn't participate in the insurance plan, you may have to pay the difference between her charge and the insurance plan's reimbursement.

Some insurers offer plans that combine hospital, medical-surgical, and major medical coverage into one policy. These combination policies are known as *comprehensive insurance.*

Most indemnity plans place no limits on the cost or quality of services. You can generally seek the services of any practitioner you choose and be charged whatever fee that practitioner feels is appropriate. If the practitioner charges more than what your insurance company believes is *usual, customary, and reasonable* and does not participate in your insurance plan, you may get stuck paying the difference.

Coverage for the Future: Managed Care

These plans are the new kids on the block, but they're rapidly gaining in popularity. In fact, the majority of Americans are now enrolled in either a managed care plan or an indemnity plan with managed care elements. Managed care offers an entirely different approach to health insurance. Its goals are to provide consumers with access to appropriate health care at a reasonable cost and to control health care spending. It achieves this goal by studying health care services and eliminating those that are unnecessary, unproven, or not cost-effective. It also focuses on preventive health care — services that keep people from getting sick or delay the onset of illnesses. But all managed care is not the same. Form and quality vary and savvy consumers need to know what to look for to make managed care work for them.

Table 3-2 explains the four main types of managed care plans.

Table 3-2	Types of Managed Care Programs
Type	**Description**
Health Maintenance Organizations (HMOs)	This is the oldest and best-known type of managed care. In exchange for your monthly premium, you receive all the medical care you need as covered by that particular plan. Many HMOs cover and pay for some services that traditional indemnity plans do not. In return, you agree to use only those doctors and hospitals affiliated with or employed by the HMO. If you use a doctor or hospital not affiliated with the HMO, you will likely pay for all or part of the cost of the service yourself.
	With an HMO, you usually don't have to worry about deductibles. However, you may have to pay a nominal co-payment (usually $5 to $20) each time you visit your doctor.

(continued)

Table 3-2 *(continued)*	
Type	*Description*
Preferred provider organizations (PPOs)	Similar to HMOs, PPOs are large networks of doctors and hospitals that are organized and owned by insurance companies or by the doctors and hospitals in the PPO. These plans usually offer consumers more choices of doctors and hospitals than are available in HMOs.
Point-of-service (POS) plans	These plans are hybrids of HMOs and traditional indemnity insurance plans: If you're in a POS plan and you use the doctors or hospitals in that plan's network, you pay nothing or just a small co-payment for each visit. If you visit a doctor or hospital that is not in the plan's network, you pay a larger share of the bill. The POS plan does pay a significant portion of your bill, however, typically 60 to 70 percent. And although you must pay the other 30 to 40 percent, the total amount you are required to pay in a year is generally capped. After you reach that cap, the POS generally pays all the bills for covered services.
Physician hospital organizations (PHOs)	Typically owned by their member doctors and hospitals, who share as many resources as possible in order to keep a lid on spiraling costs, PHOs vary in the number of providers affiliated with them. They can either contract with HMOs to treat their members or, depending on state law, sign up consumers directly.

Managed care basics

All types of managed care programs share certain features. For example, each plan provides services to its members through a network of health care providers — hospitals, doctors, and other health care workers who are selected by or contract with the plan to treat its members. Consumers who enroll in managed care plans are generally expected to obtain the majority of their health care services from network providers.

The primary care provider is the network provider consumers consult most often. These individuals, usually family physicians, internists, pediatricians, obstetrician/gynecologists, and, in some instances, nurse practitioners, are responsible for providing basic health care services, such as preventive health care and routine checkups, and for treating a wide range of illnesses and injuries. These individuals may also control consumer access to other health care providers. In other words, they may act as gate-keepers, controlling the gate through which consumers are referred to see specialists, undergo diagnostic services, or be admitted to the hospital. In this way, they make sure that consumers are not seeing specialists or receiving treatments for conditions that can be cared for in a more cost-effective manner.

Managed care plans — and even some traditional indemnity plans — also engage in *utilization review*. Utilization review programs oversee the services members get, how frequently those services are used, and how much they cost. They generally look for ways to keep consumers from using expensive services unnecessarily, to keep tabs on the number of visits consumers make to doctors, and to monitor prescription drug use. These programs can also require consumers to get permission to have a major diagnostic test or procedure or to be admitted to a hospital.

Tips to consider when shopping for a managed care plan

Here are some things to look for in choosing a managed care plan:

✔ **Carefully review the managed care plans you are considering.** Investigate the companies that own the programs. Check over the list of doctors and hospitals to see whether you are satisfied with their selections. Make sure that you understand what the plans cover and what they don't.

✔ **Stay away from brand new managed care plans.** Most experts say you should wait until the program has been available in your town for a minimum of four years.

✔ **Know the plan's policies regarding emergency care.** Although most plans will want you to visit their own emergency center or a participating hospital, they realize that an emergency is just that — an emergency. However, if you don't follow the instructions, you may find that your plan refuses to pay the bill.

✔ **Look for an accredited managed care program.** Accreditation is a voluntary review process in which a managed care plan is measured against a set of specific standards to see how well it is performing. Although accreditation cannot guarantee that a managed care plan will meet your needs, it does show that the plan is willing to let an independent third party review it. Accreditation information is available from the following sources:

American Accreditation Healthcare Commission, 1130 Connecticut Ave., NW, Suite 450, Washington DC, 20036; 202-296-0120

Joint Commission on the Accreditation of Healthcare Organizations, One Renaissance Blvd., Oakbrook Terrace, IL 60181; 630-916-5600

National Committee for Quality Assurance, 2000 L. St., N.W., Suite 500, Washington, DC 20036; 202-955-3500

Managed care versus fee-for-service

Both managed care and indemnity insurance have their pluses and their minuses.

The limitations managed care places on consumers' choices of doctors, hospitals, and treatments have made headlines, as has the accusation that managed care rations health care or encourages doctors to cut corners. Many managed care companies save money by paying participating doctors a fixed, monthly fee based on the number of enrolled patients in their care. This fee is intended to keep doctors from performing unnecessary procedures for their own financial benefit, but this same fee may provide some doctors with an incentive to withhold care or cut corners in order to save more money.

Managed care has succeeded in restraining the growth of health care costs, increased the efficiency of doctors and hospitals, lowered costs to consumers, and increased the use of preventive care.

Fee-for-service insurance offers consumers more choice — of doctors, hospitals, and treatments. This type of insurance is rarely accused of rationing health care or encouraging doctors to cut corners in patient care.

In fact, it may do just the opposite. In a fee-for-service plan, doctors are paid only when they perform a service, which may entice unscrupulous doctors to perform unnecessary procedures.

Uncle Sam's Coverage: Medicare and Medicaid

When people talk about health insurance, they generally refer to commercial insurance — the kind that you or your employer purchase. But millions of Americans get their insurance from another source — the federal government. Medicare and Medicaid are two of the largest health insurance programs around, serving an estimated 39 million and 37.7 million people, respectively.

Medicare

Medicare provides disabled individuals and people 65 and older with basic health insurance coverage.

The traditional Medicare program is made up of two parts:

  ✔ **Hospital insurance:** Also known as *Part A*, this coverage provides payment for inpatient hospital care, post-hospital extended care, and some home health care.

✔ **Medical insurance:** Also known as *Part B,* this coverage provides payment for doctor's services, home health care services, hospital outpatient services, and other medical services and items not covered under Part A.

Under the Federal Insurance Contributions Act (FICA), payroll taxes fund Part A. If you receive a payroll check, you see the deduction on your stub. Part B is financed with general revenues and with monthly premiums paid by each Medicare beneficiary. The premiums are automatically deducted from your Social Security check if you have applied for Medicare Part B.

If you are enrolled in the traditional Medicare plan, you are also subject to a deductible for both Parts A and B and a 20 percent co-payment for services you receive under Part B.

Eligibility

Medicare is available to three different groups of people:

✔ Anyone 65 years of age or older

✔ Anyone who is permanently and totally disabled

✔ Anyone who has end-stage renal disease (kidney disease severe enough to require dialysis or a transplant)

For most Americans, becoming eligible is simply a matter of turning 65 and applying. For information on eligibility, contact your local Social Security office.

Covered services

Many people mistakenly think that Medicare is comparable with the best private health insurance plans available on the market today. It's not. Although Medicare does cover physician and hospital-related services, it places limitations on days of care and comes with large co-payments if you are subjected to a lengthy hospital stay.

Medicare also places limitations on exactly what it will pay for. (For information on what Medicare does and doesn't cover, consult the official Medicare handbook, *Medicare & You.* The publication is available online at `www.medicare.gov/publications.html`).

Medicare does not cover what we usually think of as "nursing home care." It pays only for nursing home care received at the most intensive type of nursing facility after a three-day hospitalization. And it pays that in full for a limited number of days. Because of these gaps in coverage and because of the 20 percent co-payment for Part B services, many Medicare beneficiaries purchase additional insurance or enter a Medicare managed care program.

Expanding Medicare coverage

For many years, the only way to supplement or expand Medicare coverage was to buy a Medicare supplemental, or *Medigap,* policy. These policies are designed to pick up expenses Medicare does not cover, such as the deductibles and co-payments. Some also offer additional benefits, such as nursing home co-payments, prescription drugs, and preventive services.

Recently, another option has become available — managed care plans.

The most common form of managed care available to Medicare beneficiaries is the HMO. Medicare pays a premium to the HMO to cover the costs of caring for a Medicare beneficiary. The HMO is required to provide all the services you would receive in the traditional Medicare program, plus the deductible and co-payments. This arrangement virtually eliminates the need for a Medigap policy. The only cost to you may be a nominal co-payment for the services you use. Some HMOs also offer additional services — services not covered under the traditional Medicare plan. You may or may not be charged a separate premium to cover these additional services, but you will not have to pay a premium for basic Medicare coverage through an HMO other than the standard Part B premium.

HMOs generally require their members to obtain care from participating providers. But recent changes in Medicare law allow HMOs to offer a point-of-service option to Medicare beneficiaries. If you enroll in an HMO that offers this option, you can seek care from doctors or hospitals outside of your HMO, although you may pay more for this privilege.

New regulations also permit the establishment of provider-sponsored organizations (PSOs), a catchall term that encompasses a variety of managed care programs. In general, the law allows doctors, hospitals, or doctors and hospitals to offer some type of managed care program to Medicare beneficiaries. Before a PSO can operate, however, it must obtain a license from the insurance department in the state it wishes to operate. So these programs may not become available everywhere for some time.

New options

Two new options for obtaining Medicare coverage became available in 1999: private fee-for-service plans and medical savings accounts (MSAs).

Private fee-for-service plans are private insurance plans that accept Medicare beneficiaries. The plan, rather than Medicare, decides how much to reimburse health care providers for the services you receive. You pay the Part B premium, any monthly premium the plan charges, and an amount per visit or service. Health care providers are allowed to bill more than what the plan pays; you are responsible for covering these additional costs.

In a Medicare MSA, Medicare pays the premium for a policy with a high deductible and makes a deposit into your own personal medical savings account. You then use the money from this account to pay for your medical expenses. If you use all your money, you must pay your own medical expenses until you meet the plan's deductible.

For more information, check the latest edition of *Medicare & You.*

Medicaid

The Medicaid program provides health coverage to families with low incomes and to certain categories of aged and disabled individuals. The program is jointly financed by the federal and state governments. The federal government establishes the regulations and minimum standards for eligibility, benefit coverage, and provider participation and reimbursement. States can expand their programs beyond the minimum standards.

Eligibility

The federal requirements for Medicaid eligibility, which were based on income level, age, and disability, are undergoing change as a result of the Personal Responsibility and Work Opportunities Act of 1996. As a result, states are redetermining their own eligibility requirements.

To find out your state's eligibility requirements, check with the local office of your state's welfare department.

Covered services

Medicaid benefits are fairly comprehensive and include the services traditionally included in commercial group health insurance packages. As with eligibility, some benefits are federally mandated, while others are optional. The general benefit package is fairly similar from state to state.

The mandatory benefits required of all states include the following: inpatient hospital services; outpatient hospital services; physician services; laboratory and x-ray services; nurse-midwife services; family planning services; rural health clinic services; federally qualified health clinics; early and periodic screening, diagnosis, and treatment for children; nursing facility services for adults over 21; and home health care for people eligible for nursing facility services.

To find out more about the Medicaid program in your state, contact your state's Medicaid office.

Care for the Road Ahead: Long-Term-Care Insurance

At some point in their lives, many people unfortunately find themselves dealing with the financial burden of long-term care. Paying for nursing home care may cost you from $30,000 to $60,000 a year. One way to ease the pain on your pocketbook is to purchase long-term-care insurance.

Long-term-care insurance pays a fixed amount for each qualified day, whether the person receives long-term care in a nursing home or at home. These policies run for a specified period of time, typically several years.

The majority of policies sold include care in all levels of nursing facilities, home health care, adult day care, coverage for Alzheimer's disease, and inflation protection, among other benefits. But not all these features are available in all plans, and some may be available only at an extra cost.

Although long-term-care insurance can save you money and protect your assets, it's not for everybody. About half of people age 65 or older are unable to purchase coverage because of their health or their inability to afford the premiums, which are based on age and health status.

Long-term-care insurance may be necessary only if you have significant assets to protect. *Money* magazine suggests that you should consider buying it if you are around age 65, your net worth is greater than $100,000 excluding your home, and your annual income is at least $50,000. You should also be in good health; otherwise, noncoverage for preexisting conditions could mean that you never collect any benefits or that your premiums will be high.

For those who cannot afford or cannot purchase long-term-care insurance, Medicaid will pay the cost of long-term care after you meet eligibility requirements. For more information, contact your state's Medicaid office.

Chapter 4

Making Choices for Your Future

In This Chapter

▶ Exploring long-term care options

▶ Confronting death and dying issues

▶ Declaring your medical choices in advance

*A*lthough everyone wants to live a long, healthy life, life has no guarantees. You can follow a healthy eating plan, exercise regularly, and get regular checkups to keep your body in fine-tuned, working order, but you still may succumb to accidents, illness, and aging. When these unfortunate conditions occur, you may be faced with a multitude of important decisions to make, and you may not be in the best frame of mind to make them. A little bit of advanced planning can make a world of difference.

Long-Term-Care Options

At some point in your life, you may need *long-term care* — care for an extended or chronic physical or mental illness. And the time that you need it may not necessarily be when you're older. Although an estimated 7.2 million Americans age 65 or older currently need long-term care, so do 5.4 million children and working-age adults. The need for long-term care can result from an accident or a disabling illness as well as from chronic illnesses.

Long-term care is not just nursing home care, rather it's a continuum of home- and community-based services to assist people with physical and mental impairments and help them live as independently as possible. For a rundown of the services included, see Table 4-1.

Table 4-1 — Long-Term-Care Services

Medically Based Services

Hospice care	Physical therapy	Respiratory therapy
Occupational therapy (therapy to help a person carry out daily tasks and learn to cope with her limitations)	Skilled nursing	Home health
Intravenous medication therapy	Physician and other professional services	Mental health counseling and referral

Housing Alternatives

Foster care	Retirement communities	Continuing care communities
Congregate housing (a facility in which each person has her own bedroom and bathroom but other rooms are shared)	Shared housing (two or more unrelated people living in the same apartment or house and sharing space, expenses, and responsibilities)	Assisted living
Nursing facilities		

Socialization

Volunteer visiting	Telephone reassurance	Recreation

Personal Care/Assistance

Adult day care	Nutrition/diet counseling	Congregate meals
Meals on Wheels	Personal care	Shopping assistance
Chore services	Laundry	Transportation
Escort	Housekeeping	Emergency response systems
Respite care	Information and referral	Preretirement counseling

Not all these services are available in every community. Check with your local Area Agency on Aging, senior center, or other social service agency to find out if a specific service is offered in your area.

Your individual situation dictates what services you need. And your family members can take care of many of those needs. But if you or a loved one requires long-term care, you need to become familiar with the options available to you:

Determining which long-term-care option is right for you

To determine which long-term-care option — home health care, assisted living, or a nursing facility — is right for you or your loved one, you need to first determine your needs:

✔ **Make a list outlining your or your loved one's basic physical difficulties:** Do you need help with bathing, dressing, walking, eating, or using the bathroom?

✔ **Make a list of your or your loved one's needs for services:** Do you need intravenous injections; intravenous feeding; injections; wound dressing; therapy; help with bathing, dressing, or eating; or assistance with household chores?

✔ **Investigate the long-term-care options that are available in your area:** What services does each facility or agency provide? Do those services meet your needs? Does the type of facility or service that you prefer meet your needs?

✔ **Investigate facilities or agencies in your area that provide the option that you're interested in:** Find out whether they're licensed, certified, or accredited. Call your local Better Business Bureau or your state attorney general's office and ask whether any complaints have been filed. Find out about eligibility requirements, costs, and waiting lists.

✔ **Consider making an unscheduled visit to see how you are handled by the staff:** And visit during meal hours so that you can observe the menu and whether the elderly or handicapped are assisted with eating.

✔ **Home health care:** Home health care addresses the common desire to stay at home when you're ill or disabled by delivering medical and personal services to your home. Home health care services include medical services — such as doctor and nurse house calls and visits by physical therapists — and personal care services — such as help with bathing, dressing, eating, and other *activities of daily living.* Both nonprofit agencies and for-profit agencies provide these services.

People who receive long-term care at home can also benefit from community services such as Meals on Wheels, chore services, adult day care, housekeepers, and transportation. These services are available from home health agencies as well as from churches, social services, and neighborhood organizations. Depending on the service, your age, and your income level, you may qualify to receive these services for free or you can purchase them.

✔ **Assisted living residences:** Assisted living is a combination of housing and personalized health care for people who need help with activities of daily living. Assisted living residences provide housing, meals, and services, including supervision and assistance with medications, dressing, housekeeping, bathing, and other personal needs. Also known as personal care homes, family care homes, and sheltered care facilities, these facilities can be operated by either businesses or nonprofit organizations.

✔ **Nursing facilities:** Commonly called nursing homes or convalescent homes, nursing facilities provide homes for people who are chronically ill, for those whose mental state requires 24-hour supervision, and for people recovering from an illness or operation who need regular nursing and care.

Nursing homes provide two major levels of care: *skilled nursing care* and *intermediate care*. In a skilled nursing facility or unit, nursing care is available 24 hours a day. Patients who require skilled nursing are often bedridden. Patients in an intermediate care unit or facility are usually more mobile. Intermediate care features 24-hour supervision and basic nursing care and often stresses rehabilitation.

Death and Dying Issues

Although you probably don't want to think about death, it is an inevitable outcome of life. In recent years, advances in medical technology have made prolonging the inevitable possible.

In the past, if you stopped breathing and your heart stopped pumping, you were dead. Death is not so simple anymore. With the help of medical technology, doctors can maintain heartbeat and breathing functions and filter waste products even if your heart, lungs, liver, and kidneys fail. In other words, medical technology can keep your body alive.

As a result, many issues surrounding death and dying have come to light: dying with dignity, the right to die, and even controversy about the very definition of death itself.

These issues have generated legislation that gives consumers a say in the type of treatment they will receive in their final days. This section looks at your right to make decisions about the care you receive at the end of life.

Advance directives: Your right to decide

You have a right to plan and determine the type of health care that you receive.

You also have the right to determine in advance what type of treatment you will receive at the end of your life and under serious medical conditions — conditions that would prevent you from telling your doctor how you want to be treated. You exercise this right by signing an advance directive.

Advance directives are written statements that tell others how you want medical decisions to be made if you become incapacitated. The two most common forms of advance directives are the living will and the durable power of attorney for health care.

What is a living will?

A *living will* is a written statement that says you do not want life-prolonging medical procedures when your condition is hopeless and you have no chance of regaining a meaningful life.

Not only is a living will a tool to control the extent and type of medical care you receive at the end of your life, but it can also help reduce the emotional stresses and strains felt by both your family and your doctor, who must decide whether to withhold, withdraw, or continue medical treatment that cannot cure or reverse your terminal condition.

Each state has its own laws regarding living wills. If you have specific questions concerning living wills in your state, speak with your attorney (or the state bar association) and physician.

Here are some questions that you may want to ask:

- ✔ Do I need more than two standard witnesses to the document?
- ✔ Do I need to have the document notarized?
- ✔ Does the withdrawal of life-sustaining treatment include artificial feeding and hydration? (Many states prohibit the withdrawal of food and water, while others allow it.)
- ✔ Can I add any personalized instructions?
- ✔ Is my state's living will valid if I'm traveling in another state?

Depending on what state you live in, you may use a form — provided by state agencies or the organization Choice in Dying — or simply write a statement expressing your preference. (See the section "What is a durable power of attorney for health care?" for contact information for Choice in Dying.) A sample living will appears in this chapter. This is just a sample and may not be the correct or legally binding form for your needs. Check the requirements of the law in the state where you live.

Remember to inform your doctor, family, and attorney that you have a living will and tell them about its contents. Also remember that you can revoke or change a living will at any time.

One point to bear in mind: A living will has shortcomings. You have no guarantee that what you want will be carried out. In a situation when your wishes are not known to those treating you or in a situation in which a doctor does not consider your condition terminal, a doctor may initiate life-saving procedures even if you have requested that none be made. Nevertheless, a living will does make your wishes known to your family and friends, giving them guidance in making health care decisions for you.

Sample of a living will

Declaration made this ___ day of _____, 20___

I, _____, being of sound mind, willfully and voluntarily make known my desire that my dying shall not be artificially prolonged under the circumstances set forth below, and do declare:

If at any time I should have an incurable injury, disease, or illness certified to be a terminal condition by two physicians who have personally examined me, one of whom shall be my attending physician, and the physicians have determined that my death will occur whether or not life-sustaining procedures are utilized and where the application of life-sustaining procedures would serve only to artificially prolong the dying process, I direct that such procedures be withheld or withdrawn and that I be permitted to die naturally and with only the administration of medication or the performance of any medical procedure deemed necessary to provide me with comfort care.

In the absence of my ability to give directions regarding the use of such life-sustaining procedures, it is my intention that this declaration shall be honored by my family and physician(s) as the final expression of my legal right to refuse medical or surgical treatment and accept the consequences from such refusal.

I understand the full import of this declaration, and I am emotionally and mentally competent to make this declaration.

Signed

_____

Address

_____

The declarant has been personally known to me and I believe him/her to be of sound mind.

Witness

_____

Witness

_____

Source: President's Commission for the Study of Ethical Problems in Medicine and Behavior Research, "Deciding to Forgo Life-Sustaining Treatment," U.S. Government Printing Office. pp. 314-315.

What is a durable power of attorney for health care?

A *durable power of attorney for health care* (sometimes called a DPA) is a written document that names a person or surrogate who will carry out your wishes regarding medical treatment if you become incompetent and are unable to make those decisions yourself. Whereas the living will is only about the final moments of your life, you can draft the DPA to give your *agent* or *proxy* (the person that you choose to represent you) the authority to make decisions about other areas of medical treatment.

The Patient Self-Determination Act

The Patient Self-Determination Act requires workers in all federally funded institutions — hospitals, health maintenance organizations, hospices, skilled nursing facilities, and facilities accepting Medicare and Medicaid customers — to inform patients of their right to establish advance directives.

If an institution has moral or ethical codes that conflict with advance directives, it should inform you of its policies when you are admitted.

You may be familiar with durable power of attorney in its standard sense — that is, as a way of authorizing another person to make decisions or take actions on your behalf in financial or property transactions. Some states have also passed legislation creating a durable power of attorney specifically for health care decisions. Check with your state bar association for details on these laws.

Your agent is legally able to speak on your behalf. Obviously, you should choose this person carefully. Consider someone who knows you as an individual and who will respect your wishes regarding treatment. Ask yourself the following questions: Who do you trust with life-and-death decisions? Who knows you best? Who would respect your wishes?

For more information on advance directives, contact Choice in Dying, an organization that provides information and materials on death and dying, 200 Varick St., Suite 1001, New York, NY 10014; 800-989-WILL or 212-366-5540; www.choices.org.

The hospice option: Dying with dignity

If you are terminally ill, you do not have to spend your last days in a hospital or nursing home; you can choose the *hospice* alternative. Hospices deliver specialized nursing care to terminally ill patients in a less sterile environment than hospitals, allowing them to live their remaining weeks or months as free of symptoms and in as much control as possible.

Do not resuscitate orders

A *do not resuscitate (DNR) order* is another way that you can gain more control over the circumstances of your death. A DNR order means that cardiopulmonary resuscitative measures (CPR) will not be started or carried out if your heart fails or you stop breathing. It also means that you will not be placed on long-term mechanical life support equipment. These orders generally come into play when a person is terminally or critically ill; thus, most DNR orders are written when a patient is not capable of making the decision. But a serious accident or complications from surgery could put you in a situation in which such a decision must be made. If you plan ahead, you can have a say in your care. Here are some suggestions:

- Talk with your doctor and know your hospital's policy regarding DNR orders before you are admitted.

- Make sure that your family (and whomever holds durable power of attorney) knows your wishes.

- Document your wishes about emergency resuscitation and ask your doctor to make it part of your medical record.

- Be aware that you can revoke a DNR order if you change your mind.

You can receive hospice care in your home or in a special facility designed solely to provide hospice care. The hallmarks of hospice care are control of pain, relief from suffering, preparation for death, and support for survivors. Hospice care allows you to die with dignity and allows you and your family to help one another during the dying process.

The hospice team generally includes the primary caregiver, a physician, a nurse, a social worker, counselors and therapists, clergy members, and volunteers, who provide patient care and provide emotional support and assistance to the patient and her family.

Hospice organizations are located across the country. Although hospice care is not necessarily cheap, Medicare does pay the cost of hospice care for some elderly patients. Some commercial insurance companies also offer hospice benefits. Some hospices do not charge at all; they rely on donations and bequests from people and family members that they have served.

For more information on hospice care, contact the following organizations:

- National Hospice Organization, 1901 N. Moore St., Suite 901; Arlington, VA 22209; 703-243-5900; www.nho.org

- Hospice Association of America, 228 7th St., S.E., Washington, DC 20003; 202-546-4759; www.nahc.org

Part II
Righting the Wrongs

The 5th Wave   By Rich Tennant

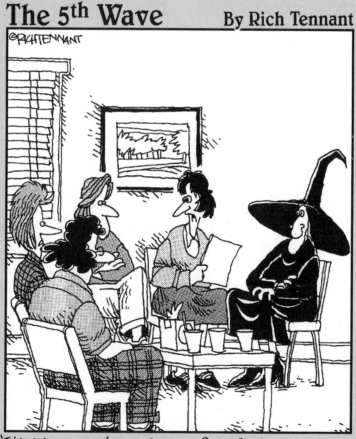

"I'd like you to welcome Grinda to our group. Grinda has issues with potion abuse, poison apples, and a history of negative relationships with men and toads."

In this part . . .

Two wrongs don't make a right. They just make things worse. So negative behavior, such as overeating, undereating, abusing drugs or alcohol, or giving in to violence, can not only have a negative impact on your health and well-being but can also compound existing problems. Learning to right the "wrongs" in your life and taking care of yourself, however, can reverse this situation.

Chapter 5

Weight Reduction

• •

In This Chapter

▶ Exploring health risks for overweight women

▶ Calculating your healthy weight

▶ Following diet and exercise guidelines

▶ Finding out about eating disorders

• •

*W*omen decide to lose weight for two basic reasons: to get thin and to improve their health. Both reasons can be valid, but women can take the first one to such an extreme that it negates the second. Just as some women's excessive weights place them at risk for heart disease, diabetes, and other serious health problems, other women's obsessive desires to be thin jeopardize their health (and sometimes, their lives).

If you want to lose weight, take a moment to analyze your reasons. Being supermodel-thin doesn't guarantee happiness. But being the right weight — that is, the right weight for you — can make you look and feel better and reduce your risk of developing certain health problems later in life.

When Your Weight Becomes a Health Risk

Being overweight is not simply an issue of how you look — it can affect what you're able to do physically, and it can affect your health. Obviously, playing a vigorous game of tennis is difficult when you're carrying 30 extra pounds. (Unfortunately, the extra weight is exactly what stops many people from enjoying exercise, which is a key ingredient to maintaining a healthy body.) Those extra pounds can also increase your risk of the following diseases:

✔ **Cancer:** The medical community has recognized for some time that if you've already gone through menopause, being overweight puts you at greater risk of developing breast cancer. The connection between weight and breast cancer is complicated and seems to involve the level of hormones (estrogen and possibly progesterone) in a woman's body.

Research also shows that gallbladder, ovarian, uterine, and pancreatic cancers are more common in women who are *obese* — those who are 20 percent or more above their ideal weight.

✔ **Cardiovascular disease:** You're probably already aware that being overweight puts you at greater risk of high blood pressure and heart disease. The excess weight puts stress on your heart, especially if you carry it around your middle.

Excess cholesterol and fat tend to build up in the walls of blood vessels, narrowing the passageways that are used to transport blood through your body. As a result, your heart works harder to pump the blood, while less blood gets carried to your body's cells. If the buildup blocks the vessels that lead to your heart, you can have a heart attack or even die.

✔ **Diabetes:** Diabetes is the result of the body's inability to produce or use *insulin,* a hormone that enables your body to use sugar for energy. Without insulin, your body can't move blood sugar into the cells, and sugar builds up in your bloodstream. This kind of "insulin resistance" gets worse as you gain weight.

The good news is that you can often control the most common type of diabetes with diet and exercise. And if you're obese, you can reduce your risk of developing diabetes by simply losing 10 to 15 percent of your body weight.

✔ **Osteoarthritis:** Being overweight puts stress on weight-bearing joints, such as your hips and knees, and over time can wear them down. This repeated stress can cause *osteoarthritis,* the "wear and tear" arthritis. When a physician encounters osteoarthritis and the patient is overweight, the doctor will likely recommend that the patient lose weight to take stress off the joints and exercise to build up the muscles that support the joints.

Calculating Your Healthy Weight

You may be wondering, what is the right weight for me?

In the past, all you had to do was look up your height on a life insurance chart and see what weight you were supposed to be. Today, research suggests that you should look at your body size and weight in several different ways, which you can do by asking yourself the questions in the following three sections.

What is your body mass index (BMI)?

The health risks of being overweight are often measured in relation to your *body mass index,* or BMI. BMI is calculated by dividing your weight in kilograms into your height in meters squared. Don't worry, you can figure your BMI by following these steps:

1. **Get out your calculator!**

2. **Divide your weight by 2.2 to get your weight in *kilograms*. (Weight ÷ 2.2 = W)**

3. **Multiply your height in inches by .0245 to get your height in *meters*. (Height × .0245 = H)**

4. **Multiply your height in meters by itself to square it. (H × H = H²)**

5. **Divide your weight in kilograms by your squared height to get your BMI. (W ÷ H² = BMI)**

According to weight guidelines released in 1998 by the National Institutes of Health, the optimal BMI is between 18.5 and 24.9. A BMI between 25 and 29.9 is considered overweight, and a BMI of 30 or above is considered obese. (A BMI below 18.5 is considered underweight.) The NIH guidelines, which lowered the threshold for what is considered overweight, were established based on the health risk additional weight places on the body. According to the guidelines, anyone with a BMI of 25 or more is at increased risk of health problems. Risk is considered high for people with a BMI above 30 and for overweight people with a large waist circumference.

What's your waist-to-hip ratio (WHR)?

Determining whether you need to lose weight isn't simply a matter of knowing your BMI. You also need to look at how your weight is distributed on your body. Research has shown that a greater risk of heart disease, stroke, and diabetes is associated with weight carried around your middle than with weight carried on your hips and thighs.

Here's how to determine if you're at increased risk: First thing in the morning (before you eat breakfast), measure your waist and your hips. Then, divide your waist measurement by your hip measurement. This number is your waist-to-hip ratio (WHR). A waist-to-hip ratio higher than .90 puts you at a greater risk of dying from heart disease, stroke, and diabetes than a ratio of .75.

If math wasn't your best subject, the NIH guidelines provide this shortcut: If your waist is 35 inches or greater and you have a BMI of 25 or more, you are at high risk of obesity-related diseases. A study reported in the December 2, 1998, *Journal of the American Medical Association* found that women with a waist circumference of 30 inches or more are at increased risk of heart disease even if their BMI is in the optimal range.

How old are you?

Your age is important because the health risks associated with weight gain change as you age. Gaining a little weight as you age is normal, and the government's current recommended weight charts, shown in Table 5-1, take that tendency into consideration. Be aware, however, that several recent studies have found that even moderate weight gains (as little as 11 pounds after age 18, according to one study) can increase your risk of heart disease and cancer. Still, many experts believe that moderate weight gain in adulthood does not present a health risk to most people. The key is moderate, and the amount of weight isn't the only question; you also need to pay attention to the area of your body where you gained the weight.

This chart should give you a general range of where your goal weight should fall. Before you select the bottom of the scale as your "ideal weight," remember that muscle weighs more than fat (so you should take your fitness level into consideration), and your bone structure and body shape affect how much weight you can carry well.

Table 5-1	Age-Adapted Healthy Weights for Women				
Height	Age 20–29	Age 30–39	Age 40–49	Age 50–59	Age 60–69
4'10"	84-111	92-119	99-127	107-135	115-142
4'11"	87-115	95-123	103-131	111-139	119-147
5'0"	90-119	98-127	106-135	114-143	123-152
5'1"	93-123	101-131	110-140	118-148	127-157
5'2"	96-127	105-136	113-144	122-153	131-163
5'3"	99-131	108-140	117-149	126-158	135-168
5'4"	102-135	112-145	121-154	130-163	140-173
5'5"	106-140	115-149	125-159	134-168	144-179
5'6"	109-144	119-154	129-164	138-174	148-184
5'7"	112-148	122-159	133-169	143-179	153-190
5'8"	116-153	126-163	137-174	147-184	158-196

Height	Age 20–29	Age 30–39	Age 40–49	Age 50–59	Age 60–69
5'9"	119-157	130-168	141-179	151-190	162-201
5'10"	122-162	134-173	145-184	156-195	167-207
5'11"	126-167	137-178	149-190	160-201	172-213
6'0"	129-171	141-183	153-195	165-207	177-219
6'1"	133-176	145-188	157-200	169-213	182-225
6'2"	137-181	149-194	162-206	174-219	187-232
6'3"	141-186	153-199	166-212	179-225	192-238
6'4"	144-191	157-205	171-218	184-231	197-244

Source: National Institutes of Health

Remember: No exact right weight exists for any person. Set a reasonable weight loss goal. This goal is easier to attain if you look at body weight in terms of a range you'd like to stay in rather than a fixed number that you must achieve.

Putting it all together

The answers to the questions in the preceding three sections can help you determine whether you need to lose weight and, if you do, give you an idea of how much you need to lose to improve or maintain your health. You may wish to consider losing weight if any of the following are true:

- Your BMI is 25 or above.
- Your WHR is .8 or more.
- Your waist circumference is 35 inches or more, and your BMI is 25 or more.
- Your weight exceeds the upper limit for your height and age group.

You also need to take personal factors into consideration. If only one of the preceding statements is true and you lead a healthy lifestyle, you may not need to change anything. But if any of the preceding statements are true and you smoke or have a family history of heart disease, cancer, diabetes, or another obesity-related disease, it is probably in your best interest to lose enough weight to bring those measures down to healthier levels.

Diet and Exercise Guidelines

After you have a weight range in mind, the question is: *How do you lose weight?* The old way of thinking was to go on a crash diet and starve yourself to lose weight. Unfortunately, this approach just didn't work. Oh, you can definitely lose weight that way. But the weight you lose from a starvation diet consists not only of fat but also of water and muscle. And after you stop the diet, your body responds as though it has been starved, instinctively causing you to binge and gain weight back. An estimated 90 to 95 percent of people who lose weight gain it back within a year. And considering the health risks discussed earlier in this chapter, you just can't afford those kinds of odds. To lose weight and keep it off, you have to make permanent changes in your diet and exercise regimen.

Before you can change your body, you must change the way that you live and the way that you think. You have to stop thinking about diets and start thinking about changing your lifestyle. You need to ask yourself two questions:

- ✔ What do lean, healthy people eat and do every day?
- ✔ What do I eat and do every day?

Your body's relative health, shape, and size is the result of

- ✔ **Genetics:** You were born with a specific bone structure and *type* of body that you aren't going to be able to change — at least not without plastic surgery.
- ✔ **Age:** As you age, your body shape and metabolism change.
- ✔ **Food:** Food is the energy that you put into your body.
- ✔ **Exercise:** Exercise is how you move and what you do every day to burn that energy.

To have a lean, healthy body, you must change the way that you live day to day. Your lifestyle must include a healthy approach to eating and regular daily exercise.

Developing healthy eating habits

Believe it or not, a healthy approach to eating and a healthy diet plan to lose weight are pretty much the same thing. You need to watch your intake of both fat and calories.

To reduce your risk of heart disease and certain cancers, you need to cut down your intake of fats from animal and dairy products (saturated fats) to 10 percent of your overall calories. All types of fats in your diet should make up no more than 30 percent of your overall daily calories.

How many calories should you eat each day? To lose weight at a rate that won't overtax the body, most experts recommend that women eat somewhere between 1,000 and 1,500 calories per day. (This daily allotment of calories should result in a weight loss of one to two pounds a week). Again, this is a *range* of calories, not a rigid amount. You may very well eat more calories one day and less the next.

Your body also needs a variety of foods to get the nutrients, vitamins, and fiber that it needs to run efficiently. Refer to the food pyramid in Chapter 1. Concentrate on whole (not processed) foods, such as whole potatoes (with the skin), whole-grain breads, rice, and whole apples and pears (not peeled or canned). Whole foods not only provide fiber, but they also satisfy and fill you up more. To avoid fats, buy fat-free dairy products and light meat (breast cuts) chicken and turkey without the skin. Try to eat fish two to three times per week, avoiding the fatty fishes like salmon and orange roughy.

Sticking with your new diet

How do you stick to your new eating approach? Here are a few strategies to help you keep on track eating-wise:

✔ **Don't skip meals:** Skipping meals just makes you ravenously hungry (and more vulnerable to fat-laden, quickie snacks) later.

✔ **Snack healthily:** Some snacks are bad, and some are good. A bad snack gives you a quick boost but then makes you crave another. A good snack, such as a bagel with all-fruit preserves, provides energy *and* fills you up.

✔ **Fill up on high-volume, low-fat foods:** Give yourself big servings of vegetables, fruits, rice, and pasta.

✔ **Try a couple of no-meat days each week:** Have pasta, try meatless chili, or put salsa or low-fat toppings on baked potatoes.

✔ **Keep your hands busy while you watch TV:** For many women, watching TV is the cue to pull out the chips. Try a new hobby to keep your hands busy. Better yet, don't watch TV; do something else.

✔ **Spice up your life:** Healthy food does not mean boring food. Use spices, (low-sodium) soy sauce, mustards, vinegars (balsamic is especially good), pickles, marinades, and lemon juice.

Weight loss medications: A weighty solution to a weighty problem

Weight loss medications have not proven to be a miracle cure. This fact became evident in September 1997, when the makers of two weight loss drugs — dexfenfluramine (Redux) and fenfluramine (Pondimen), a component of the popular "fen-phen" prescription combination — pulled them off the market at the urging of the Food and Drug Administration (FDA). The reason: The drugs were found to damage heart valves. This problem, which was not apparent during the testing that led to the drugs' initial approval, emerged after the drugs became commonly prescribed.

These drugs were designed to be used primarily by people who have a BMI of 30 or more, or those with a BMI of at least 27 and a history or family history of obesity-related disease.

And they were designed to be taken on a short-term basis as part of balanced program of diet and exercise. But many doctors and weight loss clinics prescribed the drugs for long periods of time to people who were not truly obese and, in the case of fenfluramine, in combination with other drugs.

The FDA has approved a new weight loss drug, sibutramine (Meridia), and is expected to approve a second, orlistat (Xenical), shortly. Neither of these two drugs works the same way as the ones recently pulled from the market. Nevertheless, their safety won't be clearly established until they've been used extensively, making it wise to consider them only if you are an appropriate candidate for the treatment.

Exercising the healthy way

If you are overweight and not very mobile, you're probably pretty tired most of the time. In fact, you may think that you don't have the energy to exercise. Oddly enough, exercising and building up your muscles is what gives you more energy and lessens your fatigue. Exercise also helps raise your metabolism and reduce your weight. Regular exercise really has a lot going for it.

Exercise aerobically half an hour or more each day and exercise with weights to build strength two or three times a week.

The key is to exercise regularly, gradually build up your muscles, and vary what you do so you don't get bored. See Chapter 1 for more about exercising.

Keep in mind that exercise may not result in pounds off the scale because when you exercise you burn fat *and* build muscle. Muscle weighs more than fat but takes up less space, which is why exercise can bring you down a clothing size or two even though you haven't lost weight. Instead, you are leaner: You have more muscle and less fat. Because muscle cells burn up more calories than fat cells, even when you are at rest, being more muscular means burning more calories all the time.

Eating Disorders

An estimated 7 million women in the United States have eating disorders. The three main types of eating disorders are

- ✔ Anorexia nervosa (self-starvation)
- ✔ Bulimia (bingeing and purging)
- ✔ Compulsive overeating

Anorexia nervosa and bulimia in particular are common in young women, who are the prime targets for the media's obsession with appearance and dieting. According to the American College of Sports Medicine, 62 percent of women and girls who compete in sports that stress appearance, such as gymnastics and endurance sports, such as running, have eating disorders.

The causes of eating disorders are complicated. Eating disorders have a psychological component that involves a lack of self-esteem and a warped body image; a biochemical component that results from a lack of specific chemicals in the brain; and obviously, a nutritional component. Eating disorders often start at a very young age. Compulsive overeating, for example, has its roots in childhood, and anorexia and bulimia are most common in women between the ages of 16 and 22. According to Anorexia Nervosa and Related Eating Disorders, Inc., these problems often begin when a young woman is dealing with a difficult transition, shock, or loss that makes her feel out of control, including puberty, family problems, a new job or school, the breakup of a relationship, or physical or sexual abuse.

Anorexia nervosa

An anorexic woman has a warped view of her body; she's convinced that she's too fat, even when she becomes skeletal in appearance. These distorted perceptions drive anorexic women to starve themselves and overexercise in an effort to lose weight. Dieting is one of the most common triggers of the starvation mode. Later, they become obsessed with food and develop rituals associated with preparing and eating it. As an anorexic woman's body becomes dangerously underweight, her menstrual cycle stops, her skin becomes dry and scaly (her body doesn't have enough fat to moisturize her skin), and she is cold all the time (she lacks a layer of fat to keep her warm).

Over time, the loss of nutrition can result in osteoporosis (as a lack of estrogen causes the bones to lose calcium), anemia, a weakened heart, liver and kidney damage, dehydration, and, ultimately, death from starvation.

Treatment for anorexia includes monitored or forced eating, supplements, nutrition education, and psychiatric counseling and therapy.

Bulimia

Bulimic women are much harder to spot because they often maintain a normal weight. The cycle starts with an emotional *trigger* that brings on a session of binge eating. A trigger can be a rejection, failure, depression, loneliness, anger, or even a celebration. When a bulimic woman binges, she quickly eats massive amounts of food. Then, ashamed at giving in to her need, she *purges* herself — she makes herself throw up, or takes excessive amounts of laxatives, or goes without food for a period of time.

Over time, the binge and purge cycles can lead to a loss of tooth enamel (from the stomach acids brought up by vomiting), dehydration, imbalances of electrolytes (minerals or salts in the body that keep fluids in balance), fainting spells, heart irregularities, bowel damage (from excess laxative use), possible liver and kidney damage, internal bleeding, heart attack, and death.

Treatment for bulimia includes monitored eating, dental treatment (for tooth enamel loss), nutritional education, supplements, and psychiatric counseling and therapy.

Compulsive overeating

Compulsive overeating (which is sometimes referred to as binge-eating disorder) has started to be recognized only relatively recently. The compulsive overeater either binges or eats constantly as a way to relieve stress, anxiety, or depression. Unlike women with anorexia or bulimia, the compulsive overeater is most often obese and exercises little. Where the anorexic starves herself to achieve some warped image of thinness, the compulsive overeater uses her fat to shield herself and hide. Compulsive overeating often has its roots in childhood when children first develop coping mechanisms to deal with problems and emotions.

Compulsive overeating can lead to obesity and, consequently, a higher risk of heart disease, stroke, certain cancers, diabetes, and osteoarthritis.

Treatment of compulsive overeating includes nutritional education, dieting, exercise, and counseling and often includes the use of self-help groups.

For more information on eating disorders, contact

✔ The National Eating Disorders Organization, 6655 S. Yale Ave., Tulsa, OK 74136; 918-481-4044; www.laureate.com/aboutned.html

✔ Anorexia Nervosa and Related Eating Disorders, Inc. (ANRED) at the same number or www.anred.com

Chapter 6

Understanding Addictions

● ●

In This Chapter

▶ Addictions: The basics

▶ Alcohol and your body

▶ Drug use, abuse, and addiction

▶ Up in smoke

● ●

*A*lthough more men than women smoke, drink, and use illegal drugs, the number of women engaging in these behaviors is increasing. And women are less likely to be diagnosed and treated for their addictions.

This chapter examines the issues of women and addiction, including causes and effects and the special needs of women with addictions.

What Is Addiction?

Addiction is a compulsive, uncontrollable dependence on a substance, habit, or practice — a dependence to such a degree that withdrawal from the substance or a cessation of the practice causes severe physical, emotional, or mental reactions.

People become psychologically dependent on a substance because of the way that substance makes them feel. Some people become so used to having a substance in their system that they become physically dependent.

Physical dependence is characterized by *tolerance,* in which a person needs higher doses of a substance to produce the desired effect, and by *withdrawal symptoms*. Withdrawal symptoms are physical and psychological responses (such as anxiety, vomiting, and diarrhea) that occur when a substance is eliminated from or reduced in the body.

Many factors, including biochemical factors, individual personality, and sociocultural factors, can figure into addiction, and the actual causes vary from person to person.

And although no clear "genetic predisposition" to addiction exists, research suggests that people with alcoholic relatives may be less sensitive to alcohol's effects and may be less able to estimate their level of intoxication.

Research shows that compared with men, women are more likely to have multiple addictions; suffer from sexual dysfunction or a coexisting psychological problem, such as depression; point to a particular stressful event as the onset of addiction; mimic the addictions of their partner or spouse; and have a family history of alcoholism, addiction, or childhood sexual abuse.

Shattering Lives: Alcoholism

Although alcohol use overall is decreasing, consumption is increasing among younger people — especially young women. According to the National Council on Alcoholism and Drug Dependence, 44 percent of American women drink alcohol to some extent, 10 percent are heavy drinkers or binge drinkers, and nearly 4 million women are alcoholics or problem drinkers.

The U.S. Department of Agriculture's dietary guidelines recommend that women drink no more than one drink per day and men no more than two per day. What constitutes a drink?

- 12 ounces of beer
- 5 ounces of wine
- 1 1/2 ounces of 80-proof liquor

But many women drink much more.

How alcoholism starts

Alcoholics may begin drinking as a way of escaping their problems, but ironically, their drinking creates more problems. Eventually, they may develop a physical dependency and drink to relieve or avoid withdrawal symptoms, which can include vomiting, sweating, diarrhea, trembling, cramps, seizures, and *delirium tremens (DTs)*, a potentially life-threatening collection of symptoms that includes fear, anxiety, mental confusion, hallucinations, rapid heartbeat, insomnia, fever, body tremors, sweating, and chest and stomach pain.

Women typically begin drinking at a later age than men and drink somewhat less than men. But women are more likely to develop alcohol-related medical problems sooner than men, and they need lower doses to do so. This is because women have more body fat than body water, so the alcohol is more concentrated. Women also have lower levels of the stomach enzyme that metabolizes alcohol. And hormonal changes that coincide with the menstrual cycle may affect alcohol tolerance and metabolism in women.

The signs of alcoholism

According to the National Council on Alcoholism and Drug Dependence, *alcoholism* is a progressive, potentially fatal disease characterized by

- ✔ An inability to control drinking
- ✔ A preoccupation with alcohol
- ✔ The use of alcohol despite its adverse consequences
- ✔ Distortions in thinking, notably denial

Consequences of drinking

Long-term heavy drinking, with or without alcoholism, can result in physical and social problems and even death. It can directly cause or worsen liver and heart disease, cancer, brain damage, and ulcers. Its indirect complications include automobile accidents; falls, fights, and the injuries and deaths associated with them; unwanted, unplanned pregnancies; sexually transmitted diseases; loss of employment; domestic problems; and financial ruin.

Alcohol, or ethanol, is a *depressant* — a drug that slows the central nervous system and acts like a mild tranquilizer and anesthetic. This tranquilizing effect can relax you and reduce your inhibitions; it can also depress your brain function, affecting your thoughts, emotions, and judgment. And it can slow your reaction time and impair your muscle coordination.

When you drink, alcohol is absorbed into your bloodstream (primarily through your small intestine) and transported throughout your body, where it dilates your blood vessels, causes your pulse to rise, and acts as a *diuretic*, causing your kidneys to produce more urine.

Your body uses alcohol much as it uses other food — to gain energy. It does this in large part by sending the alcohol through the liver (hence, alcohol's effects on the liver). You should know, though, that alcohol's food value is limited. The calories from alcohol are *empty calories* — they provide no vitamins, minerals, or proteins. Because people who drink heavily may obtain a large percentage of their calories from alcohol, they may develop serious nutritional deficiencies.

Effects on your body

The mortality rate for women alcoholics is higher than that for men because women are at increased risk of suicide, alcohol-related accidents, and liver diseases such as cirrhosis and hepatitis.

Alcohol-related health risks for women also include

- ✔ **An increased risk of breast cancer:** A study published in the *Journal of the American Medical Association* in early 1998 found that women who drank more than one drink per day had a 40 percent higher risk of breast cancer than women who drank one or fewer drinks.

- ✔ **An increased likelihood of miscarriage and menstrual disturbances:** Fertility and sexual function may be affected by problem drinking.

- ✔ **Vulnerability to risky behavior (for example, sex without a condom).**

Effects on your baby

You probably already know that pregnant women are advised not to drink alcohol. Moderate to heavy drinking during pregnancy can cause complications that include miscarriage, premature birth, and stillbirth. In addition, babies born to mothers who drink during pregnancy may suffer from the physical and mental defects associated with fetal alcohol syndrome, including facial and head deformities, retarded growth, and mental retardation.

The danger doesn't necessarily stop after delivery. Women who are breast-feeding can pass alcohol to their babies. Because no conclusive evidence exists on how much alcohol is harmful, for safety's sake, pregnant and breast-feeding women are advised to consume no alcohol at all.

Getting help for your problem

For many women, stopping or limiting drinking may require nothing more than becoming aware of their drinking habits and modifying them.

For others, additional assistance may be necessary, but the stigma associated with alcoholism may prevent them from getting the help they need. Studies show that doctors are less likely to recognize alcoholism in patients who do not fit the societal stereotype. In addition, some women may feel embarrassed to admit that they have a problem. Still others may fear losing custody of their children or the reactions of their families.

If you think that you have a drinking problem, talk with your family, your health care provider, or your clergyman. Enroll in a self-help program such as Alcoholics Anonymous or Women for Sobriety. For some women, enrolling in a self-help program may be enough. For those who have psychiatric problems or who need detoxification, intensive treatment is available through both inpatient and outpatient rehabilitation programs offered by hospitals.

Detoxification programs provide you with medical care and monitoring as you move through the withdrawal process. They help you counter withdrawal symptoms and treat medical problems associated with alcoholism.

For more information, look in the blue pages of your phone book under the heading for Human Services or contact

- ✔ Alcoholics Anonymous Worldwide Services Office, 475 Riverside Dr., New York, NY 10115; 212-870-3400; www.alcoholics-anonymous.org

- ✔ National Council on Alcoholism and Drug Dependence, 12 W. 21st St., New York, NY 10010; 800-622-2255; 212-206-6770; www.ncadd.org

- ✔ National Clearinghouse for Alcohol and Drug Information, Drug Abuse Information and Treatment Referral Line, Box 23345, Rockville, MD 20847; 800-662-4444357; 800-662-9999832 (Spanish); 800-222-0427 (hearing impaired); 301-468-6433; www.health.org

Drug Abuse and Addiction

You see it on television. Movie stars, rock stars, and other celebrities letting drugs turn their bright futures into dull glimmers. You may not have had first-hand experience with drug abusers . . . or so you think. More than 4 million U.S. women used illicit drugs, and more than 3 million women took prescription drugs non-medically in 1997, according to the National Institute of Drug Abuse.

Drug abuse does not refer simply to the use of illegal street drugs such as marijuana. Drug abuse is *any* deliberate misuse of a drug. All drugs — from illegal street drugs, to prescription medications, to legalized drugs such as alcohol and nicotine — have the potential to be misused and many have the potential to cause addiction.

Why do women use drugs? The answer depends on the woman. Some women use drugs to enhance their moods or perceptions of reality; others use them to calm them down or "rev" them up; still others use them to blot out physical or emotional pain. Whether a woman uses drugs is also affected by the drug's availability, the influence of her family and peers, her sociocultural environment, her personality, and her psychological health.

Beginning the trip: How drug addiction starts

Drug abuse often begins with recreational use of a drug. The user tends to periodically experiment with small amounts of a drug. But some people develop a dependency on the drug.

Commonly used — and abused — drugs

Here are some commonly abused drugs.

- **Narcotics:** Drugs such as heroin and opium can be used to alleviate pain; they can produce feelings of euphoria. They are physically and psychologically addictive.

- **Stimulants:** These drugs increase energy and alertness. They are psychologically addictive, but it is unclear whether they are physically addictive. Common stimulants are cocaine, amphetamines, caffeine, and nicotine.

- **Depressants:** These drugs slow down the nervous system and calm a person. They can cause both physical and psychological dependence. Familiar depressants include alcohol, barbiturates, tranquilizers, and sedatives such as Valium and Quaaludes.

- **Hallucinogens:** These drugs include substances such as LSD, marijuana, ecstasy, and mescaline. In low doses, they stimulate the user, but at higher doses, they may cause hallucinations and erratic, unpredictable behavior. Addiction to hallucinogens is unlikely, but they can cause effects that may not appear until long after the drug has been discontinued (the proverbial acid flashback, for example).

Dependency on a drug can be physical, psychological, or both. For example, a cancer patient may be physically dependent on — but not addicted to — a medication to relieve pain. When she stops taking the drug, she may experience withdrawal symptoms, but she is unlikely to go looking for the drug when she no longer needs to take it. On the other hand, a teenager who regularly smokes marijuana may experience problems in school but will not physically suffer if she stops smoking. Her dependence is psychological.

In psychological dependence, the user feels good when she uses the drug and she wants to continue to produce that feeling. Psychological dependence is often the only contributor to the compulsive use of a drug, which explains the attraction of psychotropic (mind-altering) drugs.

People who are physically dependent on a drug tend to repeatedly use it to avoid the discomfort of withdrawal, such as vomiting, chills, and insomnia.

The road signs of drug abuse and addiction

The symptoms and signs of drug abuse and addiction vary from person to person, but some general signs include the following:

- ✔ **Changes in behavior or personality:** Violent mood swings, apathy, depression, changes in friends, secretiveness, and lying
- ✔ **Changes in physical appearance or habits:** Weight loss, loss of appetite, change in sleeping habits, bloodshot eyes, or puncture wounds
- ✔ **A decline in job or academic performance**
- ✔ **Withdrawal from parents, family, and friends**
- ✔ **The discovery of drugs or drug paraphernalia**
- ✔ **Frequent intoxication**

You may also suspect drug addiction if lowering the dose or stopping the drug produces obvious withdrawal symptoms.

A bumpy ride: The consequences of drug abuse

Drug abuse can result in poor nutrition, liver disease, lung disease, heart disease, and psychiatric problems such as depression. Pregnant women who use drugs are likely to have smaller babies or deliver prematurely. Their babies may have long-term mental and physical defects. Some babies are born addicted and suffer withdrawal in their first days of life.

Drug use carries other risks. Women who use drugs are at greater risk of contracting AIDS because they may share needles or engage in unprotected sex while they are under the influence. And overdose can lead to death.

The road ahead: Treatment

Many women with drug problems are reluctant to seek treatment. And because women may become more quickly addicted to drugs, those who do receive treatment tend to be more severely addicted.

Women who receive drug treatment need to undergo detoxification along with psychotherapy. Treatment can take place at an outpatient or inpatient treatment facility or at a residential community, and it may include the dispensing of other drugs to prevent or relieve withdrawal symptoms.

Smoking

Americans overall are smoking less, but women are smoking more. According to the American Lung Association, more than 22 million American women smoked in 1996. Cigarette smoking is the most popular means of consuming *nicotine,* a drug that stimulates the release of *endorphins,* brain chemicals that produce pleasant feelings and give you a "kick." But that kick doesn't come cheap. Nicotine is more addictive than heroin.

Getting addicted to smoking

Nicotine addiction, obviously, is a major reason people smoke. But it is not the only one. People also smoke because they

- Achieve energetic or calm feelings
- Derive pleasure from the ritual of handling and smoking cigarettes
- Associate smoking with good times
- Use smoking as a way to cope with bad times
- Crave cigarettes

Recent studies have shown that many women may smoke for reasons other than the nicotine hit. Women may be less dependent on nicotine than men because they smoke fewer cigarettes, smoke brands with less nicotine, and may inhale less deeply. They may be more likely to smoke because of the social pleasure they derive from smoking or for sensory effects such as the sight and smell of tobacco smoke.

Teenage girls appear vulnerable to the lure of cigarette advertising, which suggests that smoking makes you thin and beautiful. Ironically, research shows that smoking causes wrinkling that can lessen attractiveness.

Looking through smoke to see the signs

Nicotine is released in cigarette smoke. Although it takes only seconds for the nicotine to reach your brain, it affects your body for up to 30 minutes. When you smoke regularly, the level of nicotine accumulates in your body.

In addition to nicotine, cigarette smoke contains gases and contaminants such as carbon monoxide and tar. Exposure to carbon monoxide increases the risk of cardiovascular disease, and tar is associated with a higher incidence of lung diseases, including cancer, emphysema, and bronchitis.

According to the American Lung Association, smoking is responsible for 87 percent of all lung cancer cases in the United States. Smoking may also increase your risk of gum disease and *macular degeneration,* an eye disease that is a leading cause of blindness; and smoking can worsen high cholesterol. Smoking is also associated with high blood pressure, stroke, and cancers of the mouth, lips, and esophagus.

Risking your health and your baby's, too!

Smoking during pregnancy can prevent oxygen from getting to the fetus, which can cause premature birth or low birth weight. In fact, 10 percent of all infant deaths can be attributed to smoking. Smoking during pregnancy may also be associated with asthma in infants and toddlers. Mothers who breast-feed also pass along nicotine to their infants.

Women who use oral contraceptives and smoke, especially those over 35, are more likely to suffer from heart disease and stroke. Smoking may also cause early menopause, which may increase risk of osteoporosis.

Putting yourself at risk: Secondhand smoke

When you are exposed to someone else's cigarette smoke, you absorb the nicotine and other compounds the smoker does. The more you are exposed to secondhand smoke, the higher concentration of these compounds you are exposed to and the greater your risk of lung cancer and respiratory diseases and infections.

Putting out the fire

Research suggests that successful smoking cessation may best be accomplished gradually. This approach appears to help minimize withdrawal symptoms, such as headache, drowsiness, and fatigue, which are the main reasons most smokers relapse.

Studies demonstrate that the best therapy for successful long-term smoking cessation is a combination of behavioral and medical therapy.

What can you do to quit? Here are some tips:

- ✔ Enlist the support of family and friends.

- ✔ Quit with a friend or join a smoking cessation program such as those offered by hospitals and your local chapters of the American Cancer Society, American Lung Association, or Smokenders.

- ✔ Exercise and eat right. Doing so will not only help you feel better but will also help keep off the weight that you may gain after quitting.

- ✔ Spend as much time as possible in places where you can't smoke.

- ✔ Don't be discouraged if you begin to smoke again. Most smokers typically try two or three times before they are successful. Just try again.

If these tips alone don't help you change your behavior, you may want to consider *hypnosis,* a trancelike state that mimics sleep and makes you more open to suggestion. If you're interested in hypnosis, ask your doctor to recommend a reputable hypnotist. But be aware that sensitivity to hypnosis varies from person to person.

In addition to behavior modification, try a nicotine patch, gum, or inhaler to temporarily replace the nicotine and help you get past the withdrawal symptoms. These aids, now available without a prescription, have been proven to ease the process and minimize the likelihood of relapse.

A new weapon in the fight to stop smoking is bupropion (Zyban), a prescription medication also used as an antidepressant. Unlike the patch and gum, which replace one form of nicotine with another, bupropion has been shown to actually reduce the craving for nicotine.

It's never too late to quit smoking. Once you stop, your body immediately begins to reverse some of smoking's harmful effects.

Chapter 7
Women and Violence

● ●

In This Chapter
▶ Taking a plan of action to avoid domestic violence
▶ Avoiding sexual assault

● ●

*W*omen may be less aggressive than men, but that certainly doesn't shield them from violence. In fact, it may put them more at risk. Women face violence on many fronts — on the streets, in the workplace, even in their homes. From rape and sexual assault to domestic violence, women not only face violence — they are its victims.

This chapter looks at the types of violence women face and what they can do about it.

Domestic Violence

It's hard to know exactly how many women are victims of domestic violence because many women don't report it. The Centers for Disease Control and Prevention estimates that 1.8 million women are assaulted by their partners each year. Other widely cited reports place the number between 2 and 4 million.

One 1996 report estimates that 25 percent of women in the United States will be abused by a current or former partner at some time during their lives. The National Coalition Against Domestic Violence places that figure higher still; it estimates that half of all women will experience some form of domestic violence from their spouses during their marriages. The only facts about which the experts agree are that the victims of domestic violence are most often women and that domestic violence is both widespread and under-reported, due in large part to fear of retaliation or to shame.

Domestic violence is a pattern of behavior that one person uses to establish control over another person by using threats and fear. Domestic violence includes not only physical beating, but also threats, intimidation, sexual abuse, and exploitation. The attacks usually begin with verbal threats, and then progress to physical violence, with results ranging from bruises and broken bones to death. In fact, approximately 30 percent of all murdered women are killed by an intimate partner. Ironically, physical violence often escalates during pregnancy. The abuse can also include sexual assault, which this chapter discusses later.

Who is involved?

What kind of people abuse their partners? Research indicates that abusers often

- ✔ Have low self-esteem
- ✔ Grew up in a violent family
- ✔ Abuse drugs or alcohol
- ✔ Tend to use force or violence to solve problems
- ✔ Are pathologically jealous
- ✔ Have traditional ideas about gender roles

Women who are abused often share common characteristics. They generally

- ✔ Have low self-esteem
- ✔ Have traditional ideas about gender roles
- ✔ Deny or minimize the abuse
- ✔ Accept responsibility for their abuser's actions

Despite the fact that abusers and victims often share these common characteristics, however, they are otherwise impossible to categorize because domestic violence occurs across all social, ethnic, economic, and religious boundaries.

Why it continues

It seems to go without saying that the solution to the problem of domestic violence is for the woman to leave the relationship. But leaving is not always possible.

Do you think you are abused?

The following are signs of abuse. You may be a victim of abuse if your partner has ever

- Threatened to harm you

- Hit, kicked, punched, or otherwise physically harmed you

- Deliberately destroyed things you care about

- Used a weapon to intimidate you

- Prevented you from leaving the house or seeing your friends

- Prevented you from getting a job

- Forced you to have sex when you didn't want to

- Blamed you for his or her abusive behavior

Some women believe that their partners can change or that the problem will go away. Many abusers are apologetic and promise to change their behavior. But even women who want to leave an abusive relationship may have difficulty.

Many women don't have the financial means to leave home, especially if they have children to support. In addition, many women may be afraid to leave — and with good reason. Leaving does not always put an end to the violence. Studies show that the violence often becomes worse for women who attempt to leave. Some abusers increase the abuse to convince the woman to reconcile with them; others to punish them. One widely reported study found that 73 percent of abused women who sought emergency medical services sustained their injuries *after* they left their abuser.

This increase in violence does not mean, however, that a woman should stay in an abusive relationship.

What to do

If you're in an abusive relationship, you need to plan ahead — both to increase your safety during an attack and to make your departure easier.

If an attack occurs, try to protect yourself. Call the police as soon as possible or inform a neighbor about the violence and ask her to call the police if she hears suspicious noises coming from your house. Know what exits are available to you and keep your purse and car keys ready so you can leave. Identify a safe place to go in such an emergency. Take pictures of your injuries for use in a possible court case.

How to protect yourself from escalating violence

You can help protect yourself from violence if you follow a few rules:

✔ **Refuse to tolerate abuse:** If you take a stand against abuse early on, you may be able to deter future incidents.

✔ **Don't excuse put-downs:** Criticism, ridicule, and name-calling constitute verbal abuse, which may lead to physical abuse.

✔ **Don't excuse a slap, shove, push, or punch:** Abuse rarely occurs only once.

✔ **Maintain contact with your friends, family, and activities:** An abusive partner may try to cut you off from friends and family and monitor and control your every move. This is a form of domination, and it can be unhealthy. Your friends and family can provide you with an outside support system, and maintaining contact with your outside activities may keep your self-esteem intact.

✔ **Tell your abusive partner to seek counseling:** If he or she doesn't, leave the relationship.

If you're planning to leave your partner, gather some money, your car keys, and valuable documents, such as birth certificates and other identification papers, and keep them in a safe, accessible place. Identify a place you can go when you leave, such as an emergency shelter, a social service agency, or the house of a friend. Leave clothes with a friend, if possible. And rehearse your escape plan.

You can also seek a protection order from your local police department. Not all batterers obey protection orders, but some do. You may need to ask the police or the court to enforce the order. Be aware, however, that the police cannot enforce the order until the abuser is disobeying it.

For help in dealing with domestic violence, contact the National Family Violence Helpline, operated by the National Council on Child Abuse and Family Violence at 800-222-2000, or the National Coalition Against Domestic Violence at 800-799-SAFE.

Sexual Assault

Sexual assault is one of the fastest growing violent crimes in the United States. *Sexual assault* is a verbal or physical attack with sexual connotations. Although rape is the most well-known type of sexual assault, the term also encompasses sexual harassment, date rape, and incest.

Because of this broad definition and the fact that so many incidents remain unreported, no firm statistics exist on how often sexual assault occurs. But the National Victim Center reports that more than 700,000 women are raped or sexually assaulted annually. And the National Organization for Women reports that half of all working women experience some form of sexual harassment. Although men can be the victims of sexual assault, women and children are the primary targets.

Sexual assault is a crime of violence, power, and control. Like domestic violence, it can happen to anyone, regardless of age, gender, race, ethnicity, or social class. Strangers, acquaintances, friends, or relatives can commit this assault. In fact, it is estimated that 80 percent of sexual assaults against women are committed by someone the woman knows.

Sexual assault can affect the victim's relationship with her family and friends as well. Many women withdraw from relationships or become clingy and needy. As a result, family members and friends may find themselves dealing not only with their own reactions to the assault on their loved one, but also with the changes they see in that person.

Rape

Rape is not about sex. This violent crime causes both physical and emotional anguish for the victim. Rape is humiliating and traumatizing and can do serious damage to a woman's sense of self and well-being. It can also do physical damage: Rape can cause acute injuries, increase the risk of acquiring sexually transmitted diseases, and increase the risk of pregnancy.

Traditionally defined as vaginal penetration of a woman without her consent, the legal definition of rape has been expanded to include oral and anal contact as well. Although the actual definition varies from state to state, the fact that it occurs without the victim's consent is a key component of the definition.

Remember: You have the right to say no to sexual contact and have your wishes honored. This right applies to sexual contact with dates, partners, spouses, and other acquaintances as well as to contact with strangers. Knowing an attacker does not constitute consent. In most instances of rape, the woman knows her attacker. This attack is known as *acquaintance rape,* or *date rape,* because it often occurs on dates.

Date rape is common on college campuses and is often linked to alcohol. It is also linked with a societal belief in men that when a woman says no, she really means yes. But if a man spends money on a date with a woman, he is not automatically entitled to sex at the end of the night. Nor is he entitled to sex based on a past relationship or sexual encounter with the woman. The woman always has the right to refuse.

What to do if you are raped

If you are raped

✔ **Contact your local rape crisis center:** Ask what course to follow for medical care, support, and police procedures.

✔ **Help preserve the evidence:** Don't shower, change clothes, or change the scene where the assault occurred.

✔ **Get medical attention as soon as possible:** A medical examination can help detect injury. Medical personnel can also test you for sexually transmitted diseases and discuss your contraceptive options.

✔ **Report the crime to the police as soon as possible:** The police may be able to arrest the rapist and preserve the evidence. You don't need to decide right away whether you wish to prosecute.

✔ **Seek post-rape counseling:** Contact your local rape crisis center. These centers are usually listed in the phone book. Your local hospital can also put you in touch with your local rape crisis center. Or you can call the Rape, Abuse, and Incest National Network (RAINN)'s 24-hour hotline, 800-656-HOPE, for a referral.

To help prevent date rape, make your wishes and desires clear to your partner. Stay in control and don't give in to the influence of alcohol and drugs. Be aware that some men have been known to slip sedatives such as rohypnol into the drinks of unsuspecting women, which makes them defenseless against assault. Don't accept a drink you didn't see mixed or have left unattended.

Incest

Incest is sexual contact between family members who are not marital partners. Although it happens most often between brothers and sisters, it is also common between fathers and daughters.

Like other forms of sexual assault, incest is often underreported. It is also traumatic for the victim. Victims of intergenerational incest often experience depression, anxiety, low self-esteem, chronic pain, personality disorders, irritable bowel syndrome, and fear of sexual intimacy.

If you are a victim of incest, seek counseling with a therapist or through a support group.

TIP

Protect yourself

You can take a number of steps to reduce your risk of becoming a victim of rape or sexual assault:

✔ Lock the doors of your home, even when you are inside.

✔ Leave lights on inside and outside the house.

✔ Don't list your full name in the phone book or on your mailbox if you live alone.

✔ Don't open your door to strangers. Ask repair, service, or delivery personnel for identification before you let them in.

✔ Have your house and car keys ready when you go from your house to your car or your car to your house.

✔ Check your car before getting in it. Keep the windows up and the doors locked.

✔ Don't accept rides from people you don't know.

✔ Don't pick up hitchhikers.

✔ Don't stop to assist stalled drivers. Drive on and call the police.

✔ Carry a whistle, personal alarm, or pepper spray. Be aware, however, that pepper spray is considered a weapon in some states and its use may be limited.

✔ Be aware of your surroundings. Know your route, stay in well-lit areas, and look behind you.

✔ Learn how to defend yourself. Your local YWCA or police department may offer self-defense classes and seminars.

Sexual harassment

Anita Hill may have brought sexual harassment into the pubic consciousness, but it has been around for years. By definition, sexual harassment is any unwelcome sexual advance — from verbal innuendoes and jokes to physical advances and rape — that occurs as a condition of employment or education.

According to law, harassment occurs when the victim must submit to sexual conduct to get a job, a promotion, admission to a school, or any related benefits. It also occurs when the conduct creates a hostile workplace or an educational environment that interferes with the victim's performance or participation.

If you feel you are a victim of sexual harassment

- ✔ Avoid the person doing the harassing.
- ✔ Tell the harasser how you feel about his behavior and ask him to stop.
- ✔ Keep records of the incidents.
- ✔ Report the action to your boss or, if the harasser is your boss, report it to his boss.
- ✔ Take legal action if necessary.

Chapter 8

Caring for Yourself

. . . .

. . . .

*Y*ou jump up to answer the doorbell and slip, spraining your ankle. As you fall, you startle your sleeping cat, who scratches your arm. Then you hit your head on the doorknob, leaving a tooth dangling from your mouth. A really, really bad day — but not necessarily one you can't handle without medical attention.

You can treat a number of these kinds of unpleasant emergencies yourself. Furthermore, you can diagnose several medical conditions — from pregnancy to high blood pressure — on your own. This chapter covers the basics of self-care — from home medical tests to CPR.

Why You'd Want to Treat Yourself

Okay, so maybe biology wasn't your best subject. But that doesn't mean that you're not qualified to "play doctor." In fact, studies show that more than 80 percent of all medical care you receive is self-care. Every time you pop an aspirin to stop a pounding headache or put a Band-Aid on a minor cut, you're acting as your own doctor.

Many of the minor aches and pains you deal with from day to day don't need a doctor's attention. Imagine the expense — in both money and time — of running to the doctor every time you have a minor cut, menstrual cramp, or sniffle. By treating these ailments yourself, you get immediate relief, save yourself money, and leave your doctor free to take care of more serious problems.

And when you or a loved one is the victim of one of those more serious problems, self-treatment in the form of first aid can mean the difference between life and death. It can buy you the time you need to get to the doctor and can help speed your recovery.

Be Prepared: What You Need to Have on Hand

Of course, to treat yourself effectively, you must be prepared. While you don't need years of medical training, you do need some basic knowledge of first aid. You need to know, for instance, what to do if you're choking, how to stop a wound from bleeding, and how to treat a burn. You also need to have supplies on hand to treat these conditions. A well-stocked first aid kit, home pharmacy, and a first aid handbook can prepare you for an emergency.

You should store first aid supplies in a small, waterproof box, and keep the box handy when you travel or participate in sports activities. Table 8-1 lists the supplies that you should include in your first aid kit. These supplies are available in most drugstores and pharmacy departments.

Table 8-1	Must-Haves for Your First Aid Kit
Adhesive tape	Adrenaline kit (if a family member is allergic to insect stings)
Alcohol wipes	Moleskin (for blisters)
Elastic bandage (for sprains)	Insect repellent
Instant cold pack (for sprains and bruises)	Needle
Pain reliever, such as acetaminophen or aspirin	Plastic adhesive strips, waterproof
Small bar of soap	Sterile gauze pads, both regular and nonstick
Bandages and tape (to close small wounds)	Sunscreen, 15 SPF or above
Syrup of ipecac (to induce vomiting)	Triangular bandage (for arm splints or tourniquet)
Tweezers	Universal antidote for unidentified poisons ($\frac{1}{2}$ ounce activated charcoal, $\frac{1}{2}$ ounce magnesium oxide, $\frac{1}{4}$ ounce tannic acid, to be added to a glass of water)

The Heimlich maneuver: The hug of life

First aid for choking can be a lifesaver.

First, make sure the victim is actually choking. If she can speak, she is getting oxygen and does not have an obstructed airway.

To perform the Heimlich maneuver on a conscious person:

1. Stand behind the choking victim, and wrap your arms around the victim just above the navel (below the lower edge of the breastbone and ribcage).

2. Make a fist with one hand.

3. Grab the fist with your other hand.

4. Exert pressure inward and upward in quick, hard thrusts.

5. Repeat until the airway is open.

If the victim is pregnant or obese, position your hands higher on her trunk — closer to the lower edge of the breastbone.

To perform the Heimlich maneuver on an unconscious person:

1. Position the victim on her back, and straddle the victim's thighs.

2. Place the heel of one hand in the middle of the victim's abdomen, below the breastbone — not on the ribs or tip of the breastbone.

3. Place your other hand on top of the first.

4. Exert pressure inward and upward in quick thrusts.

5. Repeat until the airway is open.

To perform the Heimlich maneuver on yourself: fold one fist into the other and thrust upward, just above the navel. Or drape yourself over a chair or some other firm object and press yourself firmly into it.

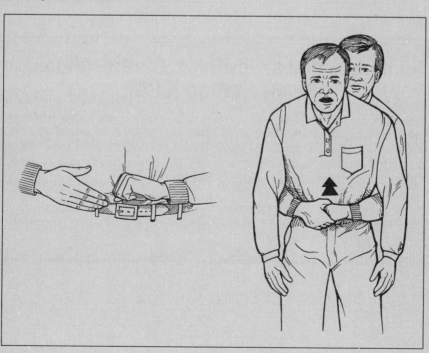

Keep the medications and supplies listed in Table 8-2 on hand, too. You should store them, as well as prescription drugs, somewhere away from the hot, humid bathroom. A child-safe container in your bedroom, away from sunlight, is best.

Table 8-2	Items for Your Home Pharmacy
Activated charcoal (antidote for certain poisons)	Antacids (for upset stomach)
Antifungal medications (for athlete's foot)	Motion sickness remedies
Calamine lotion (for sunburn and minor burns and bites)	Cough suppressant without expectorant (for dry coughs)
Expectorant with dextromethorphan (for coughs with mucus)	Flashlight
Heating pad	Hydrocortisone cream (for itching and rashes)
Ice pack	Laxatives (for constipation)
Petroleum jelly	Throat lozenges
Toothache pain reliever	

A technique that saves lives: Cardiopulmonary Resuscitation (CPR)

When someone has an accident, such as drowning or choking, or a medical emergency, such as a heart attack or cardiac arrest, the heart can stop beating. During this time, cardiopulmonary resuscitation (CPR) can save a life. CPR is a combination of breathing and chest compression that helps keep someone alive until medical help comes or the victim has resumed breathing and has a heartbeat.

The best way to learn CPR is through your local Red Cross or American Heart Association chapter, YMCA, or hospital. Contact any of these organizations to see where courses are available.

Treat Yourself — to Self-Care

While many conditions do require professional medical treatment, you can treat many conditions and accidents yourself or at least give yourself the immediate care you need until medical help arrives.

Just remember these tips:

✔ If you're treating yourself with over-the-counter medications, read and follow the instructions.

✔ Keep the supplies in your first aid kit and home pharmacy current.

✔ If you're unsure how to deal with a minor problem, consult your doctor or a family health reference book.

✔ If a treatment you are using does not work or the condition worsens, consult your doctor.

Here are some of the most common conditions that can be self-treated and what you can do to avoid or postpone a trip to the doctor:

✔ **Ankle sprains:** When you've twisted your ankle, your body lets you know. Think R-I-C-E when it comes to healing yourself: Rest, Ice, Compression, and Elevation. If putting weight on your affected foot is painful, use crutches for a few days. Start ice treatments every two to three hours for the first three days. You can use a plastic bag of crushed ice or a bag of frozen food. First, put a cloth around your ankle, place the bag over the cloth, and then wrap an elastic bandage around the bag to keep it in place. Keep the ice in place only until the skin is numb. Between ice treatments, keep your ankle wrapped with an elastic bandage. And whenever possible, elevate your foot above the level of your heart.

✔ **Bites and stings:** Bites and stings from insects and other animals are more common than you'd like them to be. Fortunately, however, they can usually be self-treated.

  • **Animal and human bites:** If Bowser bites or Fluffy scratches you, clean off the area with soap and water as with any minor scratch. If the skin is broken, contact your doctor. Some animals — wild and domestic — carry rabies and other diseases. Always have a doctor check human bites because of the high levels of bacteria in the human mouth. Make sure you have a tetanus booster shot every 10 years.

  • **Insect bites and stings:** *Ticks* should be removed with tweezers. Use the tweezers to pull the tick straight up, without crushing it. If the head remains, seek medical help to have it removed. Clean the wound with soap and water. Because some ticks can carry the bacteria for Lyme disease, a bacterial infection that can cause joint swelling, meningitis (an infection of the central nervous system), and even heart block, it's important to watch for any signs of the disease, such as a bull's eye rash around the bite and flulike symptoms.

Stinging insects can be dangerous to the one person out of ten who is allergic to the venom. If you're allergic, use an emergency adrenaline kit (a hypodermic syringe containing the hormone adrenaline, which counters dangerous allergic reactions) and seek medical attention. These kits usually require a doctor's prescription, so if you know you have this type of allergy, be prepared and always keep a kit on hand. If you're not allergic, wash the site with soap and water; scrape off any embedded stinger with a credit card, knife blade, or other straight edge; and apply an ice pack to keep swelling down. You can relieve itching and swelling with an over-the-counter topical steroid cream such as hydrocortisone.

Spiders usually are harmless; most of their bites simply cause a welt. You can treat these bites by placing a cold compress on the affected area. A bite from a black widow or brown recluse — the only common poisonous spiders in the United States — can be dangerous, however. (The black widow has an hourglass shape on its back; the brown recluse has a violin shape on its back. Both are common in the southern United States.) Use an ice pack on the site immediately (this helps prevent absorption of the poison into circulation) and seek medical care immediately.

Jellyfish or *Portuguese man-of-war* can release venom that causes considerable pain. To treat these stings, apply rubbing alcohol or vinegar to relieve the pain and inactivate any remaining stinging capsules. If neither is available, sprinkle the area with meat tenderizer or sand and gently rub it into the skin. After 15 minutes, gently wash the area with sea water, being careful not to release more venom. You can then use a local anesthetic cream or hydrocortisone cream on the wound. Aspirin or acetaminophen may be necessary to relieve pain.

✔ **Blisters:** Poke, don't cut is the rule with blisters. The outer layer of a blister protects the raw skin underneath and shouldn't be removed. You can use a sterilized needle (hold the needle tip for 20 seconds over an open flame) to make a pinprick to drain the fluid in the blister; you should then apply a sterile dressing and watch for signs of infection.

✔ **Burns:** For minor burns, immerse the burn in cold (not icy) water for at least five minutes. If you can't immerse the burned area, apply wet cloths or pour water over the area. Then cover the area with a clean gauze pad, making sure that adhesive tape doesn't touch the burn.

Acetaminophen or ibuprofen helps relieve the pain. Ibuprofen also relieves inflammation. After 24 hours, you can apply an antiseptic cream. See a doctor for any extensive or second- or third-degree burns such as a burn that blisters soon after the injury.

Never use butter or any type of grease on the burn because it holds in heat and prevents air from circulating and helping to heal the burn.

✔ **Choking:** The cough reflex usually clears the esophagus within a few seconds. If a person can't cough, breathe, or make a sound, use the *Heimlich maneuver* to remove the blockage. (See the sidebar if you're unfamiliar with the Heimlich maneuver.)

✔ **Cuts and wounds:** You should wash minor cuts and wounds with soap and water. Rinse off or remove any loose debris, but not objects that are embedded in the wound. If bleeding continues, use a bandage or clean cloth to put pressure on the injury. When bleeding stops, use a fresh bandage or dressing that is attached by tape. To prevent infection, you may want to use an antiseptic or antibiotic cream. And be careful to only *glaze* the cut with the cream, rather than *frost* it. Too much cream can suffocate the skin and delay healing. You don't have to bandage a superficial cut because air speeds the healing process.

If the cut continues to bleed, is deep, gaping, has jagged edges, or is very dirty, it may require a doctor's care.

✔ **Dental injuries:** If a tooth has been knocked out, chances are good that you can have it successfully transplanted if you get to your dentist within an hour or two. Hold the tooth by only the crown and rinse it in a bowl of tap water. Replace it in the socket and put a piece of gauze or a wet tea bag over it. Bite down to keep the tooth in place. If the tooth doesn't fit into the socket, put it into a container of milk, your own saliva, or warm water with a $1/2$ teaspoon salt added. Either way, see your dentist immediately.

✔ **Dry skin:** Even if you resist the temptation to scratch, dry skin has the ability to crack, leaving you vulnerable to infection. The most effective way to prevent dry skin is to limit the time that you shower or bath, especially avoiding very hot water. While you're washing away your cares, you're also washing away the *sebum,* the skin's protective coating. After showering, apply a moisturizer. People with sensitive skin also should use cream moisturizers with a minimum 15 SPF and use hypoallergenic cleansers.

✔ **Food poisoning:** Unwashed or improperly handled food, raw or undercooked meat, and food contaminated by uncooked poultry juices left on your chopping board are common sources of food poisoning. The body's way of getting rid of the contaminated substance is through vomiting and diarrhea — usually within 3 to 12 hours after you've eaten the food. Let these actions run their courses, which should be over in several hours. Follow up with clear liquids and bland foods for the next day. And be careful: Keep food properly refrigerated and don't prepare meals without scrubbing utensils used on raw poultry. If you have a headache, stiff neck, and fever; nervous system symptoms, such as difficulty speaking or swallowing, visual changes, or paralysis; blood in the vomit or stool; a fever that lasts more than 24 hours; vomiting that lasts for more than 12 hours; or diarrhea that lasts for more than three days, see your doctor. You could be experiencing a more severe form of food poisoning, an infection, dehydration, or some other condition requiring medical treatment.

✔ **Frostbite:** If you've been out in the cold too long, especially on windy days, the underlying tissues of your skin may become mildly frostbitten. If you experience frostbite, put the affected areas in lukewarm (not hot) water. Keep changing the water to keep the temperature between 100 and 105 degrees F. For the nose, ears, and face, warm cloths are easier to use. Keep warming the area until the skin becomes soft and you feel sensation in the affected area. Avoid movement of affected parts; massage is not helpful. If pain becomes severe or circulation doesn't return to the affected areas (in the form of color or sensation), see a doctor.

Never rub snow on a frostbitten area or use direct heat, such as that from fires or heating pads, to thaw it out. This action can further damage tissues.

✔ **Leg cramps:** If you exercise strenuously, you can lose water and salt (electrolytes) through sweating. Sometimes this loss of water and salt causes body cramps. To treat heat cramps, drink fluids with $1/4$ to $1/2$ teaspoon salt per pint added. Sports drinks are also fine.

You can eliminate ordinary muscle cramps, often felt at night, by stretching the cramped muscle. If the cramp is in your calf muscle, flex your foot upward, or get out of bed and do a gradual deep knee bend. Adding potassium (bananas, oranges, and potatoes) and calcium to your diet before going to bed may also help.

✔ **Hemorrhoids:** Often a result of giving birth or frequent straining during a bowel movement, hemorrhoids are one of life's little trials. These inflamed or swollen veins, located inside or outside the anus, can result in bleeding, pain, and itching. You can treat the annoying itching and tenderness with warm sitz baths. Simply fill your tub or a basin with warm (not hot) water and sit in it. Using premoistened towelettes after a bowel movement may be helpful. To relieve itching, you can use petroleum jelly, zinc oxide, and medicated creams and suppositories, such as Preparation H. For more information on hemorrhoids, see Chapter 9.

✔ **Hypoglycemia:** Hypoglycemia means an abnormally low blood sugar that may cause irritability, hunger pangs, sweating, clamminess, or a rapid heartbeat. Sugar — such as that in fruit juice, honey, or soft drinks — relieves the symptoms quickly, but because it is absorbed and metabolized quickly, may start the cycle again. Avoiding sweets, soft drinks, and caffeine, and getting proper exercise help prevent this cycle from occurring. If you have diabetes and you experience these symptoms, you should seek medical attention. For more information on diabetes, see Chapter 17.

✔ **Ingrown toenails:** Use a wooden toothpick to carefully lift the ingrown nail. Then slip a tiny piece of gauze under the nail. You may want to add a bit of antibacterial ointment to reduce the chance of infection. You can replace the gauze daily and leave it off when the inflammation subsides.

✔ **Morning sickness:** Some women find that eating small, frequent meals and drinking water and juices throughout the day helps alleviate morning sickness. Ginger, taken as a tea or in capsules as soon as you get up, may also help. Bland foods, such as saltine crackers, are also good.

✔ **Nosebleed:** To stop the bleeding, sit down and lean slightly forward. Use your thumb and index finger to pinch the lower portion of your nostrils while you breathe through your mouth. Hold it for at least five minutes. If the bleeding hasn't stopped, pinch your nose for another ten minutes. If you're experiencing frequent nosebleeds that are not associated with a cold or other minor nasal irritation, consult your doctor. Your doctor may want to screen you for high blood pressure or a bleeding disorder.

✔ **Smashed fingers:** Have you ever closed the car door with your fingers still in it, winding up with a blood clot under the nail? To treat smashed fingers, use an ice pack to reduce swelling for the first 24 hours. After that, warm soaks or heating pads will gradually help dissolve the clot and relieve joint stiffness. If you think you may have broken one of the bones in your finger, ask your doctor about getting an x-ray. You probably also will need a pain reliever such as aspirin or acetaminophen.

✔ **Sore throat:** Try this remedy: Combine $1/4$ cup vinegar with 1 cup water, add a dash of salt, and gargle. If the sore throat persists, see your doctor to rule out strep throat or other infections that require medical treatment.

✔ **Splinters:** Tweezers do the job if you haven't already tried to pull the splinter out with your nails, breaking it off. If the splinter is under the skin, you can take a clean needle and carefully cut away the upper, dead layer of the skin. After the splinter is exposed, use the tweezers.

✔ **Stress incontinence:** As many as 9 million women suffer from urine leakage when they laugh, exercise, cough, or sneeze. This condition often is a result of childbirth, when the vagina stretches the structure that supports the bladder and the tube leading to it. Can anything short of surgery be done? Kegel exercises are effective for mild cases, experts say. See Chapter 23 for more information about Kegel exercises.

✔ **Sunburn:** Cool baths, calomine lotion, or cool compresses should help relieve sunburn pain. You can use these methods of treatment several times a day. Pain relievers such as aspirin or acetaminophen reduce the discomfort. Corticosteroid creams also help with pain and inflammation, and calamine lotion is soothing.

If a severe sunburn is accompanied by vomiting and fever, seek medical attention to rule out sunstroke.

Never use petroleum jelly or butter on a sunburn because it prevents air from helping to heal the burns. Also, avoid creams or sprays with benzocaine, which often causes allergic reactions. And remember that the best way to treat a sunburn is to avoid getting one in the first place!

Testing, Testing: Using Home Medical Tests to Your Advantage

Home medical tests help you stay on top of a medical condition without spending lots of money or time cooling your heals at a doctor's office. The home tests listed in this section help you diagnose and monitor several conditions. Most of these tests are available at your local pharmacy.

Just remember that no test — whether performed at home or in a laboratory — is 100 percent accurate. You can enhance the accuracy of a test, however, by following the directions exactly as they are printed.

Here are some of the more common home tests:

✔ **AIDS test:** A home test that screens for HIV — the virus that causes AIDS — is now available. You simply prick your finger to get a blood sample, then send the sample to a lab to be tested. The testing process is completely confidential, and so are the results, which you receive by phone. You can purchase a test kit at a pharmacy, or you can order one by calling 800-448-8378. For more information about AIDS, see Chapter 22.

✔ **Body temperature test:** You've had your temperature taken since you were a kid. The trusty thermometer is probably the easiest home medical test available. You can choose from several kinds of thermometers to test for the normal body temperature of 98.6 degrees F. These thermometers include the traditional oral glass bulb as well as electronic, disposable, and earlobe versions.

✔ **Home blood pressure monitor:** If you have high blood pressure (hypertension) or are at risk for this condition, a home blood pressure cuff is an important way to monitor the pressure of your blood as it is pumped through your circulatory system. You can buy kits in digital wristwatch or finger styles or the traditional type of cuff used in health care facilities. (The traditional cuff is the most accurate, but it's also the most difficult to use.) Before buying a home blood pressure monitor, make sure you can use it easily and properly. And once you've bought it, it's a good idea to take it to your doctor's office and compare the readings of your device with those of your doctor's device.

Don't rely on one reading to determine if you have — or don't have — high blood pressure. (For more information about blood pressure, see Chapter 15.)

✔ **Home cholesterol test:** Fifteen minutes is all you need to get a cholesterol reading from a home kit. If you have high cholesterol, the test may help you see how successful you are at lowering it. A simple pinprick provides the drop of blood the kit needs to analyze the total cholesterol. (A reading of 200 or less is best; 200 to 240 is borderline high, depending on your health history; and 240 and above is considered too high.) Confirm a high reading by repeating the test at your doctor's office after a 12-hour fast. Cholesterol can fluctuate depending on what you've eaten recently and other factors, so don't rely on just one reading. For more information on cholesterol and cholesterol levels, see Chapter 15.

✔ **Pregnancy testing:** Why wait for the good news? A home pregnancy kit quickly analyzes your urine and confirms pregnancy. For more information on pregnancy, see Part V.

✔ **Occult blood screening test:** The occult (meaning hidden) blood screening test checks a small sample of fecal material for hidden blood that can be a warning sign of colon and rectal cancers — both of which are highly treatable if detected early. The American Cancer Society, the American Gastroenterological Association, and other groups recommend that healthy people take this test every year starting at age 50. The easiest home version of this test involves dropping a test pad in the toilet after a bowel movement. If blood is present, the pad changes color. Please note, however, that a positive result does not indicate the presence of cancer, only the presence of blood within the gastrointestinal tract. Still, a positive result does warrant a consultation with your doctor.

✔ **Ovulation prediction kits:** If you want to know when you're ovulating — either in order to get pregnant or as a natural birth control method — you may wish to try an ovulation prediction kit. These tests, like home pregnancy tests, involve urine analysis.

Not all tests are the same

When you're shopping for medical testing kits and medical testing devices, be aware that accuracy, cost, and procedure vary from test to test. Some pregnancy tests, for example, require you to collect your urine in a cup, while others simply ask you to hold a stick under your urine stream. Likewise, some occult blood tests come with dietary restrictions, while others do not. Compare the kits you are considering before you buy them.

Emergency! When You Shouldn't Treat Yourself

Although you may be quite adept at taking care of everyday aches and pains, there are instances in which you need professional medical help — fast.

First aid measures can staunch severe bleeding, and CPR can resuscitate someone who has stopped breathing. But such measures are only temporary fixes. These conditions and others, such as heart attack, stroke, poisoning, and shock, require prompt medical attention.

If you are experiencing any of the following warning signs, do not try to treat yourself. Get help immediately! Call 911, call an ambulance, or drive (or have someone drive you) to the emergency room:

- ✔ Sudden severe pain anywhere, especially in the chest or upper abdomen
- ✔ Sudden severe dizziness, headache, or vision change
- ✔ Difficulty breathing
- ✔ Sudden severe or intense weakness
- ✔ Severe diarrhea
- ✔ Heavy bleeding, for any reason
- ✔ Sudden inability to move all or a part of the body
- ✔ Suicidal feelings

Part III
All That Ails You

The 5th Wave   By Rich Tennant

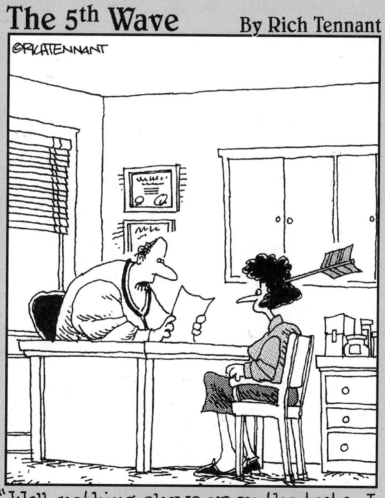

"Well, nothing shows up on the tests. I think your headaches are probably just stress related."

In this part . . .

You really can't predict *all* that can ail you, but if you have a good idea of problems that commonly affect women, you can prepare yourself to deal with — and possibly prevent — many of them. Your preparation begins in this section, in which you learn the basic causes, symptoms, diagnosis, treatment, and prevention techniques for a wide variety of conditions common to women.

Chapter 9
Passing Pains

- -

In This Chapter

▶ Dealing with colds and flu

▶ Heading off headaches

▶ Understanding heartburn and indigestion

▶ Living with hemorrhoids

- -

*T*his chapter talks about *acute* conditions — those annoying health problems that come on suddenly and usually stick around only a short while. Depending on their severity, you may or may not consult a doctor for these kinds of problems. But in this chapter, you'll see how to spot the symptoms, how the problem is diagnosed, what you can do to ease the discomfort, the warning signs that should cue you to seek medical help, what your doctor may do to make these pains go, and what you can do to prevent them from coming in the first place.

Colds and Flu

Every woman has experienced a cold at one time or another. Statistics indicate that each person experiences between two and four colds a year. Fortunately, influenza, or the flu, which is generally more severe than a cold, is less common, although it's certainly not rare. Public health officials estimate that 40 million Americans develop the flu each year.

Viruses cause both colds and flu. A *virus* is a parasite, which means that it can't live on its own. It needs a host to carry it and be its "body," so to speak. Viruses, which are spread by direct contact with a contaminated object or person and by air (through sneezing and coughing), invade host cells and take over their genetic material to reproduce themselves. In the process, the virus damages the host cell and sometimes kills it. Viruses invade host cells and replicate extremely quickly, which is why you can come down with a cold or the flu and feel lousy literally overnight. Your immune system immediately kicks in to kill off the virus, prompting symptoms such as coughing or sneezing (to rid your body of the attacking virus) and perhaps fever (to kill the virus), and shuts down everything except essential operations to concentrate on its battle. This effort can take a toll on your energy level — making you feel tired — and on your pain threshold, making you more sensitive to pain.

The reason colds are more common in the cool weather is because that's when people move indoors where viruses can more easily spread from person to person.

Recognizing the signs

Cold symptoms vary depending on the virus that causes them. They include a runny nose, nasal congestion, sneezing, sore throat, mild-to-moderate cough, mild fatigue, achiness, and, on rare occasions, fever or headache. Flu symptoms include all the nasal symptoms of colds, as well as a sore throat, severe coughing and chest discomfort, a high fever and chills, headache, aches and pains, and fatigue.

Generally, the onset of a cold comes one to two days after exposure; onset of the flu generally begins one to four days after exposure. Colds usually last three to four days and flu three to five days, but both can last longer. If a cold persists for more than two weeks, or the fever of the flu lasts longer than three days, you should see your doctor to make sure that you have not developed a complication such as pneumonia.

Knowing for sure

If you go to a doctor (most people won't for colds but may for the flu), your doctor will most likely listen to your symptoms, review your medical history, and examine you, checking your nose, ears, throat, and lungs.

Making it better

Just about everything you can do to relieve the symptoms of a cold or flu is available over the counter or is already in your kitchen cupboard. Try these tips:

- ✔ **Drink plenty of fluids:** Doing so helps prevent dehydration, soothe inflammation, relieve nasal congestion, and create a productive cough.

- ✔ **Get wet:** Use a humidifier, take a hot shower, or inhale steam to keep your nasal passages moist, allowing them to constantly clean themselves and letting the mucus drain more easily.

- ✔ **Use saline spray or a syringe filled with saline to relieve nasal congestion:** To make up the salt water solution, mix ¹/₂ teaspoon of salt with a pint of lukewarm water. Hold one nostril closed, squirt the saline into the other nostril, let it drain, and repeat two or three times. Do the same for the other nostril. You can do this several times a day.

- ✔ **Don't medicate unless necessary:** Some of your symptoms (such as fever) may play a role in expelling the virus from your body.

- ✔ **When you do medicate yourself, avoid multisymptom cold relievers:** They may have medications that you don't need. If you're congested but don't have a runny nose, you don't need an antihistamine, for example. Use cough suppressants only on dry, hacking coughs that prevent you from sleeping (using a cough suppressant on a productive cough hinders your body's action to rid itself of the illness). Avoid antihistamines: They can dry out your mucous membranes just when your immune system needs the mucus to clear out the virus.

- ✔ **For a sore throat, gargle with salt water solution:** Between gargles, suck on menthol-benzocaine, or phenol-based lozenges.

Though most colds and flu can be handled at home, see a physician if you have labored or rapid breathing, chest pains, shortness of breath, wheezing, or other symptoms of pneumonia, if your cold has lasted longer than two weeks, if your fever has lasted longer than four days, or if you show signs of a secondary infection (see the sidebar, "Complicating the matter").

With the exception of amantadine, an antiviral medicine that has proven effective at reducing the symptoms of Type A flu (the type that causes epidemics) if given early, very few medications are available to treat viruses. Don't ask your doctor for an antibiotic. Antibiotics fight bacteria, not viruses. And by taking antibiotics when you don't need them, you contribute to the rise in antibiotic-resistant bacteria, which means that antibiotics may not work as well for you when you really need them.

One happy note — your doctor may be able to prescribe a nasal spray for the treatment of colds and flu in the near future. This spray would prevent some viruses from binding with the hosts, reducing the length of your illness.

Complicating the matter

Most colds, and even most cases of the flu, are not serious. Sometimes, however, a cold or the flu can lead to more serious complications, such as

✔ **Bronchitis:** An inflammation of the air passages of the throat and chest, bronchitis is characterized by a productive cough, fever, and shortness of breath.

✔ **Ear infection:** Most common in young children, bacterial ear infections, characterized by earaches, often follow a cold. Most ear infections disappear on their own, but some do not. Multiple ear infections can lead to hearing loss and other problems.

✔ **Meningitis:** This severe infection of the membranes covering the brain and spinal cord can be fatal.

✔ **Pneumonia:** This infection, which can be either bacterial or viral, inflames the bronchial tubes and air sacs of the lungs. It is dangerous and potentially fatal, particularly in those over 65 or those with a chronic heart, lung, or organ disease or an immune disorder. If you experience labored or rapid breathing, chest pains or shortness of breath, wheezing, faintness, shaking chills, a bad sore throat along with extreme fatigue or irritability, a cough that raises foul-smelling green or brown phlegm, and a high fever that doesn't abate within two or three days, see your doctor.

✔ **Sinusitis:** Sinusitis, the inflammation and infection of one or more of the sinuses, can occur as a complication of colds or flu or can begin at the same time. Because most cases can be treated with antibiotics, you should contact your doctor if you experience the symptoms of sinusitis: nasal congestion plus a headache with pain or pressure around the face, excessively sensitive upper teeth, and yellow or green nasal drainage.

✔ **Strep throat:** A common throat infection caused by the Streptococcus bacterium, strep throat can only be firmly diagnosed with a throat culture. Treating this infection — which is marked by sore throat, fever, chills, swollen lymph nodes in the neck, and, occasionally, nausea and vomiting — is important because complications of strep throat can lead to scarlet fever and kidney problems.

An ounce of prevention

Although medical science has not yet found a cure for the common cold, it has found several ways to prevent you from developing colds (and flu):

✔ **Get a flu shot:** Your best prevention against the flu is an annual flu shot, which is quite effective in preventing Type A and Type B flu. The elderly, people with impaired immune systems, and people with severe medical disorders such as chronic heart or lung disease are at greater risk of developing complications and should be vaccinated.

✔ **Wash your hands often:** Most cold and flu viruses are spread by direct contact — when you touch a contaminated object or person and then touch your eyes, nose, or mouth before you wash your hands.

- ✔ **Eat healthily:** Proper nutrition keeps your body and immune system in good working order. In addition to following the recommendations in Chapter 1, consider eating yogurt and garlic, which have been shown in some studies to help reduce susceptibility to colds. And make sure to get adequate amounts of vitamin A, vitamin C, the B vitamins, and zinc.

- ✔ **Reduce your stress level:** Studies show that when people are more stressed, they are also more susceptible to illness. See Chapter 1 for stress reduction suggestions.

Headaches

Approximately 60 percent of all headaches are caused by tense muscles. These headaches are known as *tension headaches,* or *muscular-contraction headaches.* They occur when the muscles in the shoulders, neck, face, or scalp are contracted for a long period of time, which can impinge on blood vessels, reducing blood flow. As a result of the reduced blood flow, the muscles become short of oxygen and full of pain-producing toxins. The nerves within the muscles become irritated, and you feel pain.

Abnormal expansion or contraction of blood vessels inside the skull (on the brain's surface and within its protective covering) and in the tissues of the face, scalp, mouth, throat, sinuses, and neck is the cause of approximately 30 percent of all headaches. The pain of these headaches, known as *vascular headaches,* occurs because the expansion or contraction of the blood vessels irritates nerves wrapped around the vessels, resulting in pulsating pain. Perhaps the best-known type of vascular headache is the migraine headache, which is suffered by about 11 percent of the U.S. population — the majority of them women.

In a migraine headache, the brain's blood vessels undergo a sudden expansion, stretching and irritating the nerves wrapped around them. Migraine pain can last anywhere from 1 to 72 hours and be so severe and so encompassing that it involves other parts of the body. Women between the ages of 30 and 49 are the most likely to experience these headaches, which tend to run in families and may have specific triggers. Fluctuations in estrogen seem to be one of these triggers. Other triggers can be certain foods, such as chocolate, cheese, caffeine, and red wine.

A less common type of vascular headache is the *cluster headache,* so named because they occur in clusters of several per day for days or even weeks at a time and then disappear for months or even years.

The remaining 10 percent of headaches are symptoms or side effects of other conditions.

Recognizing the signs

Here are the specific symptoms for the most common types of headache:

- ✔ **Tension headache:** This type produces a dull or pressure-like pain in the scalp, temples, or the back of the neck that usually affects both sides of the head equally. It can be associated with premenstrual syndrome in some women. Other factors that contribute to tension headaches include stress, anxiety, eyestrain, poor posture, excessive squinting or jaw clenching, and neck and spinal injuries and conditions. Tension headaches generally subside on their own within a few hours, although some can linger for days depending on the cause.

- ✔ **Migraine:** A migraine produces very intense, throbbing head pain that is often more prevalent on one side of the head or face than the other. It is often accompanied by nausea and vomiting and a heightened sensitivity to light and noise and can be made worse by physical movement. In some people, the headache is preceded by sensory disturbances such as blurred vision, flashing lights, blank spots in their field of vision, and temporary hearing impairment. These disturbances are known as *auras.*

- ✔ **Cluster headache:** A cluster headache produces a steady, boring pain in and around one eye. Cluster headaches often start at the same time of day or night and may be accompanied by tearing or reddening of the eye and nasal congestion on the same side of the face. These headaches generally last from 15 minutes to an hour each and may occur in groups of between four and eight per day.

Knowing for sure

Your doctor will diagnose the type of headache you're getting based on your medical history and physical exam. Describing the pain more clearly helps your doctor diagnose the problem. Is the pain dull, throbbing, or sharp? Where is the pain? In the front of the forehead? Behind the eyeballs? In a band around your head?

Making it better

For a regular everyday headache, such as those caused by stress or staring too long at the computer screen, and even for some migraine pain, you may be able to find relief from the following:

- ✔ **Over-the-counter pain relievers:** Aspirin, acetaminophen (Tylenol), ibuprofen (Advil), and other over-the-counter pain relievers may help alleviate both tension and migraine headache pain. If you're pregnant, use only acetaminophen until you consult with your doctor.

- ✔ **Fire and ice:** Heating pads help relax muscles and blood vessels, thus increasing blood flow through the vessels of the head and scalp and relieving tension headaches; ice packs can help blood vessels constrict, easing migraine pain.

- ✔ **Rest:** Rest is good for tension headaches.

For chronic headaches and headaches that don't respond to over-the-counter painkillers, consult your doctor. He may prescribe the following:

- ✔ **Nonsteroidal anti-inflammatory drugs (NSAIDs):** These drugs relieve pain by reducing inflammation. Examples are naproxen (Naprosyn) and prescription-strength ibuprofen.

- ✔ **Ergotamine derivatives:** These drugs, which include Ergostat and Wigraine, help swollen blood vessels return to normal and are used to treat migraine and cluster headaches.

- ✔ **Isometheptene:** This drug, which is present in the prescription drugs Midrin and Isocom, constricts blood vessels and can be used in conjunction with NSAIDs to treat severe migraines.

- ✔ **Sumatriptan:** This vessel-dilating drug (Imitrex) is used to treat both migraine and cluster headaches. It is available as an oral tablet, a nasal spray (for faster onset), and as a self-administered injection.

When you have to call a doctor

A small percentage of headaches (10 percent) are the result of other diseases or conditions — some of which, including brain tumor, bleeding within the skull, *aneurysm* (a permanently and abnormally swollen blood vessel), glaucoma (an eye disease), and meningitis (a potentially fatal infection of the brain's protective covering) — are serious. You should see a doctor if you have headaches that

- ✔ Have recently come on in an unusually severe form

- ✔ Are accompanied by neurological problems such as numbness, weakness, loss

of muscle control, or visual or speech disturbances

- ✔ Follow an injury to the head

- ✔ Are accompanied by memory loss or confusion

- ✔ Are accompanied by fever, stiff neck, nausea, vomiting, or sensitivity to light

- ✔ Are accompanied by unusual symptoms you have not experienced before

Your doctor can also prescribe *prophylactic medications,* medications to prevent headaches from recurring. These include beta-adrenergic blockers, such as atenolol and propranolol (which are used to prevent vascular headaches); calcium channel blockers, such as nifedipine, which can be prescribed to people who can't take beta-adrenergic blockers; tricyclic antidepressants, such as amitriptyline and nortriptyline, which stabilize blood levels of the brain chemical serotonin (shortages of serotonin are thought to contribute to the blood vessel expansion that causes migraine headaches); and fluoxetine (Prozac), an antidepressant that prevents serotonin depletion.

An ounce of prevention

Although you feel headache pain only in your head, factors affecting other parts of your body can contribute to headache development. If you want to prevent headaches, heed the following advice:

- **Get regular sleep:** Changes in your sleep habits can trigger migraines and cluster headaches.

- **Get adequate exercise:** Regular physical activity can help prevent vascular and tension headaches by improving circulation, strengthening the muscles responsible for good posture, reducing muscular and psychological tension, and increasing the body's levels of *endorphins,* or feel-good chemicals.

- **Avoid foods and beverages known to trigger headaches:** These include foods containing *amines* (biological substances that cause blood vessels on the surface of the brain to constrict and then expand), such as cheese; vinegar; alcoholic beverages; foods containing the flavor enhancer monosodium glutamate (MSG), such as Chinese foods, processed meats, and TV dinners; foods containing nitrates, which are used as a preservative in lunch meats and hot dogs; and beverages containing caffeine.

- **Adopt proper working habits:** If you have a desk job, make sure that you stretch frequently and take regular breaks. Make sure that you have a comfortable chair and good posture when you're sitting, and don't stare at your computer screen for extended periods of time.

- **Reduce your level of stress:** Stress has physical effects on your body, including tensing the muscles that can result in a tension headache. See Chapter 1 for stress reduction tips.

Nausea and Vomiting

If you're experiencing *nausea,* you'll feel the sensation that accompanies the urge to vomit. Vomiting is the expulsion of your stomach contents through the esophagus and out of the mouth. Neither nausea nor vomiting itself is pleasant, but both are quite common.

You may have experienced nausea or vomiting early in a pregnancy (morning sickness), during a boat trip or car ride (motion sickness), after eating contaminated food (food poisoning), or as a result of a gastrointestinal virus. Certain foods or medications, unpleasant odors or sights, and emotional distress can also trigger nausea and vomiting. Nausea and vomiting can also be symptoms of more severe illness, such as heart attack, kidney or liver disorders, infections, and some types of cancer.

Occasional bouts of nausea and vomiting are rarely cause for concern — particularly if you can link them to a specific trigger. In fact, vomiting sometimes eases stomach discomfort and helps your body rid itself of harmful toxins, such as contaminated food. But if nausea and vomiting are prolonged or recurrent or are accompanied by other symptoms, such as a high fever, abdominal pain, severe intestinal cramping, or diarrhea, you should see a doctor. Prolonged vomiting can lead to dehydration, a dangerous condition in which your body runs low on fluids.

Making it better

In many cases, nausea and vomiting must run their course. But you can take some self-care measures to help you feel better and prevent vomiting from recurring. They include the following:

- ✔ **Seek over-the-counter relief:** Over-the-counter antacids such as Tums and Mylanta can relieve nausea associated with heartburn and acid indigestion from overeating.

- ✔ **Don't eat solid food until you stop vomiting:** Eating solid food can cause vomiting to continue. After you stop vomiting, start with clear liquid foods such as broth and gelatin and then progress to milk and soft foods such as bananas and toast.

- ✔ **Drink clear liquids:** These liquids should be at room temperature, and you should take small sips.

Depending on the cause of your nausea and vomiting, your doctor may be able to provide some type of relief. Treating the cause of these symptoms usually alleviates the symptoms themselves. And if your symptoms are side effects of a medication, your doctor may prescribe an alternative or prescribe a second medication to control the side effects.

An ounce of prevention

If you know what triggers your nausea and vomiting, you may be able to take steps to prevent them from happening. If, for example, you always react to a certain food, you can avoid that food. If you get carsick, you can take over-the-counter remedies such as Dramamine before you even get into the car to prevent nausea from developing.

Heartburn

You deserved that dinner at the fancy restaurant. You didn't deserve that burning, nauseous feeling that arrived hours later. Heartburn is well named for its stinging sensation right behind the breast plate, or *sternum*.

Heartburn occurs when acid-containing stomach contents back up into the esophagus and literally burn the lining. Normally, the stomach is closed off from the esophagus by a circular muscle called the *lower esophageal sphincter*. This muscle works in the same sort of way that you bend a garden hose to close off the flow of water. Esophageal reflux is pretty common, experienced by one in ten adults once a week. About one-third of all adults suffer with esophageal reflux at least once a month. Heartburn is also common in women in their last three months of pregnancy.

Recognizing the signs

The classic symptom of heartburn is a burning or stinging feeling in the upper abdominal or chest area, particularly after meals. You may also experience the regurgitation of sour-tasting materials in your throat or mouth, especially if you are lying down.

Knowing for sure

If you are noticing recurring pain, see your doctor. She may diagnose you with *gastroesophageal reflux disease (GERD),* a chronic heartburn condition that requires careful monitoring of symptoms, prescription medications, and, in some cases, surgery. Usually a complete description of symptoms is enough for your doctor to make an accurate diagnosis. But a chronic problem such as GERD or one that doesn't respond to normal treatment may make your doctor refer you to a gastroenterologist.

A gastroenterologist may recommend a *barium x-ray,* in which you swallow a white, chalky liquid containing barium; an x-ray is taken shortly thereafter. The barium shows up on the x-ray, giving your doctor a clear view of your digestive pathways. Or the doctor may recommend an *endoscopy,* in which an *endoscope,* a flexible fiber-optic viewing tube, is inserted into your esophagus. This way, your doctor can view the inside of your stomach to check for any abnormalities. In addition, your gastroenterologist may request blood tests to check for other problems such as infection, liver or thyroid dysfunction, or other diseases or conditions.

Making it better

Depending on the severity of your heartburn, you may be able to relieve it with lifestyle changes and over-the-counter medications. Prescription drugs may be necessary for severe cases.

You may wish to try the following:

- ✔ **Try an over-the-counter antacid or acid controller:** In many cases, they may relieve your discomfort. But make sure that you read the label: Some medications, such as Tagamet and Pepcid AC, actually reduce the amount of acid your stomach produces, so you need to take them before meals. You should take others, such as Pepto-Bismol, Alka-Seltzer, Tums, and Mylanta, at the first sign of heartburn.

- ✔ **Walk away your heartburn:** A casual walk after meals actually aids digestion.

- ✔ **Wait before exercising:** A regular exercise program moves digestion along, but wait one to two hours after a meal to do your workout (that's about how long it takes to completely digest a meal).

- ✔ **Reconsider using dairy products as antacids:** Milk contains fat that requires a different stomach acid to digest than say, water. And you may be lactose intolerant, a condition in which you don't have enough of the right digestive juices to digest dairy fats.

- ✔ **Don't smoke:** Nicotine relaxes the lower esophageal sphincter, which allows acid to back up into your esophagus.

Serious, chronic burning in the stomach area could indicate a more serious condition, such as an ulcer or even a heart attack. Your doctor may tell you to reduce the dosage or amount of medications you're taking. Birth control pills, antihistamines, and nonsteroidal anti-inflammatory drugs, such as aspirin, can all cause heartburn. If your heartburn doesn't respond to regular treatment, your doctor may suggest stronger prescription medication to ease your symptoms. If you've been diagnosed with GERD, you may want to discuss the possibility of a new minimally invasive surgical procedure that allows the gastroenterologist to "tighten" the lower esophageal sphincter muscle.

An ounce of prevention

To prevent heartburn

- ✔ **Limit the size and content of your meals:** High-fat or large meals require a lot of acid to digest. Eat three balanced meals a day, and eat your vegetables — fiber helps digestion.

- ✔ **Go to bed with your stomach on empty:** An empty stomach doesn't have any digestive acids to regurgitate into your esophagus.

- ✔ **Reduce your stress level:** Anxiety has a direct effect on your stomach: Those gnawing feelings in your belly are actually your stomach reacting to stress through acid production and *peristalsis* (the churning motion of the digestive system).

- ✔ **Cut the coffee:** Your morning cup of coffee may send your stomach into double-overtime acid production. If you can't totally cut it out, eat something with your java.

- ✔ **Cut back on alcohol and peppermints:** Mint and alcohol relax the sphincter muscle, allowing acid to back up into your esophagus.

- ✔ **Loosen your belt:** Tight clothing may force stomach acid back up into your esophagus.

- ✔ **Keep your head up:** Elevate the head of your bed with blocks, use good posture, and sit upright at meals. An upright posture helps gravity keep stomach acids where they belong — in your stomach.

Hemorrhoids

Because nobody ever talks about them in polite conversation, you may not know that *hemorrhoids* are inflammations of the veins in the rectum or around the anus known as the hemorrhoidal blood vessels. Depending on which veins are affected, hemorrhoids can be either internal (located inside the anus or rectum) or external (under the skin around the anus). These veins are thin and easily ruptured. They are common during pregnancy because increased pressure from the weight of the baby and uterus on the veins causes them to swell.

Sometimes the internal veins can become so enlarged that they protrude from the rectal opening, resulting in *prolapsed* hemorrhoids. Prolapsed hemorrhoids can become irritated and bleed. They don't hurt, though they may feel full and itch and can create a watery discharge.

External veins swell as well. The real problem with the external hemorrhoid veins is that blood clots can develop from prolonged sitting or straining when you have to go to the bathroom. These hemorrhoids are referred to as *thrombosed.* A thrombosed hemorrhoid feels like a hard marble and, unlike an internal hemorrhoid, can be *very* painful.

Recognizing the signs

You may have hemorrhoids if you see bright red blood on your toilet paper, in the water of your toilet bowl, or on the stool itself; if you feel tenderness, particularly during bowel movements; and if you can see or feel a protrusion of soft tissue at your anus.

Knowing for sure

Whenever you have bloody stool, definitely see your doctor. Your doctor will do a rectal exam, using a gloved lubricated finger to feel for abnormalities. And he or she may look for internal hemorrhoids by using a lighted tube called an *anoscope.*

To rule out other sources of bleeding, your doctor may perform a *sigmoidoscopy,* in which she views the lower colon through a flexible lighted tube, or a *colonoscopy,* a similar procedure in which she can see the entire colon.

Making it better

Over-the-counter preparations are available "to relieve the itching and burning of hemorrhoids." But you may also want to try the following tips:

- Sit in plain warm water for 10 to 15 minutes several times a day.
- Put a little petroleum jelly around your anal opening to reduce friction when having a bowel movement.
- Use hemorrhoid creams or suppositories to reduce friction and reduce swelling.
- Dab the area with Tucks or cotton pads soaked in witch hazel to reduce itching.

Most hemorrhoids go away in a week or two, though they may recur.

If your hemorrhoids keep coming back or are so painful that you can't sit, walk, or go to work, see a doctor. Your doctor may need to perform a minor surgical outpatient procedure. She can lance the thrombosed hemorrhoid to remove the clot and provide relief, using a laser or infrared energy to seal off the blood vessels. For internal hemorrhoids, she can inject a shrinking agent into the hemorrhoid (a procedure known as *sclerotherapy*) or tie off the hemorrhoid with a rubber band to cut off circulation (a procedure known as *rubber band ligation*). *Hemorrhoidectomy,* a procedure in which the hemorrhoids are cut away, is generally a last resort.

An ounce of prevention

To prevent hemorrhoids, take steps to prevent constipation:

- ✔ **Make sure to get enough fiber and water in your diet:** Aim for 25 to 30 grams of fiber and at least 8 cups of water a day.

- ✔ **Exercise:** Regular exercise promotes digestion.

- ✔ **Go when you feel the urge:** And don't strain. Take your time and let things happen naturally.

- ✔ **Take an over-the-counter stool softener:** These gelatin capsules contain docussate (colace) and keep water in the stool, making it softer and easier to pass. Other fiber stool softeners, such as Metamucil and Citrucel, are also useful.

Chapter 10

Digestive System Disorders

- -

In This Chapter

▶ Getting the lowdown on gallstones

▶ Coping with indigestion

▶ Surviving the irritations of irritable bowel syndrome

▶ Understanding ulcers

- -

*T*his system, which includes your esophagus, stomach, intestines, liver, gallbladder, and pancreas, as well as enzymes and acids, transforms food into a form your body can absorb. This chapter looks at four conditions that commonly affect the digestive system — gallstones, indigestion, irritable bowel syndrome, and ulcers — outlining the causes of and treatments for each, and, whenever possible, telling you how to prevent them. In some cases, you may wish to contact a *gastroenterologist,* a doctor who specializes in treating conditions of the digestive system.

Gallbladder Disorders

The gallbladder hides beneath the liver, perched on top of the intestines. It is no bigger than a small pear, but in the case of gallstones or inflammation, this organ "speaks up" in a very painful way. The main function of your gallbladder is to store bile from the liver, and then discharge it through the bile duct into the intestines. Bile helps break down fats so your body can absorb them.

Unfortunately, bile is made up of some pretty temperamental stuff. Calcium salts and cholesterol in bile can crystallize or harden to form "stones." Gallstones are three to four times more common in women than men, usually occurring between the ages of 35 and 60. In most cases, they cause no symptoms. But in severe cases, stones can form blockages in the duct and leading from the gallbladder to the bile duct or they block the bile duct itself, causing infection, inflammation, and pain.

Recognizing the signs

Gallbladder attacks normally begin suddenly and may last for 30 minutes to several hours. The pain, which is severe and constant, generally appears in the upper-right side of the abdomen, underneath the rib cage, but it may radiate to the right shoulder and lower back and may be accompanied by nausea and vomiting. If a high fever or shaking chills accompany the pain, the gallbladder could be inflamed or the bile duct could be obstructed or infected.

Knowing for sure

Your doctor may perform a physical exam to check for swelling or *jaundice*, a condition caused by the buildup of bile acids in the body that gives the skin a yellowish tint.

If your doctor believes that you may have gallstones, she can order an ultrasound examination, in which a radiologist or a radiology technician rubs a wandlike device called a *transducer* on your abdomen to send and receive sound waves. A computer then uses the sound waves to create an image of your gallbladder. Your doctor can also perform blood tests to detect bacteria so that she can tell whether the gallbladder is infected.

Making it better

If your gallstones cause no symptoms, your doctor or gastroenterologist may not recommend any treatment: The stones may pass through your digestive system by themselves.

If you are experiencing pain, your doctor may prescribe medication to dissolve the stones or use a technique called *biliary lithotripsy,* which breaks up stones with high-frequency sound waves. *Medical dissolution,* in which a medication is given orally or injected directly into the gallbladder by means of a catheter, works only on stones composed of cholesterol.

If your gallbladder is infected or doesn't respond to medication or normal treatment, your doctor may recommend surgery to remove the gallbladder, called a *cholecystectomy.* In many cases, this procedure can be performed laparoscopically, meaning that the incision will be quite small. You can live normally after a cholecystectomy, but you may be given medication or dietary restrictions, such as lowering your fat intake.

An ounce of prevention

To help prevent the onset of gallstones

- ✔ **Eat a low-fat diet:** Gallbladder attacks are often preceded by eating fatty meals.
- ✔ **Exercise:** A regular exercise program can also help reduce the amount of fat by using it as fuel.

Indigestion

Indigestion is a nonspecific term used to describe a number of abdominal symptoms, including heartburn, nausea, and bloating, particularly after eating. (See Chapter 9 for more information about these passing problems.) Indigestion is not in itself a disease but rather a common symptom that most people have at some time or another. It can also be a symptom of a serious condition such as peptic ulcer or gallbladder disease.

If you have occasional bouts of indigestion, particularly after you eat certain foods or drink excessive amounts of alcohol, you probably have nothing to worry about. But if you have problems regularly or your discomforts do not respond to medication, you should see your doctor.

Recognizing the signs

You may experience one or more of the following: upper abdominal discomfort or a feeling of fullness, bloating and belching, nausea, and heartburn.

Knowing for sure

Indigestion is a very vague description, so if you see a doctor, try to be very specific when you describe your problem. Where does it typically occur? When does it occur? Does it occur before, during, shortly after, or several hours after a meal? Where do you feel discomfort? Answering these kinds of questions clearly allows your doctor to pinpoint where the problem is originating.

Your doctor will inspect your abdomen, listen with a stethoscope for abdominal noises, feel your stomach area, and search for areas of pain and tenderness. She may ask for a stool sample to search for hidden blood in stool (a sign of colorectal cancer) and may draw blood to check for anemia.

Your abdominal symptoms can also be evaluated with barium x-ray studies of the esophagus, stomach, small intestine, and colon. Your doctor could also conceivably do an ultrasound or CT scan of your pancreas, liver, and gallbladder, or an endoscopic exam, in which a small viewing scope is inserted through your mouth into your esophagus, stomach, and duodenum to enable the doctor to view the interior of your digestive tract.

Making it better

Depending on the cause of your abdominal discomfort, you may find relief through lifestyle changes or, if necessary, through medication. If your doctor pinpoints a specific cause, she will suggest an appropriate therapy.

Here are a few things you can do on your own:

- ✔ **Maintain a food diary and track your symptoms:** Keeping a journal can help you determine whether your symptoms are associated with any particular foods, as well as give you valuable information to present to your doctor if you seek her help.

- ✔ **If you smoke, stop:** It may be contributing to your abdominal discomfort.

- ✔ **Cut down on alcohol:** Alcohol, especially hard liquor, can be a cause of indigestion.

- ✔ **Take steps to reduce stress:** Stress can contribute to indigestion. See Chapter 1 for ways to reduce stress.

- ✔ **Seek over-the-counter relief:** A variety of over-the-counter medications are available for indigestion, including antacids, such as Tums, Rolaids, Maalox, and Mylanta, and acid-reducers, such as Zantac.

You should see a doctor if your indigestion appears suddenly, becomes chronic, is accompanied by black or bloody stools, or if you have persistent or severe symptoms that don't get better with over-the-counter remedies. These signs can be a warning of a serious underlying illness.

Indigestion can be the result of a variety of prescription drugs. Your doctor can help you identify the culprit and propose a solution — either changing your prescription, helping you time your prescription to prevent its effects on your stomach, or offering remedies to deal with the indigestion it produces.

Your doctor can also prescribe stronger antacids or acid controllers, such as cimetidine, ranitidine, nizatidine, or famotidine or medications, such as sucralfate, which coats and protects the lining of the stomach.

An ounce of prevention

Depending on the cause, you can take steps to prevent your symptoms from occurring. See the previous section "Making it better" for additional advice.

Irritable Bowel Syndrome (IBS)

Irritable bowel syndrome (IBS), also known as *spastic colon,* affects an estimated 15 percent of the American population and is more common in women than men.

You may have had IBS for a while but never knew the cause of your seemingly constant abdominal pain, gas, constipation, or diarrhea. If chronic diarrhea or other symptoms, such as abdominal pain that's relieved after you have a bowel movement, the presence of mucus in your stool, bloating, and gas, continue for more than two or three months, you need to make an appointment with your doctor. Although IBS does not predispose you to complications or other conditions, its symptoms can mimic more serious problems.

IBS usually makes its appearance between the ages of 15 and 35. Although the cause of the condition is not completely understood, experts believe it is the result of abnormal muscular activity in the intestinal walls. This activity is triggered by certain foods, stress, or depression.

Recognizing the signs

The symptoms of IBS include chronic diarrhea, intermittent constipation, bowel irregularities, abdominal pain and spasms, bloating, and gas.

Knowing for sure

Your doctor or gastroenterologist will take a detailed history and perform a physical examination. She may perform a *sigmoidoscopy* or *colonoscopy,* in which she inserts a flexible viewing scope into your rectum to check the lower portion of your digestive tract. Sigmoidoscopy is used to examine the lower part of the colon; colonoscopy to examine the entire colon. Your doctor may also order a barium enema. For this test, the doctor inserts a liquid containing barium into your rectum, then takes an x-ray. The doctor may also request blood tests that check for any problems with your thyroid or liver and ask you for a stool sample.

Making it better

IBS can be treated with a combination of lifestyle changes, medications, and, in some instances, psychological counseling.

If you have IBS, you may wish to

- ✔ **Keep a dietary diary:** A *dietary diary* — keeping track of the food you eat and your reaction to it — can help you spot your "trigger" foods.
- ✔ **Drink lots of water:** If you suffer from chronic diarrhea, you're at risk for dehydration and vitamin or mineral deficiencies.
- ✔ **Increase your fiber intake:** Doing so can help relieve constipation and diarrhea. The recommended daily amount of fiber is 20 to 30 grams.
- ✔ **Try over-the-counter medications:** Your doctor may recommend an antimotility medication, such as Imodium, to help control your diarrhea, or laxatives, such as Milk of Magnesia, to control your constipation.
- ✔ **Take steps to reduce stress:** Stress and anxiety can aggravate IBS and trigger symptoms. Try to identify the sources of stress in your life and reduce them if possible.

If your symptoms don't improve with dietary modification, over-the-counter medications, or counseling, your doctor may recommend stronger drugs, including prescription stool softeners and antimotility medications, antispasmodic medications, antidepressants, and antianxiety medications. Her choice of medication will depend largely on the symptoms you experience.

An ounce of prevention

You can decrease your risk of suffering from IBS by remembering the three E's: Eat right; exercise daily; and erase stress.

Ulcers

Ulcers are simply holes in your digestive system. You can develop an ulcer just about anywhere you have digestive acids. Most ulcers occur in adults ages 40 to 50.

The most common kind of ulcers are called *peptic ulcers*. Peptic ulcers, which affect an estimated 25 million Americans, are formed when the acid "burns" or wears away a weakness or hole in the lining of the digestive tract. Normally, the balance of mucus and acid is kept in check, but when things get out of balance, the constant exposure to stomach acid creates a raw, often bloody patch in the stomach lining. Peptic ulcers can occur in the stomach *(gastric ulcers)*, esophagus *(esophageal ulcers)*, or the *duodenum,* the beginning of the small intestine, below the stomach *(duodenal ulcers)*. The small intestine is where most of the digestion and absorption of food takes place, so acid content is pretty intense there.

The majority of ulcers are now believed to be caused by infection with the bacterium *Helicobacter pylori (H. pylori)*, which alters the stomach lining's *pH balance* (the ratio of acid to base chemicals). Another cause of ulcers is the overuse of nonsteroidal anti-inflammatory drugs such as aspirin and ibuprofen. Heredity and excessive stomach acid also appear to play roles.

Contrary to popular belief, high stress levels and hurried, irregular meals have not been proven to cause ulcers.

Recognizing the signs

Common ulcer symptoms include a burning, aching, or hungry sensation in the upper abdomen or lower chest; abdominal pain; black, tarry, foul-smelling stools; bloated feeling after meals; and nausea and vomiting.

Knowing for sure

Your doctor or gastroenterologist may perform a barium x-ray, in which you swallow a chalky white liquid containing barium. An x-ray is performed shortly thereafter. The barium shows up on the x-ray, giving your doctor a clear view of your digestive pathway, including any obstructions or ulcers.

If the x-ray is inconclusive or your doctor needs more information, she may perform an endoscopy. This technique, which involves viewing the inside of your stomach through a flexible tube inserted into your esophagus, enables the doctor to see the extent and size of your ulcer. During an endoscopy, your doctor may use an instrument inserted through the scope to remove a small sample of ulcer tissue to examine for the presence of *H. pylori*.

Your doctor can also test for the presence of *H. pylori* by using a breath test. A blood test can also be used to detect *H. pylori,* as well as to rule out more serious conditions such as *Zollinger-Ellison Syndrome,* in which ulcers are caused by stomach tumors. Your doctor may also test your stool to check for blood, which could indicate a more serious breakdown in the lining of the stomach or intestines. Blood in the stool may also indicate cancer.

Making it better

Your doctor may recommend a restricted diet and ask you to avoid anti-inflammatory drugs, especially aspirin — taking more than three or more per day may worsen your existing ulcer (or it may have caused it in the first place). She may also prescribe medication to decrease the amount of acid present in the digestive system. Antihistamines known as H_2 blockers, including ranitidine (Zantac), cimetidine (Tagamet), nizatidine (Axid), and famotidine (Pepcid AC), are often prescribed to decrease the amount of acid produced in the stomach. Another acid-inhibiting drug used to treat ulcers is omepazone (Prisolec). These medications help control your symptoms.

If your ulcer is the result of an *H. pylori* infection, your doctor will prescribe antibiotics, such as amoxicillin, as well. If your ulcer doesn't respond to this treatment, your doctor may prescribe a combination of medications, including different antibiotics.

An ounce of prevention

To help prevent an ulcer

- **Eat right:** Make sure that your diet is low in fat, but high in fiber; eat regularly; stay away from food loaded with fat and sodium; and eat slowly. If you're eating on the run, you can force your stomach into excess acid production.

- **Incorporate a stress reduction program:** Deep breathing techniques or simple stretches may help reduce stress.

- **Go easy on the aspirin and other nonsteroidal anti-inflammatory drugs:** They can cause ulcers.

- **Don't smoke:** Smoking may contribute to the development of ulcers and may slow healing of existing ulcers.

You can do very little to prevent ulcers caused by the bacterium *H. pylori*. Fortunately, however, although the majority of adults in the United States have been infected with this bacteria, they don't all develop ulcers.

Chapter 11

Urinary System Disorders

. . . .

In This Chapter

▶ Dealing with incontinence

▶ Understanding urinary tract infections

▶ Recognizing kidney stones

. . . .

*A*ny well-built mansion has a first-rate plumbing system. Your body does too. Your urinary tract is a very complex but efficient waste management system. But like the components of a sewer or septic system, the components of your urinary tract can fail, resulting in infection, incontinence, and kidney problems.

Your urinary system is designed to filter toxic waste from your blood. This process starts in the *kidneys,* a pair of organs that also act in conjunction with other systems in your body to produce hormones that regulate blood pressure and even help in the formation of bone. The kidneys are shaped like large kidney beans. They sit upright, opposing each other on either side of your spine, above your hips and below your ribs. Attached to your kidneys are long tubes called *ureters* that transport urine to the *bladder,* a temporary holding tank, if you will. Although a small organ, the bladder is sheathed in muscles. It's in front of your vagina and on top of your pubic bone. Urine exits the bladder via the *urethra,* a narrow tube in front of your vagina. Problems with any part of this complex system can spell trouble. This chapter looks at several common problems: incontinence, urinary tract infections, and kidney stones.

Incontinence

No matter what they call it — overactive bladder, uncontrolled bladder, or incontinence — the subject is still embarrassing to talk about. *Incontinence* is the inability to control the flow of urine. The most common types of incontinence are

- ✔ **Stress incontinence:** This type results from sudden pressure — such as that from a laugh, sneeze, or cough — on the bladder.
- ✔ **Urge incontinence:** This type is the overwhelming urge to urinate when hearing, seeing, or touching water.
- ✔ **Overflow incontinence:** This type results when the body produces more urine than the bladder can hold.
- ✔ **Mixed incontinence:** This type is a combination of the types mentioned above.

An estimated 20 million people in North America suffer from incontinence, the majority of them women.

The causes of incontinence are many, and most are treatable. In some women, it's caused by muscles weakened by childbirth or surgery. The delicate nerves become stretched and injured and don't respond to the normal messages the brain sends for the body to relieve itself. For others, the problem may be due to a lack of estrogen. As women age, estrogen levels plummet and so does the elasticity of the smooth muscle in the vagina, bladder, and other urogenital organs. Obesity, urinary tract infection, constipation, side effects of common medications, and sensitivity to certain foods, including caffeine, are additional causes.

Recognizing the signs

The symptoms of urinary incontinence are rather obvious — sudden leakage of urine, especially after laughing, sneezing, coughing, lifting heavy objects, or running, and feelings of a full bladder or not being able to make it to the bathroom in time.

Knowing for sure

Your doctor may be able to diagnose incontinence with just a medical history, including any medications you're on and your surgical history. Your doctor may want to test for urinary tract infection, which involves taking a urine sample. (Urinalysis detects high levels of bacteria in the urine.) She may want to do an x-ray to rule out other conditions such as cancer, or possible damage from prior surgery you may have had. Damage to muscles and nerves can be a cause of incontinence.

Making it better

You can do a few things on your own to get yourself back to a normal routine:

✔ **Exercise:** Kegel exercises (see Chapter 23) help work the pelvic floor muscles, which, among other things, help control the flow of urine.

✔ **Train your bladder:** In some cases, you can train your bladder by making frequent trips to the bathroom.

✔ **Experiment with your diet:** With your doctor's okay, try eliminating foods that irritate the bladder, such as alcohol, acidic fruits and juices, caffeine, spicy foods, and dairy products, for a few weeks.

✔ **Plan ahead:** You can plan a strategy that will minimize the frequency and embarrassment of incontinence. If your incontinence is infrequent, for example, you may want to wear sanitary napkins or pads especially designed to absorb urine flow.

Your treatment regimen depends on your diagnosis. If your incontinence is caused by a urinary tract infection, for example, you may be put on a regimen of antibiotics. (For more information, see "Urinary Tract Infections.") If you've only experienced incontinence during menopause, your doctor may recommend hormone replacement therapy (HRT), which helps keep the bladder elastic and thick. (For more information on HRT, see Chapter 20.) If your incontinence is not the result of another condition, your doctor may suggest self-care techniques such as those listed above or prescribe medication or one of several prescription devices designed to alleviate the problem. These may include

✔ **Medications:** Prescription drugs are available to relax the bladder muscles and stop abnormal contractions. Most of these drugs are approved only for the treatment of urge incontinence because they have numerous side effects. But a new drug, tolterodine tartrate (Detrol), was approved by the Food and Drug Administration (FDA) in 1998 specifically for the treatment of overactive bladder. This drug works by blocking the nerve endings that cause premature contractions of the bladder leading to urine leakage.

✔ **The urethral plug:** Sold under the brand name Reliance Urinary Control Insert, this device is a small plastic balloon that you insert into the urethra to block the flow of urine. This tool is especially helpful for women with unusually shaped bladders.

✔ **The patch:** This tiny pad, about the size of a quarter and coated with a special gel, forms a seal over the urethra and is peeled off when you have to urinate. The pad is marketed under the brand name Miniguard Patch.

When other treatments fail, your doctor may recommend surgery. Surgery can correct anatomical problems, improve the position of the neck of the bladder, remove blockages, enlarge the bladder, or support the surrounding structures to strengthen the urethra. Surgical procedures can also be used to implant a device to stimulate faulty bladder nerves or to implant a *catheter,* a tube through which urine can drain.

An ounce of prevention

Kegel exercises can be helpful in preventing incontinence. You can also help prevent incontinence by avoiding clothing that restricts or weakens the pelvic muscles. Girdles, tight pants or shorts, extra-support pantyhose, and even high heels force the body into unnatural positions that weaken muscles. Other prevention tips include maintaining the proper weight (extra body weight puts additional pressure on the bladder and weakens muscles that support the pelvis and lower back), drinking plenty of water, and making frequent pit stops during travel.

Urinary Tract Infection

The urinary tract is susceptible to infection, largely because bacteria from the rectum can gain easy access to the tract through the urethra. Under normal circumstances, these bacteria are flushed out when you urinate. But certain factors increase the likelihood that these bacteria will take up residence in your urinary tract, causing an infection. Most urinary infections affect the lower urinary tract — the bladder and urethra. But the kidneys can also become infected. The medical term for a bladder infection is *cystitis;* for an infection of the urethra, *urethritis*; and for a kidney infection, *nephritis.*

Cystitis is often referred to as *honeymoon cystitis* because it is commonly a result of bacteria introduced into the bladder through the urethra during sexual intercourse. Some experts believe that some contraceptives, such as spermicides or an ill-fitting diaphragm, may also promote the growth of bacteria in the urinary tract, as may trauma to the urethra.

Urethritis, which often occurs in conjunction with cystitis, may have similar causes or may be caused by a sexually transmitted disease, such as gonorrhea, trichomonaisis, herpes, or chlamydia (for more information on sexually transmitted diseases, see Chapter 22).

Most serious is nephritis, which may infect a portion or all of one or both of the kidneys and, if not treated properly, can progress to kidney disease. Fortunately, damage caused by nephritis is usually reversible.

Recognizing the signs

For cystitis and urethritis, the symptoms include a burning sensation when urinating; frequent urges to urinate; bloody, cloudy, or discolored urine; and pain or pressure in the lower abdomen or back. A high fever or chills may indicate a kidney infection.

Knowing for sure

Your doctor will want a complete medical history, including any surgery or previous conditions. She'll also want to know the frequency of intercourse as well as what type of contraception, if any, you use. She will likely perform a *urinalysis,* in which a urine sample is tested for high levels of bacteria. She will give you a clean plastic container with a lid and ask you for a urine sample. Be sure to handle the sample properly; contaminated urine may give you false test results. Your doctor may also want to do an x-ray to rule out any serious disorders of the urinary tract. If she suspects kidney damage, she may recommend a biopsy.

Making it better

Here are a few things you can do for yourself. Be aware, however, that if your symptoms don't resolve within 24 hours or get worse, you should contact your doctor:

- ✓ **Think herbal:** Some women have found that herbal remedies ease the symptoms and recurrence of urinary tract infections (UTIs). Spices such as cinnamon and a tincture of the herbs buchu, uva ursi, and juniper berries supposedly act as antiseptics and clean out the kidneys and bladder.

- ✓ **Drink cranberry juice:** This juice increases the acidity of urine, making it an unfriendly environment for infection-causing bacteria. It also coats the cells in the lining of the bladder, protecting them from bacteria.

- ✓ **Drink plenty of fluids and urinate as frequently as possible:** Don't let work or chores around the house force you to put off bathroom trips.

Depending on your symptoms, your doctor may recommend over-the-counter urinary pain relief tablets, antibiotics, and plenty of fluids. Finish all your medication — especially antibiotics. Naturally, you want to stop taking medication when your symptoms disappear, but that doesn't mean the infection is gone. Your doctor may prescribe medications that change the pH or acidity of your urine.

An ounce of prevention

To reduce your risk of contracting a urinary tract infection, drink plenty of fluids and make regular trips to the bathroom. During long trips, make frequent pit stops — holding urine increases your chances of developing UTIs because the bladder's lining has prolonged exposure to bacteria. To keep your genital area clean, wipe from front to back, change sanitary napkins frequently during your period to discourage bacteria from traveling up into the urethra, and urinate before and after sexual intercourse. If you are using contraceptives, make sure that they fit comfortably.

Kidney Stones

Imagine how forcing a stone the size of a golf ball through your nose would feel. That painful picture gives you just an inkling of how it feels to experience kidney stones. Not really stones per se, but crystals of a mineral such as calcium or potassium, kidney stones can even be made of hardened cholesterol. These stones form in the fluid in the kidneys when the urine is too concentrated. And when these stones try to "pass" through the delicate (and microscopic) filtration system in the kidneys — the result is pain. This pain is experienced by an estimated 3 to 5 percent of all women at least once by the time they reach age 70. And those who have had one stone are likely to have another. The tendency to develop kidney stones appears to run in families.

Recognizing the signs

The symptoms of kidney stones include pain in the lower back below the rib cage, changes in the color and consistency of urine (such as bloody urine), a persistent urge to urinate, and pain during urination. The pain may be so intense when you pass a kidney stone that you may pass out.

Knowing for sure

Your doctor may be able to diagnose your condition based on your symptoms and blood and urine tests that show high levels of salts and minerals. Or she may want to want to refer you to a urologist, a specialist in the treatment of urinary tract problems. If you have a stone, the doctor will want to determine its composition so that she can take action to avoid the development of future stones.

Making it better

Depending on the severity of your condition, your urologist may prescribe medication to help you pass the stone(s). Self-care techniques may also be a part of your treatment. In serious cases, surgery may be necessary.

Your doctor may tell you to care for yourself in these ways:

✔ **Drink water:** If you are diagnosed with small kidney stones (less than 1 centimeter) and do not require hospitalization, you'll be encouraged to drink about 2 quarts of water per day to help them pass.

✔ **Hold the salt shaker:** Reduce the salt or sodium in your diet.

✔ **Avoid calcium-based antacids:** Ask your doctor for an alternative if you experience indigestion or heartburn.

If your kidney stones are larger than 1 centimeter, you may have to stay in the hospital until the stones are passed through your urine. Pain caused by the movement of the stones through your urinary tract can require serious pain-killing medications that may knock you out. You'll be asked to drink plenty of water and to urinate through a strainer to save your stones for analysis. If you do not pass the stones, your doctor may give you medication that will help shrink the stones or recommend *lithotripsy.* The procedure dissolves stones by sending ultrasonic waves through your body. Your body systems will not be disturbed, but kidney stones are so brittle that they crumble or shatter when the waves make contact. The remnants of the stones will then pass through your urinary tract. For larger stones, your doctor may recommend a surgical procedure known as *ureteroscopy,* in which a fiber-optic instrument is threaded through the urethra and bladder and into the ureter to grasp the stone and pull it out.

An ounce of prevention

To prevent kidney stones from occurring, drink plenty of fluids. It may sound like a scientific paradox, but increasing calcium-rich foods in your diet may help prevent stones, while calcium supplements increase your risk of stones.

You can also prevent kidney stones by watching your diet. Avoid meats that are smoked or cured (bacon, ham, and many deli meats), canned soups, and fast foods. They have large amounts of sodium that can lead to the formation of stones.

Chapter 12
Skin Disorders

• •

• •

*Y*our skin is your body's largest organ. It covers and protects all the other organs, helps you regulate your body temperature, and helps your body produce vitamin D. Your skin's health is much more important to the health of your body than to the health of your vanity. Nevertheless, any problems that develop on your skin affect your appearance, too. So, for both your physical and emotional well-being, taking care of your skin makes sense. This chapter examines four conditions that commonly affect the skin's function and/or appearance.

Eczema

Eczema, or *dermatitis,* is a catchall term for inflammation, irritation, and itching of the skin. The cause can be anything from heredity to poison ivy, although the term eczema is often used to refer to atopic dermatitis.

Atopic dermatitis generally begins in infancy and usually disappears by age 15. In atopic dermatitis, the skin is unable to retain moisture, so it becomes red, scaly, and itchy. Weeping blisters sometimes develop, the skin may crack, and the rash may be followed by the development of scaling, thickened skin. This condition has no known cause and no known cure, but it is often associated with allergies and tends to run in families.

Contact dermatitis, another common skin rash, can also be associated with allergies — or with irritants. *Allergic contact dermatitis (ACD)* is caused by your skin's reaction to allergens such as nickel-plated jewelry, fragrances, and poison ivy, oak, and sumac. Not everyone is allergic to these allergens, however. An ACD outbreak may start with mild redness and itching, and then progress into swelling and blistering of the skin. (For more information on allergies, see Chapter 17.) *Irritant contact dermatitis (ICD)* is caused by irritating agents, such as harsh soaps and chemicals, and strong substances.

Recognizing the signs

General eczema symptoms include an area of itchy, often scaly, rash or redness on the skin; skin swelling and irritation; and blisters. In atopic dermatitis, the skin may thicken and crack; in contact dermatitis, the rash is limited to the area that has come in contact with the allergen or irritant.

Knowing for sure

Your doctor may be able to identify the problem (eczema, or dermatitis) simply by examining you, but identifying the cause — particularly of contact dermatitis — may be easier said than done. If you don't know what may have triggered your rash, make a list of all the things you came into contact with over the course of the past few days. Your doctor or dermatologist will review this list and perhaps perform a patch test, in which small amounts of suspected allergens are placed on your skin and covered with patches, then examined 48 hours later to see whether they prompted a rash.

Making it better

The primary treatment for eczema, or dermatitis, is to stop scratching: Scratching aggravates rashes and may lead to infection if you scratch the skin till it breaks open.

If you're suffering from eczema

- ✔ **Seek over-the-counter itch relief:** Apply calamine lotion or a hydrocortisone cream to the affected area. If your rash is allergic in nature, you may want to try an over-the-counter antihistamine such as diphenhydramine (Benadryl).

- ✔ **Try a home remedy:** An oatmeal bath may help soothe the itch: Fill an old nylon stocking with 1 cup of colloidal (ground) oatmeal, put it in the tub with you, and soak for a while. You can also apply a paste of baking soda and water.

- ✔ **Moisturize:** Choose oil-rich moisturizer rather than one that contains alcohol.

- ✔ **Shorten your shower:** Don't take frequent hot or long showers or baths. Water can dry the skin.

If your rash doesn't respond to self-care, your doctor may prescribe a stronger cortisone cream or another steroid, such as prednisone, which you can take orally or as an injection. Steroids reduce swelling, redness, and inflammation. She may also prescribe antihistamines to reduce itching.

An ounce of prevention

You can't prevent atopic dermatitis, but you can prevent contact dermatitis by keeping your skin out of harm's way. If you know that something causes you to break out in a rash, avoid it. Barrier creams are now available to prevent poison ivy. These creams, which are available in most drugstores, are applied like sunscreen — before exposure. If you do touch poison ivy or another substance to which you are allergic, wash your skin thoroughly with soap and water as soon as possible.

Psoriasis

Psoriasis normally takes about a month for a new skin cell to move from its birthplace in the lowest layer of skin to the outermost layer, where it dies and sloughs off. Figure 12-1 shows an example of healthy skin. But in people with psoriasis, this process takes only three or four days. These precocious dead skin cells accumulate on the surface of the skin, producing a buildup of scaly, red cells. This chronic condition, which affects an estimated 6.4 million Americans, usually appears on the scalp, elbows, knees, and trunk in cycles; it flares up and then goes into remission.

Although experts aren't sure what causes psoriasis, they do know that stress, skin injuries, infections, and certain medications may trigger or aggravate flare-ups. Psoriasis can strike at any age, but it usually begins between the ages of 15 and 35. Many people with psoriasis develop fingernail problems, such as pitted or thickened nails. A small number of those with psoriasis — mostly women — will develop a form of arthritis that resembles rheumatoid arthritis (for information on arthritis, see Chapter 17).

Recognizing the signs

The symptoms of psoriasis include patches of dry, red skin covered with silvery scales, especially around the elbows, knees, trunk, and scalp; itching; and cracking or bleeding skin.

Knowing for sure

Your doctor can usually diagnose psoriasis by a physical examination. In some cases, she may refer you to a dermatologist, a specialist familiar with disorders of the skin, or obtain a skin sample, which can be examined under a microscope to rule out other disorders.

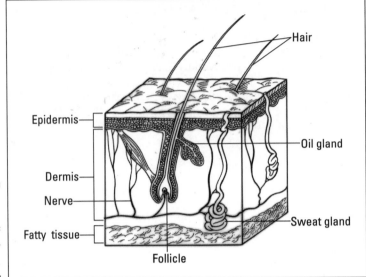

Figure 12-1:
Cross
section of
healthy
skin.

Making it better

Psoriasis has no cure, but you can relieve flare-ups with self-care techniques and medications.

If you have psoriasis, you might want to

- ✔ **Forgo scratching:** Scratching can cause the patches to thicken.

- ✔ **Take a bath:** Bathing in hot water to which you have added oil, powder, or table salt can help soften the scales. Soak for 15 to 20 minutes, and then wash away the scales.

- ✔ **Use moisturizers:** Using a moisturizer is particularly important during the winter months.

- ✔ **Sit in the sun:** Sunlight helps clear psoriasis in some people, but don't allow your skin to burn.

- ✔ **Steer clear of stress:** Let your mother-in-law stay only for a few days, not a whole month. Stress aggravates psoriasis.

Depending on the severity of your psoriasis, your dermatologist may prescribe any of a number of medications. Topical medications include the following:

- ✔ Steroids such as cortisone, which reduce inflammation

- ✔ Calcipotriene (Dovonex), a medicated ointment containing a derivative of vitamin D

Oral medications include the following:

- ✔ Methotrexate, an oral anticancer medication that slows the production of skin cells

- ✔ Vitamin A-derived medications such as etretinate (Tegison), acitretin (Soriatane), and isotretinoin (Accutane)

- ✔ Psoralen, a photosensitizing medication that is given before a dose of ultraviolet A light, in what is known as psoralen and ultraviolet light A (PUVA) therapy

Methotrexate is usually prescribed as a last resort; long-term use may cause liver damage. Vitamin A-derived medications may cause birth defects and should not be used by women who are pregnant or trying to conceive. And PUVA therapy may increase the risk of skin cancer (see Chapter 16), although many experts feel its benefits outweigh its risks.

Therapy with ultraviolet light B (UVB) is also used to treat psoriasis.

An ounce of prevention

You can't prevent psoriasis, but you can reduce your risk of flare-ups by using the self-care tips listed in the earlier section.

For more information, contact the National Psoriasis Foundation, 6600 SW 92nd Ave., Suite 300, Portland, OR 97223; 503-244-7404.

Rosacea

Rosacea is a serious skin disease that involves a whole lot more than pimples. Rosacea affects areas of the face that blush — mostly the cheeks. Many people with rosacea think they have a bad case of sunburn or windburn. In the beginning stages, as larger amounts of blood quickly flow through the blood vessels, they expand under the skin, giving it a reddish, flushed, or "burned" appearance. As the disease progresses, the skin becomes dry and pimples appear. Eventually, the expanded blood vessels show through the skin as tiny red lines. In the most severe cases, nasal bumps or an enlarged nose appears. Women are more likely than men to develop rosacea, which usually begins after age 30 and is more common in fair-skinned people who have a tendency to blush easily. The cause of rosacea is unknown, but early treatment does help control the condition and keep it from progressing.

Recognizing the signs

The symptoms of rosacea include red, inflamed areas on the face, particularly the cheeks, nose, forehead, and eyelids; pimples; the development of tiny red lines; and, in severe cases, a bumpy, swollen nose.

Knowing for sure

Your doctor or dermatologist can probably give you an accurate diagnosis without performing any invasive tests. Provide her with details about your facial flushing, eating and drinking habits, family history, and any medications you're taking. These things all have an effect on rosacea.

Making it better

In many cases, lifestyle changes and prescription medications can bring rosacea under control.

Facial flushing can make rosacea worse, so avoid spicy foods, alcohol, intense exercise, and other factors that trigger flushing. Limit your exposure to the sun, and stay warm on cold days. Use only mild soaps or cleansers and nonirritating moisturizers. Practice relaxation techniques (see Chapter 1) and learn to control your response to situations in which you may find yourself blushing.

Your doctor can prescribe topical antibiotics, such as metronidazole (Noritate), or oral antibiotics, such as tetracycline, to control rosacea. (**Remember:** You should not take tetracycline if you are pregnant or trying to conceive.) Topical steroid creams can control redness and swelling, but you should not use them long term. After the condition is under control, laser surgery can be used to treat tiny blood vessels visible through the skin and excess tissue on the nose.

An ounce of prevention

Because research has not yet found the cause of rosacea, there is no hard and fast way to prevent it. But early detection can help keep it under control.

For more information, contact the National Rosacea Society, 800 S. Northwest Highway, Suite 200, Barrington, IL 60010; 888-NO-BLUSH.

Varicose Veins

Varicose veins, those ugly spidery veins that get worse with age, pregnancy, or weight gain, strike many women at some time or other — often during pregnancy and menopause. Varicose veins are really swollen veins that usually appear on the legs. They're are caused by the failure of small valves in the veins. Normally these valves keep blood from flowing in the wrong direction; when they fail, the blood pools in one spot, causing *dilation,* or enlargement, of the vein. The condition is also common in people who are overweight and people who stand for long periods of time.

Recognizing the signs

Varicose veins appear as purple or bluish-tinged, gnarled-looking lines, usually on the legs. With these lines, you may also experience muscle cramps, swollen ankles and legs, a feeling of fatigue, and soreness in your calves. In serious cases, you may experience a patch of dry or ulcerated (sore and bleeding) skin, which means the blood supply to that area has been interrupted.

Knowing for sure

Your doctor can make an accurate diagnosis by checking your family medical history and examining the areas in question.

Making it better

Varicose veins do not disappear on their own, but if they don't cause pain, you may not need treatment. If, however, you wish to improve the appearance of your veins or if they cause discomfort, you may wish to try self-care or seek medical treatment:

- ✔ **Lift your legs:** You can ease pain and swelling by elevating and icing your legs.

- ✔ **Wear support hose:** Elastic support hose or an elastic bandage compresses your veins and provides them with the support they need.

- ✔ **Don't wear tight clothing:** Tight socks, shoes, and girdles may interfere with circulation.

- ✔ **Avoid standing for a long period of time:** If you must stand, move around as much as possible.

- ✔ **Exercise regularly:** Exercise helps push blood toward the heart.

Your doctor or dermatologist may recommend *sclerotherapy*. The procedure involves injecting an irritating solution into the vein to cause inflammation and block blood flow, which usually eliminates the discoloration within two months. Laser treatments, in which light beams are used to burn and close off the walls of a vein, are another possibility. If your case is severe, your doctor may suggest surgery to strip and remove the problem veins.

An ounce of prevention

The self-care tips listed earlier can help you keep the blood circulating and may reduce the risk of developing varicose veins.

Cosmetic procedures

An estimated 600,000 cosmetic procedures are performed each year. Here are a few common procedures and their risks:

✔ **Liposuction:** Liposuction involves sucking out the fat under the skin through a thin tube inserted into the treatment area. On the face, liposuction is used to eliminate double chin, puffy neck, or jowls. On the body, it is used to reduce fat in problems areas such as the hips, thighs, buttocks, or stomach. *Risks:* Dimpled skin, diminished sensation in the treated area, scarring, infection.

✔ **Dermabrasion:** Used to improve the texture and tone of the skin, dermabrasion involves brushing or "sanding" the skin to remove the top layers. On the face, it can remove age spots, fine wrinkles, and acne scars. *Risks:* Swelling, skin lightening or pigmentations, scarring, infection.

✔ **Chemical peels:** In this procedure, chemicals are applied to the skin to burn off its top layers. Chemical peels alleviate fine wrinkles, mild scars, and pigmentation problems. They can be painful and skin may remain reddish for several months. *Risks:* Increased pigmentation, infection, scarring.

✔ **Collagen injections:** Used to fill in wrinkles such as crow's feet, laugh lines, nose-to-mouth lines, and furrowing between eyebrows, this procedure involves injecting a collagen into the skin. The primary risk is allergic reaction.

✔ **Lifts:** Surgical lifting of the face, brow, or eyes involves incision, the removal of excess skin and fat, and the repositioning of sagging skin and facial muscles. It is performed to eliminate wrinkles and sagging. *Risks:* Bruising, scarring, infection, *hematomas* (swellings containing blood), loss of sensation in the face, loss of skin caused by lack of blood flow to the surgical site, and death.

Chapter 13
Sleep Disorders

*F*orty percent of American women have trouble sleeping at least some of the time. Working, taking care of your family, and spending time on church, community, or school activities can pile on the stress. On top of that, your monthly hormone fluctuations can affect your sleeping patterns.

But you can fight back. This chapter looks at two common sleep disorders: insomnia and sleep apnea.

Insomnia

Everyone has trouble sleeping at some time or another. Excitement, stress, changes in your schedule, or anything that makes you alter your regular sleep habits for a while can keep you awake. This condition is called *transient insomnia,* and it usually goes away in a few nights.

Short-term insomnia lasts two or three weeks and can be due to stress, a medical or mental health problem, or the late stages of pregnancy. It goes away when the underlying problem is solved.

Chronic insomnia lasts more than a month, and you probably need medical help to break its bonds. That's because it either has an underlying physical or psychological cause or because you get so used to the idea that you're not going to sleep that you have to be coached into how to do it again.

What happens when you sleep

Your body goes through two major classes or periods of sleep: REM (rapid eye movement) and NREM (nonrapid eye movement). REM sleep is a shallow sleep associated with dreaming. During REM sleep, body temperature and blood pressure rise, breathing becomes shallower and faster, and brain function is active. REM sleep is needed to sort through short-term memory storage, delete unnecessary information, and store important information in your long-term memory. NREM is the deep, restorative sleep necessary to your physical well-being. During NREM sleep, your body synthesizes protein, maintains immune function, and manufactures hormones. These two types of sleep alternate in 90-minute cycles throughout a typical night.

Recognizing the signs

Insomnia is characterized by difficulty falling or staying asleep, waking up too early, waking up unrefreshed, and feeling tired during the day.

Knowing for sure

Diagnosing insomnia is relatively easy. More difficult is determining the cause, which, in turn, helps determine treatment.

If you've had trouble sleeping for a week or two, take a look at your daytime life. Keeping a diary of what you do and when may be helpful. For about a week, record what time you get up and go to bed, what you eat and drink and when and so forth. Jot down how you're feeling both physically and emotionally. At the end of that week, look for anything that may be interfering with your sleep, such as drinking more caffeine than normal, watching a scary movie on late-night TV, or menstrual cramps.

You may have to live with some things, such as menstrual cramps, for a few days, but others may be within your complete control.

Many over-the-counter and prescription drugs can interfere with sleep. Check the package insert, but don't stop taking a prescribed medicine without talking to your doctor first.

You should talk with your doctor if your symptoms have lasted for a month or more. Sleep problems can be a symptom of several serious physical ailments, including kidney disease, asthma, Parkinson's disease, and thyroid disorders. You obviously want to catch such illnesses early, and treating them will most likely relieve your insomnia, too.

Your doctor is likely to ask you to keep a diary such as the one previously mentioned. She may also ask you about your sleeping partner, who may be a contributing factor to your insomnia or may offer more insights into your sleeping patterns.

Making it better

If you've been able to pinpoint the cause of your sleeplessness and the cause is something you can control or eliminate, take steps to do so.

Resorting to nonprescription sleep aids may not be a good idea. Many of them contain antihistamines, which put many people to sleep at first but cause anxiety and nervousness later in the night. The best way to banish short-term insomnia is to deal with the cause of your sleeplessness.

Another way to deal with insomnia is to develop good sleep habits (see "Developing good sleep habits").

For occasional sleeplessness, you may want to try to eat your way to sleep. Some foods, notably complex carbohydrates, promote calm by stimulating the conversion of the amino acid tryptophan into serotonin, the brain chemical that regulates sleep. A light snack of complex carbohydrates, such as crackers, toast, or cereal, may do the trick, but stay away from sugary or salty foods.

Developing good sleep habits

One of the best ways you can counter insomnia is to develop good sleep habits, or as the experts call it, *sleep hygiene*. Here are some suggestions:

✔ Go to bed and get up at the same time every day (seven days a week).

✔ Cut out or greatly reduce caffeine.

✔ Don't drink alcohol, especially four hours or less before bed.

✔ Don't smoke, especially four hours or less before bed.

✔ Don't work, read, watch TV, or do anything in bed except sleep and make love.

✔ Stick with light to moderate exercise in the evening.

✔ Establish a relaxing prebed routine that signals your body and brain that it's time to go to sleep.

✔ If you can't get to sleep after 30 minutes, get up and do something relaxing or even boring.

After your doctor rules out a physical or psychological cause for your insomnia, you'll probably get a list of things to do — and not do — to help you get back to sleep. The list will probably look something like the one shown in the sidebar "Developing good sleep habits."

Often insomnia becomes a self-fulfilling prophecy. You expect you won't sleep, so you don't. Many doctors use sleep-restriction therapy to break that mind-set. You start with the average time you sleep. For one week, you are limited to spending only that amount of time in bed. If you're awake, you have to get up. The next week, you can add 15 minutes to your in-bed time by going to bed 15 minutes earlier, and so on. It takes a few weeks, but most people who follow this therapy eventually achieve a full night's sleep.

Nowadays, many doctors won't prescribe sleeping pills until you've tried some lifestyle modifications and/or relaxation techniques first. But if those don't help, your doctor may tell you to take one of a class of drugs called hypnotics. These include diazepam (Valium) and lorazepam (Ativan). She may suggest you take them only every other night, and perhaps for only a few weeks because these drugs do carry some risk of making you dependent on them, and in many cases, a short course is enough to help you get back to sleeping regularly.

If you do get a prescription, follow the directions carefully. Don't drink alcohol while taking the drugs or combine them with any other drugs unless your doctor knows about it.

If your insomnia persists, your doctor may refer you to a sleep disorders center. There, a specialized staff reviews your symptoms and treatment and probably interviews your bed partner and other family members as well. Then, you'll be asked to spend a night or two in the clinic, where the staff attaches sensors to your body and head to measure brain activity, muscle and limb movement, heartbeat, respiration, and other functions. This procedure is called a *polysomnogram*. The staff also monitors how long you take to get to sleep.

This intensive monitoring often uncovers a physical problem that had gone undetected.

An ounce of prevention

You can reduce your chances of suffering from insomnia by following the good sleep hygiene practices in the sidebar, "Developing good sleep habits."

Sleep Apnea

Sleep apnea is a serious, potentially fatal condition that is almost always associated with heavy snoring. Because of this, it is often considered a "man's" condition, with the result that sleep apnea is probably greatly underdiagnosed in women.

A woman with sleep apnea literally stops breathing momentarily because her nose or mouth is blocked from inside. This blockage is usually because the muscles of the soft palate at the base of the tongue and the *uvula* (the "punching bag" visible at the back of the throat) relax and sag, blocking the airway. The shortage of oxygen and increase in carbon dioxide alert the brain to resume breathing. The brain sends a message to the airway muscles to open the airway, and breathing is resumed, often with a snort or gasp.

Some people have these involuntary breathing pauses — and the resulting arousal as the brain signals the body to breathe — as often as 20 to 30 times or more per hour, but they never know about it. What they do know is that they wake up tired and have trouble staying awake. People with apnea may also be depressed, irritable, forgetful, unable to concentrate, accident-prone, and prone to sexual problems — all because they never get a good night's sleep. Worse, half of all people with apnea have high blood pressure and appear to be a greater risk of heart disease and stroke.

Recognizing the signs

If most people with apnea don't know they have it, their sleeping partners most certainly do. The combination of heavy snoring and struggles to breathe usually interfere with the sleep of anyone nearby.

Obesity is another common characteristic of people with sleep apnea. But body weight appears to be less decisive of a factor than neck size — women with a neck circumference of 16 inches or more are more likely to have apnea. So are women with double chins and/or fat abdomens.

Knowing for sure

Your doctor will likely refer you to a *pulmonary* (lung) specialist or an *otolaryngologist* (ear, nose, and throat doctor). Most likely he will closely question both you and your sleeping partner and then send you to a sleep disorders clinic for several nights of evaluation.

This evaluation will include polysomnography, a collection of data taken while you sleep with sensors attached to your body and head. The sensors monitor brain waves, body temperature, respiration, heart rate, and several other factors. This test tells your doctors whether you have apnea and how severe it is.

Another diagnostic test for sleep apnea and other sleep disorders is the Multiple Sleep Latency Test, which measures how fast you fall asleep during the day.

Making it better

Treatment of sleep apnea needs to be carefully tailored to the individual. In some cases, only behavioral modification is needed; if the apneic person loses weight, stops smoking, avoids alcohol and sleeping pills, and shifts to sleeping on her side, the number of apneic episodes drops dramatically.

But sometimes more drastic measures are necessary. Though simple oxygen administration does not appear to help, you may undergo *continuous positive airway pressure,* or *CPAP,* in which you wear a mask over your nose and mouth that forces air through the nasal passages under pressure. The pressure is adjusted so that the throat does not close up during sleep. If CPAP doesn't work for you, you may benefit from dental appliances much like orthodontic retainers, which reposition the jaw and tongue and prevent snoring. These work best in cases of mild apnea.

Surgery to increase the size of the airway is considered a last resort. Though several techniques have been developed, none is entirely successful and all have risks and side effects. Many people need to undergo several kinds of surgery before their apnea is relieved.

An ounce of prevention

Although sleep apnea tends to run in some families, you may be able to reduce your risk by maintaining a proper weight. If you have sleep apnea, you may be able to reduce the frequency and duration of breathing pauses by avoiding alcohol and sleeping pills.

For more information on sleep apnea, insomnia, and other sleep disorders, contact

- ✔ The National Sleep Foundation, 729 15th St., Washington, DC 20005; 202-347-3471; www.sleepfoundation.org
- ✔ The American Sleep Disorders Association, 6301 Bandel Rd., Suite 101, Rochester, MN 55901; 507-287-6006; www.asda.org

Chapter 14

Mental and Neurological Disorders

*M*ental disorders, which occur in an estimated one-quarter of Americans at some point during their adult lives, can take the form of altered emotions, behavior, or thinking processes and can be accompanied by physical symptoms. They can be temporary or long term. Many can be treated effectively, but many go unrecognized or untreated because people are often reluctant to seek help for their mental needs.

Mental disorders generally fall into one of the following categories:

✔ **Personality disorders:** These disorders, which often stem from emotional problems during childhood, are characterized by an inability to accept the demands and limitations of the outside world. They may interfere with your behavior and your interactions with other people.

✔ **Anxiety disorders:** These disorders, which include neuroses such as panic attacks, phobias, post-traumatic stress disorder, and obsessive-compulsive disorder, are characterized by a painful or apprehensive uneasiness about something and may manifest themselves in a variety of physical symptoms, including rapid heartbeat, perspiration, and digestive problems, as well as altered behavior.

✔ **Mood disorders:** The various forms of depression, including major depressive disorder, and bipolar (or manic-depressive) disorder, are known as mood disorders because they affect your mood. They may also affect your behavior.

✔ **Thought disorders:** These are disorders in which your thinking is impaired and your interpretation of reality is abnormal. The most common of these is schizophrenia.

Neurological disorders, too, plague many Americans. ***Remember:*** Your brain is complex. The key components in this complex machine are the nerve cells, or *neurons,* which send and receive chemical signals among one another, which they then translate into electrical signals. Through this chemical and electrical network, the nerve cells convey all information necessary to keep your body functioning properly. When something interrupts this network — for example, a disease or injury kills nerve cells or a problem occurs with the electrical signals — you may experience impaired thinking; impaired movement, vision, or speech; or a problem that affects your entire body. The part of your body that is affected depends on the part of the brain that is affected.

This chapter looks at some of the most common mental and neurological disorders.

Depression

Everyone is bound to feel a little depressed from time to time. But depression goes beyond periodic bouts of hating your job, grieving, and loneliness. *Major depressive disorder,* or *major depression,* is a more prolonged and overwhelming feeling of helplessness. Major depression doesn't let you heal mentally or move on with your life. It affects every aspect of your being — your weight, appetite, libido, thinking, feeling.

Depression strikes about 17 million American adults each year, according to the National Institute of Mental Health (NIMH), and women are twice as likely to be affected as men.

According to the American Psychiatric Association, 80 to 90 percent of all cases can be treated effectively, yet the NIMH estimates that only one-third of people with depression get the help they need. Some people fail to recognize their symptoms or attribute them to something else, such as a lack of sleep. Others are kept from seeking help because of the social stigma of mental illness. They are ashamed of what they perceive as a weakness. But depression often originates in biological problems.

Many depressed people have imbalances in the brain's *neurotransmitters,* the chemicals that allow the nerve cells to communicate. Depression appears to be related to a deficiency of the chemicals serotonin and norepinephrine. Women have naturally lower levels of serotonin than men, which could be one reason that they experience depression more often. Other causes of depression include the following:

- Illnesses and diseases, such as thyroid dysfunction, diabetes, kidney, liver or heart disease, stroke, chronic pain, and certain types of cancer
- The birth of a child *(postpartum depression)*

- Fluctuating levels of hormones

- Biochemical imbalances within the body, such as high levels of carbohydrates, low levels of minerals and vitamins such as B₆, B₁₂, and folate

- Head injuries or disruption of brain chemicals

- Surgery

- Long-term use of certain drugs

- Emotional trauma, such as incest, abuse, and rape

- Past events, such as combat duty, chronic illness, the death of a parent, or parental divorce

And because family histories often show a recurrence of depression from generation to generation, it's possible that a genetic predisposition may exist.

Recognizing the signs

Some symptoms of depression are easy to spot — feeling "blue" for a long period of time, for example. But you may have difficulty attributing physical symptoms, such as weight loss or gain, to depression. The symptoms of depression include the following:

- Diminished interest in social activity

- Fatigue or loss of energy, feelings of worthlessness

- Irritability

- Diminished ability to think or concentrate

- Change in appetite

- Change in sex drive

- Insomnia or hypersomnia (too much sleep)

- Excessive guilt for little or no reason

- Frequent thoughts about death or suicide

Knowing for sure

Your doctor may want to perform a blood test to rule out serious conditions such as cancer. You may wish to seek a referral to a mental health professional, such as a psychologist or a psychiatrist, so that she can properly diagnose depression. A thorough physical exam and an honest discussion with your doctor or mental health professional about your life's changes may be the best way to detect depression. Your doctor may ask you to fill out a General Health Questionnaire, a Beck Depression Inventory, or the Zung Self-Rating Depression Scale, which can help determine the level and seriousness of depression.

Making it better

Although most episodes of depression end within six months to a year — even without treatment — seeking help is important because depression can be debilitating and can lead to suicide. And once you've had a major depressive disorder, you're at risk of recurrence.

If you are depressed, take steps to combat negative thinking and reduce stress:

- ✔ **Participate in activities that may make you feel better:** Go to a movie or concert or get together with friends.

- ✔ **Postpone major life decisions:** If you must make such a decision, such as changing a job or getting a divorce, consult others who know you well.

- ✔ **Don't set difficult goals:** Break large tasks into smaller ones and establish priorities.

- ✔ **Practice stress reduction techniques:** See Chapter 1 for some suggestions.

The two most common types of treatment for major depression are *psychotherapy,* or talk therapy, and *pharmacotherapy,* or drug therapy. These two types of therapies are often used in combination.

In psychotherapy, you and your therapist, perhaps a psychiatrist or a psychologist, discuss your problems, and the therapist interprets your problems and suggests different ways to cope with them. The two major types of psychotherapy are

- ✔ **Psychodynamic therapy:** This type of therapy helps you understand the psychological forces that motivate your actions in the hope that these insights can help you change.

- ✔ **Behavior therapy:** This type of therapy uses specific techniques to change your behavioral symptoms.

Pharmacotherapy relies on medications known as *antidepressants,* which elevate your mood. These drugs include tricyclic antidepressants, or TCAs (Tofranil and Elavil), selective serotonin reuptake inhibitors, or SSRIs (Prozac and Zoloft), and monoamine oxidase inhibitors, or MOAIs (Parnate and Nardil). A combination of medication and therapy is thought to be the most effective treatment for major depression.

If your depression is serious (you have attempted suicide, for example, or are unable to function and can't make yourself leave the house), your psychiatrist may recommend hospitalization to monitor your condition. She may even recommend *electroconvulsive therapy*. The procedure involves sedation, and then the application of light electrical impulses to the brain to interrupt the brain's own electrical impulses, inducing a mild convulsion. This treatment is given 8 to 12 times over a period of three weeks. This therapy, which is somewhat controversial because of its potential side effects, is only recommended for the most severely incapacitated patients with depression, generally those for whom antidepressants have not worked or who cannot take antidepressants.

An ounce of prevention

You can't predict whether you'll develop depression, but you can change the way you react to negative events. Staying healthy through exercise, a balanced diet, and stress-reducing techniques can go a long way in keeping your mind healthy. Research also suggests that women with close friends and good relationships are themselves mentally healthy.

Bipolar Disorder

Bipolar disorder is a relatively common and well-named mood disorder. You literally live life from one end to the other. Bipolar disorder, or manic-depressive disorder, is characterized by patterns of emotional highs and lows that may occur alone or alternate. These are not everyday mood swings in reaction to changes in your environment, but extreme mood swings unrelated to your circumstances. These episodes may alternate rapidly, within days, or slowly, with five or more years in between. Studies show that rapid cycling is more common among women than among men. Some experts attribute this to the woman's reproductive cycle and the influences of hormones on emotions. Women may also have more depressive episodes and fewer manic episodes than men.

The average onset of bipolar disorder is between the ages of 15 and 25. Bipolar disorder occurs more often in immediate relatives of people with bipolar disorder than in the general population.

Nonhereditary causes include metabolic and endocrine changes. Some experts believe that events such as childbirth, grieving over the death of a loved one, and frequent travel through time zones resulting in jet lag, which deprive the body of sleep, may contribute to bipolar disorder. Lack of sleep disrupts the body's metabolic balances and takes its toll on levels of brain chemicals called *neurotransmitters*. Biological factors such as multiple sclerosis, brain damage, lesions or tumors in the brain, epilepsy, and an overactive thyroid or adrenal glands can trigger bipolar disorder, as can long-term use of drugs such as steroids.

Recognizing the signs

In a manic cycle, or high, symptoms include inflated self-esteem and self-aggrandizement, agitation, decreased need for sleep, pressured or loud speech, a flurry of ideas without connection, rapid thoughts, easy distractibility, excessive involvement in pleasurable activities (sex, eating, spending money), euphoria, and irritability. In a depressed cycle, or low, the symptoms include sad mood, fatigue, anxiety, change in appetite, weight loss or gain, inability to sleep or sleeping too much, loss of interest in eating, sex, and other pleasurable activities, difficulty concentrating, memory impairment, guilt, and thoughts of suicide.

Knowing for sure

Your primary care physician should start by taking a full medical history. Be sure to tell your doctor about any physical and mental illnesses that appear to run in your family. If your doctor suspects bipolar disorder, she may refer you to a *psychiatrist,* a medical doctor who specializes in the treatment of mental illness The psychiatrist may perform an electroencephalogram to detect abnormal brain waves in order to rule out a seizure disorder. In this procedure, small metal pads connected to wires are placed on your head and connected to a meter.

Making it better

Depending on the severity of your condition, your doctor may prescribe drugs that even out your mood swings. It is important to take all medications and report side effects. You must also have your thyroid, kidney, and liver functions monitored; the side effects for some mood stabilizing drugs can alter the function of these organs. You must also tell you doctor if you're pregnant or planning to become pregnant because many of these drugs can harm the developing baby.

Depending on which part or cycle of bipolar disorder you are in, your doctor may prescribe medications called *mood stabilizers,* such as lithium, valproate, or carbamazepine. For very mild agitated episodes, she may prescribe benzodiazepine, which calms and produces sleep without the side effects of other, stronger drugs.

In severe cases, hospitalization may be necessary.

Obsessive-Compulsive Disorder

In a condition such as obsessive-compulsive disorder (OCD) the brain works like a pit bull with a kitten in his mouth — one thought occupies it and won't let go. It's not clear whether OCD is a product of — or a precursor to — major depressive illness. About half of those with OCD have other mental illnesses, including depression.

Recent research suggests that OCD has a biological origin. Levels of a brain chemical called serotonin become erratic, and the brain cannot adequately function in the abnormal levels of this neurotransmitter. Serotonin helps with the body's sleep-wake cycle as well as with regulation of hormones. The incidence of OCD is higher in women than men, and in most cases, OCD is detected in adolescence or early adulthood. The onset of symptoms is more gradual than sudden. For the most part, victims of OCD recognize that their compulsions and obsessions are unreasonable but feel powerless to make themselves stop or otherwise control their behavior. They often withdraw from friends and can become totally incapacitated at work.

Recognizing the signs

Obsessive-compulsive disorder is characterized by obsessive thoughts, impulses, images, or ideas that are intrusive and inappropriate and cause you to become anxious or distressed. Some of the most common obsessive thoughts are those of becoming contaminated by not washing your hands, repeated doubts as to whether you locked a door, the need to have things in a particular order, and severe distress when they are out of place. Less commonly, people experience aggressive or horrific impulses, such as hurting loved ones, and recurring sexual imagery that cannot be put out of their minds easily. Compulsion is the action that follows to alleviate the obsession. For example, an obsession of doubt about a locked door would be followed by the compulsion to repeatedly check the door lock.

Knowing for sure

A diagnosis of obsessive-compulsive disorder starts with a full medical history. Be sure to tell your doctor of your thoughts and actions. Most women who suffer from OCD are embarrassed about their behavior, but because a dermatologist may recognize overwashed hands or a dentist may recognized overbrushed teeth, hiding the results of the compulsion is difficult. Your doctor may recommend a brain imaging test, such as an electroencephalogram or single-photon emission computerized tomography (SPECT) or positron emission tomography (PET), to assess your brain function. Many patients with OCD have abnormal activity in parts of the brain called the caudate nucleus, cingulate cortex, and orbito-frontal cortex.

Making it better

As with depression, the two major types of treatment for OCD are psycho-therapy and pharmacotherapy, which are often given in combination.

Treatment guidelines released in 1997 indicate that for mild cases, the first line of treatment should be cognitive behavior therapy, a type of psycho-therapy in which the abnormal thinking pattern is examined, addressed, and changed by way of behavior. For moderate and severe cases, the guidelines recommend a combination of cognitive behavior therapy and antidepres-sants. The antidepressants used to treat OCD include the selective serotonin reuptake inhibitors (SSRIs) Prozac, Paxil, and Zoloft and the tricyclic anti-depressant clomipramine Anafranil.

Alzheimer's Disease and Dementia

Alzheimer's disease is a progressive, degenerative disease that destroys brain cells, impairing memory, thinking, and behavior. These impairments, which can be accompanied by physical decline, lead to an inability to function normally. They also lead to a susceptibility to a variety of illnesses and complications that can lead to death. Alzheimer's disease affects an estimated 4 million people, many of them women. Researchers believe that women are affected more than men because they generally live longer, and the risk of Alzheimer's disease increases with age. The disease can, however, strike people in their 40s and 50s.

Alzheimer's disease is the most common cause of *dementia*. Dementia is a loss of intellectual function that includes impairment of more than one cognitive (or intellectual) ability (such as memory, orientation, judgment, or perception), is persistent, is severe enough to interfere with daily function-ing, and is often progressive. Dementia is a hallmark of Alzheimer's disease, although Alzheimer's is not the only condition that can cause it. In fact, more than 70 disorders and diseases can cause dementia.

When dementia is caused by depression, drug or alcohol problems, nutri-tional disorders, brain tumors, metabolic conditions, or organ dysfunction, it may be reversible. Experts estimate that dementia symptoms are poten-tially reversible in 10 to 20 percent of people who experience them. In other cases, the damage is permanent, although treating the underlying condition may slow or stop dementia's progression. These cases include the two most common causes of dementia — Alzheimer's disease and vascular dementia. In vascular dementia, blood vessels in the brain become narrowed or blocked, cutting off the oxygen supply to the brain and causing nerve cells to die. Vascular dementia is caused in large part by atherosclerosis and hypertension, both of which we discuss in Chapter 15.

The exact cause of Alzheimer's disease remains unknown. What is known is that the disease damages neurons in the areas of the brain that are responsible for thought, memory, speech, and emotions. In addition, the brain experiences a depletion of the neurotransmitter *acetylcholine,* a brain chemical crucial to memory and learning. Researchers believe the amount of acetylcholine diminishes because the neurons that produce it die, but the many factors that cause neuron death have not been fully examined.

Among the many theories are: a deficit in a brain hormone known as nerve growth factor, exposure to a viral or infectious agent, exposure to environmental toxins such as aluminum or zinc, a defect in the body's immune system, destruction caused by free radicals (unbalanced molecules generated by naturally occurring oxidative reactions in the body), and genetic defects or predispositions to the disease. Researchers have identified mutations of several genes as causes of early-onset Alzheimer's disease, and a variation of another gene has been identified as a risk factor for both early-onset and late-onset disease. Researchers identified what may be a second risk factor gene in early 1998. But because not all people with Alzheimer's have these genes, other factors likely contribute to the development of the disease.

Recognizing the signs

The symptoms of dementia (and of Alzheimer's disease) include cognitive symptoms such as impairment, slowing, or loss of memory, orientation (of time, place, and people), logic, judgment, perception, the ability to calculate, the ability to learn new things, and the ability to use language; emotional symptoms such as depression, anxiety, irritability, insecurity, fear, hostility, agitation, jealousy, and paranoia; and behavioral symptoms such as lack of initiative, loss of interest, impulsiveness, temper tantrums, social withdrawal, restlessness, disorientation, and obsessiveness. Other symptoms of dementia may include socially inappropriate behavior, communication difficulties, and a decline in coordination. Not all people with dementia experience all these symptoms.

The symptoms and their severity depend in large part on what is causing dementia and on how far that disease or condition has progressed. In the early stages of Alzheimer's disease, for example, symptoms may be limited to short-term memory loss and difficulty learning new information. These symptoms may not even be noticeable. In the moderate stage, long-term memory and judgment may also be affected, the person may become disoriented, have trouble communicating, or develop behavior or personality changes. And in the severe stage of Alzheimer's disease, the person may fail to recognize friends and relatives, have poor memory, become more restless and less able to control her movements and speech, and, ultimately, may become mute, immobile, and incontinent.

Knowing for sure

Because dementia can be reversed in some cases and because its progression can be slowed or stopped in others, it is important for the cause to be diagnosed. Making the diagnosis of dementia is basically a process of elimination. Because symptoms for many of the diseases that cause dementia are similar and no specific diagnostic tests exist for some of those diseases, your doctor or neurologist must eliminate the possibilities one by one with a succession of examinations and tests. This succession may include a physical exam, medical history, and blood, urine, and other laboratory tests to narrow down the cause, as well as brain imaging and function tests to see what is going on in your brain. These tests may include

- ✔ **Electroencephalography (EEG):** This test shows the brain's electrical activity and can indicate whether brain damage has occurred.

- ✔ **Computerized tomography (CT), or computerized axial tomography (CAT):** This test provides a computerized, cross-sectional x-ray of the brain and can demonstrate brain injuries, tumors, stroke, and vascular dementia.

- ✔ **Magnetic resonance imaging (MRI):** This test uses an electromagnetic field to produce an image of the brain, which can reveal the same things as CT.

- ✔ **Positron emission tomography (PET), or single-photon emission computerized tomography (SPECT):** These tests show how the brain is using oxygen and glucose and how blood is flowing through the brain and can indicate whether the brain's normal functioning has been affected.

If these tests don't reveal the cause of dementia, your doctor has to make an educated guess. The only way to diagnose Alzheimer's with certainty is to examine a sample of brain tissue under a microscope — and this is generally not done except at autopsy.

Making it better

Your treatment depends on the cause and symptoms of dementia. In some cases, the goal is to treat the cause of dementia and reverse dementia symptoms. In others, the goal is to slow progression of dementia; and in still others, the goal is to control as many symptoms as possible. If your problems are caused by a medication, for example, your doctor will likely take you off that medication and prescribe an alternative. If a nutritional deficiency is the problem, you'll likely be prescribed specific doses of the nutrient in question. If you suffer from vascular dementia, your doctor may suggest antihypertensive medications to keep your blood pressure under control or anticoagulants or platelet inhibitors, so-called blood thinners, to reduce the risk of further damage. And if you suffer from agitation, anxiety, or hallucinations, your doctor may prescribe a tranquilizer. If you suffer from depression, you may be given an antidepressant.

The treatments for Alzheimer's disease itself are somewhat limited, although research is moving at a brisk pace. Two drugs — tacrine (Cognex) and donepezil (Aricept) — are currently available to treat the cognitive symptoms of Alzheimer's disease, such as thinking and reasoning. Neither drug cures the disease, however, and the disease continues to progress during treatment.

Researchers are hopeful, however, that the next generation of treatments will delay the onset or slow the progression of Alzheimer's disease. Vitamin E, nonsteroidal anti-inflammatory drugs (NSAIDs), and estrogen have shown some promise in delaying the onset of the disease in recent studies. Vitamin E may work by countering oxidative damage, NSAIDs by countering inflammation in the brain, and estrogen by allowing brain cells to form better connections and promoting the formation of acetylcholine.

For more information on Alzheimer's disease, contact the Alzheimer's Association, 919 N. Michigan Ave., Suite 1000, Chicago, IL 60611-1676; 800-272-3900; www.alz.org

Parkinson's Disease

Muhammad Ali, Katharine Hepburn, and Janet Reno have more in common than celebrity status. They're famous people with an infamous disease — Parkinson's. Parkinson's disease is a progressive disorder that affects a small area of cells (called the *substantia nigra*) in the brain. These cells normally produce *dopamine,* a chemical necessary for transmitting messages in the brain. In Parkinson's disease, these cells degenerate and die, causing a deficiency of dopamine. Without this chemical messenger, the body gets strange signals (or none at all), resulting in the impaired muscle movement. Because these symptoms include tremor and muscle stiffness in large joints, Parkinson's disease was once known as shaking palsy or paralysis agitans.

Parkinson's usually starts in middle or late life and develops very slowly. It tends to be progressive, which means that the symptoms gradually worsen over time. The amount of time the disease takes to progress varies significantly from person to person. In its later stages, however, Parkinson's can be incapacitating.

Although some people link the onset of Parkinson's symptoms with acute trauma, such as an accident or surgery, most people who experience these traumatic events do not develop Parkinson's disease. And although isolated instances of families with a high incidence of Parkinson's disease do exist, researchers have not yet identified a genetic cause. While experts have not yet been able to determine the cause of Parkinson's disease itself, they do know that certain medications, such as haloperidol (Haldol) and other medications used to treat hallucinations, antihypertensive drugs containing reserpine, and the antinausea drug metoclopramide (Reglan), can interfere with the brain's metabolism of dopamine. One side effect of taking these drugs long term is that they may produce symptoms similar to those of Parkinson's disease, although they do not cause the disease itself.

Recognizing the signs

Symptoms of Parkinson's disease include shaking of the hands or head called tremors, stiffness in the limbs and joints, a masklike facial expression, stooped posture, poor coordination and balance, a slow, monotone voice, difficulty initiating physical movement, a shuffling gait due to stiffness in the large joints, and, eventually, dementia.

Knowing for sure

Your doctor may refer you to a neurologist, a specialist in the diseases of the nervous system. In addition to performing a physical exam and taking a medical history, the neurologist may want to perform several tests, including urine tests to detect low levels of dopamine. She may also want to perform brain imaging tests, such as an magnetic resonance imaging (MRI), to detect damage in the brain and rule out other problems.

Making it better

Parkinson's disease has no cure, but medications are available that improve the symptoms.

The most commonly prescribed medication for Parkinson's disease is levodopa, which restores the brain's supply of dopamine and can improve some of the physical symptoms of the disease, including movement and balance. To reduce the side effects of levodopa, which include nausea, low blood pressure, and hallucinations, this drug is often given in combination with another drug, carbidopa. Because levodopa does not actually decrease the destruction of nerve cells, however, it can become less effective at relieving the symptoms after several years of treatment. Other medications used to treat Parkinson's disease include amantadine, pergolide, and bromocriptine, which mimic the action of dopamine. New on the market are pramipexole (Mirapex) and ropinirole (Requip), which were approved by the Food and Drug Administration (FDA) in late 1997 for treating early and advanced Parkinson's disease. They, too, mimic the action of dopamine. And anticholenergic drugs such as benztropine are prescribed to relieve certain symptoms of Parkinson's, specifically tremor.

In late 1997, the FDA also approved a surgical implant to treat Parkinson's symptoms — notably tremor. The device, called the Activa tremor control system, operates on the same principle as a pacemaker, sending electrical impulses to the affected area of the brain. Though the device is not for everyone, it enables patients with severe tremor to perform tasks, such as feeding and dressing themselves, that they weren't able to do without help prior to the surgery.

Other surgical procedures have also been used to treat Parkinson's disease, including surgery to destroy brain tissue in the thalamus and globus pallidus, areas critical to preventing involuntary movement. Transplantation of adrenal gland, and other tissues, including fetal tissue, into the brain to restore lost brain circuits have also been used. Controversy surrounds the use of transplanted fetal brain cells for the treatment of Parkinson's. In initial tests, fetal brain cells from the part of the brain called the adrenal medulla have been transplanted into the brains of patients with severe Parkinson's. But this procedure has not been shown to cure — only to treat a few of the symptoms of Parkinson's. Researchers are also experimenting with the removal of the pallidum or cerebral cortex of the brain to treat the disease. Called a *pallidotomy,* this procedure is only for severe cases, after long-term drug treatment has been found ineffective.

For more information on Parkinson's disease, contact the National Parkinson Foundation, Bob Hope Parkinson Research Center, 1501 N.W., 9th Ave., Bob Hope Road, Miami, FL 33136-1494; 305-547-6666; 800-327-4545; www.parkinson.org

Chapter 15
Cardiovascular Disease

• •

In This Chapter

▶ Understanding coronary artery disease
▶ Recognizing heart attack symptoms
▶ Dealing with stroke
▶ Treating high blood pressure

• •

*B*ecause heart disease is a man's disease, women have nothing to worry about. Wrong!

Until recently, women and their doctors held this belief. A woman with heart disease often went undiagnosed and untreated. No one counseled her to reduce her risk factors, despite the fact that heart attack is more deadly in women than in men. According to the American Heart Association, in 1995 more than 505,440 women died from all forms of cardiovascular disease, compared with 455,125 deaths in men; strokes killed 96,428 women, compared with 61,563 men; and 23,321 women died from hypertension, compared with 16,660 men. (Compare those numbers with the 43,844 women who lost their lives to breast cancer!)

This chapter discusses three different types of *cardiovascular disease* (diseases that affect the heart and blood vessels). For each of these disorders, this chapter describes what it is, its symptoms, tests used to diagnose it, how it's treated, and how you can reduce your risk.

Coronary Artery Disease

The heart is a muscular organ whose job is to pump oxygen-rich blood to the entire body via the arteries. The heart itself is nourished by special blood vessels, called *coronary arteries,* that deliver oxygen-containing blood into all areas of the heart muscle.

As early as childhood, the arteries in your body may begin to accumulate globs of cholesterol (a fatty substance), fats, excess *fibrin* (normally used to make blood clot effectively), and other materials. Over time, this buildup (called *plaque*) causes the walls of your arteries to become narrower, thick, and hard. This condition, known as *atherosclerosis,* can slow down or even stop the flow of blood. When atherosclerosis affects the coronary arteries, it decreases the delivery of oxygen-rich blood to the heart and is known as coronary artery disease. Figure 15-1 illustrates the difference between a normal artery and an artery affected by atherosclerosis.

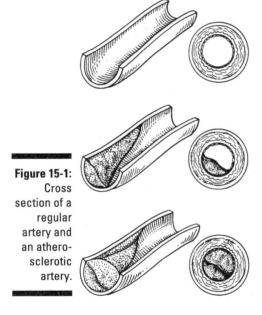

Figure 15-1: Cross section of a regular artery and an atherosclerotic artery.

You may not know you have coronary artery disease until it leads to chest pain. Chest pain is a symptom of two underlying conditions:

- **Angina pectoris:** Angina occurs when your heart doesn't get enough blood. You feel fine at rest, but when you stress your heart, spasms from the stress may cause your coronary arteries to constrict and your heart may not receive enough blood through its narrowed coronary arteries. Your heart lets you know that it's oxygen-starved by sending you a very clear message that's hard to ignore — chest pain!

  Some people have chest pain when they're resting, caused by spasm of a narrowed area of the coronary artery rather than a blockage. This type is called *Prinzmetal's angina,* and it's more likely to occur in women.

✔ **Heart attack, or myocardial infarction:** This more serious condition occurs if one or more of your coronary arteries becomes totally blocked, say from a blood clot. The part of your heart muscle fed by this blocked artery doesn't receive any blood and begins to die. A heart attack may be mild if only a small amount of your heart muscle is damaged; but if enough heart muscles dies, you can, too.

Women are built differently than men. Besides the obvious differences in anatomy, women have smaller coronary arteries, which can become blocked more easily and can make diagnostic tests, bypass surgery, and catheter procedures more difficult to perform and less successful. Nevertheless, as a woman, your risk factors for heart disease are essentially the same as for a man. What is different is how strongly these risk factors affect you:

✔ **Age and gender:** As you age, your risk for a heart attack increases. Women tend to be 10 years older than men when they have their first heart attack. But by age 75, the incidence of coronary artery disease in women exceeds that in men.

✔ **Family history:** Having a close relative who died of coronary artery disease before age 55 increases your risk by five of having coronary artery disease at an early age.

✔ **Race:** African-American women have a greater risk of heart disease than Caucasian women, possibly because they also tend to have high blood pressure. On the other hand, Hispanic women have a lower risk of heart attack than Caucasian women.

✔ **Cigarette smoke:** Chances are high that a woman who's had a heart attack before age 40 is a smoker. Don't be fooled into thinking that because you're a light smoker (that's one to four cigarettes a day) you're not at risk. You still have twice the risk of a nonsmoker. But don't despair. If you quit now, you can reduce your risk to that of a person who never smoked within three to five years. Even inhaling secondhand smoke puts you at an increased risk if you're exposed for a long period of time.

✔ **Hypertension:** *Hypertension,* high blood pressure, increases the risk of coronary artery disease in both men and women. In fact, more than 60 percent of women over age 65 have hypertension. (See the "Hypertension" section later in this chapter.)

✔ **Cholesterol levels:** As your total blood cholesterol level increases, so does your risk for heart disease. Younger women have higher high-density lipoprotein (HDL, the "good" cholesterol) and lower low-density lipoprotein (LDL, the "bad" cholesterol) levels than men. But by the time you reach menopause, your LDL and triglyceride levels start to rise, and by age 55, exceed those of a man. High LDL and triglyceride levels increase heart disease risk. And in women, low HDL levels — less than 35 mg/dl — do the same.

- ✔ **Inactive lifestyle:** Couch potatoes have twice the risk of heart disease as people who exercise. Get going: Even low and moderate levels can reduce your risk. (For more information on exercise, see Chapter 1.)

- ✔ **Body weight:** Obesity increases your risk of coronary artery disease, especially if you have more upper-body fat. In fact, even being only mildly to moderately overweight doubles your risk. More specifically, your risk is higher if you have a waist-to-hip ratio greater than 0.8. (See Chapter 5 for instructions on how to figure your waist-to-hip ratio.)

- ✔ **Diabetes:** Diabetes carries a greater risk of heart disease in women than in men. And if you have diabetes, your chances of dying from heart disease are three to seven times greater than that of a woman without diabetes. Diabetes also doubles your chances (but not a man's) of a second heart attack. Diabetes damages the small blood vessels in the entire body (especially the heart, kidneys, and eyes), although not in the same way that atherosclerosis does. Unfortunately, the two separate conditions add up the damage and worsen the end result.

- ✔ **Stress:** Scientists aren't entirely sure of the role that stress plays in heart disease. There appears to be a relationship between having a heart attack and a person's life stresses, behavior habits, and socioeconomic status. (For information on how to reduce stress, see Chapter 1.)

- ✔ **Oral contraceptives:** In the past, taking older, higher dose oral contraceptives, which are no longer available, increased a woman's risk for cardiovascular disease. (Research indicates that women who took these pills in the past are not currently at increased risk of heart disease.) The new, lower dose oral contraceptives carry less of a risk of coronary artery disease. But if you smoke and take the Pill, your risk of heart attack is significantly increased.

- ✔ **Menopause:** Thanks to the female hormone estrogen, women develop coronary artery disease approximately 10 years after men. After menopause, you lose the protective effect of estrogen, and your risk of coronary artery disease increases dramatically. By the time you're 75 years old, your risk is the same as a man's.

Recognizing the signs

You may not suspect that you have coronary artery disease unless you experience chest pain — the result of either angina or heart attack. Here are the characteristics of each.

Anginal pain typically lasts less than 15 minutes and should go away if you sit, rest, and take a nitroglycerin tablet. Anginal pain often occurs when you stress your heart. But women who have had angina for a long time have a greater tendency than men to have chest pain at rest, during sleep, and when they are under emotional stress.

The real heart "burn"

Most adults are familiar with heartburn. When you get it, you reach for the antacid. Unfortunately, they write off one of the most common symptoms of a heart attack — the burning or pressure in the upper abdominal or chest area. The feeling of a heart attack can be similar to heartburn. To make matters worse, heart attacks can follow a large meal. So if you have a history of heart disease, don't ignore the symptoms of heartburn. Report them to your doctor immediately.

Heart attack pain, on the other hand, generally persists or only goes away temporarily and then returns and is not relieved by nitroglycerin. One of the classic images that most people identify with a heart attack is a person — most likely a man — in excruciating pain with a fist clenched to his chest. Typically, this pain has a pressure, fullness, or squeezing quality and may radiate to the shoulders, neck, or arms, especially on the left side of the body. The person may also feel short of breath, lightheaded, faint, sweaty, or nauseated.

As a woman, you're more likely to experience some not-so-classic — and even subtle — signs of a heart attack. In fact, 46 percent of women who have a heart attack have no chest pain at all. For example, you may have what's called *atypical chest pain* — pain right under the sternum, or breastbone, in your stomach, upper abdomen, neck, or shoulders. You're also more apt to have less specific symptoms as nausea, vomiting, dizziness, and difficulty breathing. You may feel *palpitations* (your heart pounding in your chest), break out in a cold sweat, and look ghostly pale. And women are also more likely to have feelings of unexplained anxiety, weakness, or fatigue. Knowing all the signs of a heart attack possible for women can save your life.

If you suspect that you are having a heart attack, immediately call emergency medical services to take you to the emergency department. Heart muscle doesn't die right away, and every moment you delay seeking treatment means the death of more heart muscle. Getting to the hospital within six hours can mean the difference between whether you can receive life-saving thrombolytic therapy to dissolve the culprit blood clot that may have caused your heart attack. This therapy is more likely to be successful in the early hours of a heart attack, so don't delay.

Knowing for sure

A woman tends to have chest pain for a longer period of time than a man before her doctor diagnoses that she has coronary artery disease. This delay may be due to the more subtle symptoms a woman experiences. Or it may be because some diagnostic tests aren't as accurate in women. For instance, your breast tissue can affect your doctor's interpretation of some heart scans.

If your doctor suspects that you have coronary artery disease, she may recommend some of these tests:

- ✔ **Electrocardiogram (ECG or EKG):** In this simple test, electrical leads are placed on the skin of your chest wall to record the electrical activity of your heart. Your doctor can determine whether your heart muscle is receiving enough oxygen or whether it has been damaged. This test may not always pick up problems that do exist (called a *false-negative* result), or it may suggest problems where they don't exist (called a *false-positive* result).

- ✔ **Exercise stress test:** While you exercise on a specific type of treadmill, your doctor monitors your ECG to see whether your heart is receiving enough oxygen when it has to work a little harder. A drug may be used to raise your heart rate if you can't exercise enough to do this by yourself.

- ✔ **Echocardiography:** Echocardiography uses sound waves to make a videotape image of the beating heart. It may be combined with exercise stress testing to check the flow of blood to the heart muscle during the exercise period.

- ✔ **Radionuclide tests:** During radionuclide tests, such as a thallium scan, technetium Sestamibi, or single-photon emission computerized tomography (SPECT), a radioactive substance is injected through a vein and detected in your heart by a scanner. These tests tell your doctor information such as whether your heart muscle is receiving enough blood, how well your heart is pumping, and the location and severity of a heart attack. The accuracy of these tests in women is being studied. For example, breast tissue can interfere with the results of some radionuclide tests.

- ✔ **Cardiac catheterization and coronary angiography:** These two tests are usually performed together after a small *catheter* (hollow tube) is inserted into a blood vessel and advanced to the heart. Dye is injected as a series of x-rays are taken to show the location and severity of any narrowings or blockages in your coronary arteries and how well the chambers of your heart pump blood. Although the numbers are now increasing, women with signs of coronary artery disease aren't referred for these tests as often as men with signs of coronary artery disease.

✔ **Lipid profile:** This blood test determines your total cholesterol, triglyceride, and HDL and LDL levels. LDL particles in the blood deposit cholesterol on the walls of your arteries, while HDL removes cholesterol. High cholesterol, triglyceride, and LDL levels and low HDL levels increase your risk of developing coronary artery disease. Check out the National Cholesterol Education Program guidelines, as shown in Table 15-1, for desirable cholesterol levels, and see where your cholesterol levels fall.

Table 15-1	National Cholesterol Education Program Classification Guidelines for Adults
Cholesterol level (mg/dl)*	*Classification*
Total cholesterol	
Less than 200	Desirable
200–239	Borderline
240 or higher	High
HDL Cholesterol	
50–75 or higher	Desirable
35–49	Borderline low
Less than 35	Low
LDL Cholesterol	
Less than 130	Desirable
130–159	Borderline high
160 or higher	High
Triglycerides	
200 or less	Safe
200–400	Borderline
400–1,000	High
1,000 or above	Very high
* mg/dl = milligrams per deciliter	

Making it better

When it comes to your heart, you can do a lot of things on your own to improve its health and keep it ticking. But when self-care isn't enough, your doctor has a wide variety of drugs and interventions at her disposal to help you out. She may also refer you to a *cardiologist* (a heart specialist).

To help prevent and treat coronary artery disease, follow these tips:

- ✔ **Put out those cigarettes:** Quit smoking and avoid breathing second-hand smoke.

- ✔ **Get off the couch:** If you're in good health, the American Heart Association recommends that you exercise for at least 30 minutes a day, three or four days a week, at 50 to 75 percent of your maximum heart rate. (See Chapter 1 for tips on exercise.) See your doctor before starting an exercise program if you have heart disease, other health problems, or have been inactive for a long time.

- ✔ **Eat wisely:** The American Heart Association recommends that you limit your fat intake to no more than 30 percent of your total calories, with saturated fats making up only 8 to 10 percent of total calories. If you have coronary artery disease, limit saturated fats to less than 7 percent of total calories. Your cholesterol intake should be less than 300 milligrams a day and no more than 200 if you have coronary artery disease. (For more information on fats, see Chapter 1.)

- ✔ **Shed those extra pounds:** Losing weight will lower your cholesterol and put less stress on your heart. (See Chapter 5 for tips on weight loss.)

- ✔ **Stop and smell the roses:** Learn to relax — try progressive muscle relaxation, guided imagery, or a good massage, for starters. Consult your doctor if you need help with reducing stress. (For more information on stress, see Chapter 1.)

- ✔ **Monitor your blood pressure:** If you eat wisely, lose weight, and exercise regularly, you're already on your way to a healthy blood pressure. Cutting out excess salt in your diet and limiting alcohol also help.

- ✔ **Control your blood sugar:** If you have diabetes, work closely with your doctor to eat right, control your weight, exercise, and adjust your medications, if necessary.

- ✔ **Drink only in moderation:** Drinking low to moderate amounts of alcohol — for a woman that's one or two drinks a day — can protect you from coronary artery disease. But avoiding alcohol also has health benefits, so discuss alcohol use with your doctor.

Your doctor has a wide variety of drugs to choose from to treat coronary artery disease. Here are some of the most commonly prescribed:

- ✔ **Vasodilatory drugs:** These drugs help the blood vessels relax and expand so that the heart muscle receives more oxygen-rich blood and doesn't have to work as hard to pump. Nitroglycerin is one of the most commonly used vasodilatory drugs and comes in several forms, including an oral spray, skin patch or ointment, and pills that dissolve under the tongue. Nitroglycerin is taken "as needed" to relieve anginal pain. Another vasodilator your doctor may prescribe is isosorbide (Dilatrate-SR, Isorbide, and Isordil are a few brand names).

- ✔ **Beta-blockers:** Beta-blockers, such as atenolol (Tenormin), metoprolol (Lopressor), and propranolol (Inderal), ease the workload of your heart by lowering your heart rate and blood pressure. Doctors prescribe them to treat angina. Or, if you've had a heart attack, you may take one of these drugs to prevent another heart attack.

- ✔ **Calcium channel blockers:** These medications reduce your heart's need for oxygen, increase its blood supply, and lower blood pressure. They can also prevent coronary artery spasm if you have Prinzmetal's angina. Some common calcium channel blockers are nifedipine (Procardia), verapamil (Calan, Isoptin), and diltiazem (Cardizem).

- ✔ **Antilipemic drugs:** If you have high levels of cholesterol or triglycerides that diet can't lower, you may benefit from antilipemic drugs, which reduce blood cholesterol levels. Your doctor will recommend one or more of many, many drugs, such as niacin, or nicotinic acid, (Niacor, Nicolar), cholestyramine (Questran), colestipol (Colestid), gemfibrozil (Lopid), and simvastatin (Zocor).

- ✔ **Angiotensin-converting enzyme (ACE) inhibitors:** Your doctor may prescribe one of these drugs, such as captopril (Capoten) or enalapril (Vasotec) after a heart attack to reduce your risk of death and of having another heart attack.

- ✔ **Aspirin:** Aspirin prevents *platelets* (special blood cells necessary for blood clotting) from "sticking" together and forming a deadly blood clot. Your doctor may recommend aspirin to prevent a heart attack if you have *unstable angina* (worsening angina that is caused by less and less activity) or after a heart attack to prevent another one. Even though aspirin is an over-the-counter drug, the decision to take it should be a joint one between you and your doctor. Don't take it on your own without consulting your doctor. Aspirin may interact with other medications your doctor has prescribed, possibly resulting in a tendency for your blood not to clot properly.

- ✔ **Thrombolytic therapy:** If you are having a heart attack, a clot-dissolving drug, such as streptokinase, urokinase, or tissue plasminogen activator (TPA), can break up the blood clot in your coronary artery and restore blood flow to your heart muscle. But to be effective, these drugs must be given within six hours of a heart attack.

Medications may not be enough if you have disabling angina or if your coronary arteries are dangerously blocked. Your doctor may recommend that you undergo aggressive procedures to improve blood flow to your heart. Some doctors, however, may be less likely to recommend these procedures to you or treat you as aggressively as a man, although this trend is now changing. Be assertive and ask your doctor to describe all options to you. These procedures may include the following:

- **Balloon angioplasty (also called percutaneous transluminal coronary angioplasty, or PTCA):** During angioplasty, a catheter is inserted into the narrowed or blocked coronary artery, and a balloon at its tip is inflated, stretching the artery and improving blood flow. Although women don't fare as well at first, over the long run, women who have angioplasty seem to do as well as men.

- **Laser angioplasty:** A laser at the tip of a catheter uses pulsating beams of light to vaporize the plaque that lines the inner surface of the coronary artery. It is more successful with mild blockages than with severe ones. It can be used alone or with angioplasty.

- **Atherectomy:** A catheter with a rotating shaver at its tip is inserted into a coronary artery to grind up the plaque along the inner lining of the coronary artery. Atherectomy may be done alone or with balloon angioplasty.

- **Coronary stents:** These tubelike structures may be placed into a coronary artery following one of the above catheter procedures to keep the artery open.

- **Coronary artery bypass surgery (CABG):** The surgeon takes a vein from your leg or an artery from your chest and sews it into the coronary artery to make a detour around the blockage, allowing blood to be delivered to the area of heart muscle that was formerly deprived of oxygen. Because this requires open-heart surgery, it is less frequently performed if a less invasive procedure is likely to have similar success rates. Although women have more complications after bypass surgery, in the long run survival is about the same as men. Women, however, aren't as likely as men to get relief from angina or to return to work after surgery.

After a heart attack or a procedure to restore blood flow such as bypass surgery, a cardiac rehabilitation program can help increase your level of activity, reduce risk factors, and provide emotional support and education.

Another option for postmenopausal women

If you're a postmenopausal woman, check with your doctor to determine whether she feels hormone replacement therapy (HRT) is appropriate for you as a means of lowering your risk for coronary artery disease. Postmenopausal women who receive estrogen can lower their risk of heart disease up to 50 percent. Why? Because HRT increases HDL, the "good" cholesterol, and reduces LDL, the "bad" cholesterol. Estrogen also makes coronary blood vessels dilate, which allows more blood to reach your heart. It also has a direct effect on the lining of the coronary arteries, making them less "sticky" and less susceptible to plaque buildup.

But a recent study indicates that HRT may not be helpful for women who already have heart disease, and HRT does have side effects.

For more information on HRT, see Chapter 20.

An ounce of prevention

Reducing your risk factors lowers your chances of developing coronary artery disease or slows down the rate of plaque buildup if you already have atherosclerosis. Although you can't change some risk factors, you can reduce or eliminate other risk factors just by changing some of your habits. See the section "Making it better" for the tickets you can trade in for good health.

Stroke

A *stroke,* or brain attack, is an event that causes loss of circulation and oxygen to the brain, and, thus, the death of brain tissue and the loss of the function brain tissue normally supervises. It may be caused by a blood clot in an artery that supplies blood to the brain (an *ischemic stroke*) or by the rupture of a blood vessel in the brain (a *hemorrhagic stroke*). Either way, having a stroke can be devastating to you. Stroke is the leading cause of serious disability and the third leading cause of death for women in America after heart disease and cancer — that's about one 1 of every 14.6 deaths.

Ischemia means death of vital tissue due to a lack of circulation and oxygen. Ischemic strokes come in two varieties:

  ✔ **Cerebral thrombosis:** This type of ischemic stroke occurs when a blood clot blocks an artery already narrowed by atherosclerosis.

  People with this type of stroke often have warning ministrokes called *transient ischemic attacks (TIAs)* days, weeks, or even years before their stroke. A TIA is caused by a very tiny clot that only temporarily blocks a small, narrow artery before it is dissolved or carried away by the circulation. During a TIA, blood flow to the affected area of the brain is only temporarily halted, and symptoms go away within 24 hours. Unfortunately, many people do not heed the warning and do not seek medical attention in order to prevent a major stroke in the future.

✔ **Cerebral embolism:** This type of ischemic stroke occurs when a blood clot *(embolus)* or another type of particle, such as a plaque fragment from a major artery, travels through the blood stream and lodges in an artery in the brain. The result is the same: No circulation to the brain tissue and loss of oxygen.

Hemorrhagic (bleeding) strokes are caused by rupture of a blood vessel, with bleeding into surrounding brain tissue and disruption of the oxygen supply. They may be caused by a head injury that causes trauma to a blood vessel or the rupture of an *aneurysm* (a ballooning of an artery wall) or a malformed blood vessel in the brain. In a *subarachnoid hemorrhage,* bleeding occurs from a blood vessel on the surface of the brain; in a *cerebral hemorrhage,* bleeding occurs inside the brain. Bleeding into the brain causes pressure that interrupts brain function, as well as clot formation.

Whether the stroke is ischemic or hemorrhagic, the brain doesn't get enough blood and brain cells begin to die within minutes. The effects of a stroke depend on the type of stroke and which part of the brain was affected and can include paralysis or weakness on one side of the body, slurred speech, or difficulty understanding what's said to you. Weakness on one side of your mouth can cause difficulty chewing and swallowing and put you at risk for choking. You may also have problems with your vision, thoughts, behaviors, and emotions.

Doing what you can to prevent the disability — and even death — that can occur with a stroke is very important. You can't change some risk factors, others you can reduce on your own, and still others you need to work in partnership with your doctor to improve. These risk factors include the following:

✔ **Age:** Just as with heart disease, your risk of a stroke rises as you approach menopause and continues to rise with each passing year.

✔ **Gender:** The risk of stroke is about 19 percent higher in men than women. But women are more likely to die from a stroke.

✔ **Family history:** If you have a close relative who's had a stroke, your risk of having one rises.

✔ **Race:** If you're an African-American woman, your risk of having a stroke is greater than that of a Caucasian woman, partly because African Americans tend to have higher blood pressures — another risk factor for a stroke. African Americans — both male and female — are more likely to die from a stroke than Caucasians. Hispanics also have a greater risk of having a stroke than Caucasians.

✔ **Hypertension:** Having high blood pressure is the single most important risk factor for a stroke. Isolated systolic hypertension, in which just the systolic (the top number) is high, is of concern in older women because it increases the risk of death from stroke.

✔ **Diabetes:** Having diabetes increases the risk for stroke, particularly in women. This is because diabetes affects small blood vessels, weakening and narrowing them and making them more susceptible to injury.

✔ **Cholesterol levels:** The relationship between high cholesterol levels and stroke is unclear. But there does appear to be a positive relationship between high total cholesterol and LDL levels and the development of atherosclerosis in the carotid arteries in your neck that nourish the brain.

✔ **Smoking:** Smoking is a strong risk factor for stroke. And if you smoke and take oral contraceptives, your risk is considerably greater.

✔ **Alcohol:** Although drinking moderate amounts of alcohol may reduce your risk of an ischemic stroke, heavy use can increase the risk of a hemorrhagic stroke.

✔ **Heart disease:** Your risk of having a stroke is doubled if you have heart disease. Atrial fibrillation, in which the *atria* (the upper chambers of the heart) have an abnormal or irregular heartbeat, is one of the strongest cardiac risk factors for a stroke.

✔ **Illegal drug use of all "recreational" drugs:** Cocaine is most commonly associated with stroke, but other drugs, such as heroin, amphetamines, marijuana, and LSD, may also increase the risk.

✔ **Migraine:** Although the risk is small, a young woman with a migraine has an increased risk of stroke.

✔ **Oral contraceptives:** Your risk of stroke is increased if you use oral contraceptives and you smoke.

✔ **Carotid artery bruit:** A *carotid artery bruit* is an abnormal sound your doctor hears when she listens with a stethoscope over your carotid artery in your neck and is a sign of atherosclerosis. Having a bruit increases your risk of a future stroke.

✔ **Transient ischemic attack (TIA):** If you've experienced a TIA in the past, you have a significantly increased risk of stroke.

✔ **Lifestyle factors:** Being obese, having a sedentary lifestyle, poor nutrition, and emotional stress are associated with an increased risk of stroke.

Note: Living in certain states in the Southeast, known as the Stroke Belt, may increase your risk of stroke. These states are Alabama, Arkansas, Georgia, Indiana, Kentucky, Louisiana, Mississippi, North Carolina, South Carolina, Tennessee, and Virginia.

Recognizing the signs

You may be experiencing a stroke if you are having any of the following warning signs:

- Sudden paralysis, weakness, numbness, or any other unusual feelings in your face, or in an arm or leg on one side of the body
- Sudden dimming or loss of vision in only one eye
- Inability to talk or difficulty talking or understanding what's said to you
- Sudden, severe headache for no reason
- Dizziness, unsteadiness, or sudden falls for no reason, especially if you have any of the other symptoms

If you suspect you are having a stroke, call emergency medical services or have someone drive you to the hospital immediately. If the warning signs go away and you feel fine, you still may have had a TIA. You still need to seek medical attention to prevent a fatal or disabling stroke.

Knowing for sure

Your doctor may order any one of a number of tests if you've had a TIA or stroke. Here are some of the more common tests:

- **Computed tomography (CT scan) or magnetic resonance imaging (MRI):** The first test you may have is a CT scan, which uses radiation to take three-dimensional pictures of the brain and tells about the location, severity, and cause of a stroke. An MRI, which uses magnetic rays, gives the same information.
- **Electroencephalogram (EEG):** Electrodes are placed on your scalp to record electric activity from the brain and determine the stroke's location.
- **Evoked response:** You are presented with different sounds, sensations, or images while electrodes on your scalp record the brain's electrical impulses to determine the effects of a stroke.
- **Ultrasound tests:** In these tests, which include carotid artery duplex or transcranial Doppler ultrasound, a probe that emits high frequency sound waves is placed over the arteries in the neck or on the skull to check out blood flow and look for blockages in the arteries that feed the brain.
- **Cerebral angiogram:** A catheter is inserted into a blood vessel, and dye is injected while x-rays are taken of the brain to outline the vessels and show the size and location of blockages, aneurysms, or other malformations.

Making it better

If you've had a TIA or stroke, your treatment will focus on damage control, rehabilitation, and prevention.

Your doctor may recommend one or more of these medications and interventions to treat or prevent stroke:

- ✔ **Hormone replacement therapy (HRT):** If you are postmenopausal, estrogen replacement can reduce your risk of stroke. (See Chapter 20 for more information on HRT.)

- ✔ **Antiplatelet drugs:** Aspirin keeps platelets in your blood from "sticking" together to form blood clots. Your doctor may prescribe aspirin if you're at high risk for a stroke or have had a warning TIA. Ticlopidine is another effective antiplatelet drug. *Anticoagulants* (blood thinners), such as warfarin (Coumadin), may also be prescribed. If you are on warfarin, your doctor will have to carefully monitor your blood levels of the drug because an excessively high level can cause an abnormal tendency to bleed. You must also not take aspirin with warfarin because the two drugs add up and may actually cause a hemorrhagic stroke.

  You are at risk for bleeding if you are taking aspirin. Alert your doctor or dentist if you require surgery or dental extractions.

- ✔ **Thrombolytic therapy:** Just as with a heart attack, tissue plasminogen activator (TPA) may be given to dissolve blood clots in an ischemic stroke, but only if you reach the hospital within a few hours of your stroke.

- ✔ **Carotid endarterectomy:** When a narrowed carotid artery in the neck is the cause of your stroke, your doctor may recommend a *carotid endarterectomy.* In this surgical procedure, the surgeon removes atherosclerotic plaque from the artery to restore its normal diameter and, thus, its blood flow. The surgeon inserts a small instrument through a tiny incision to scrape out the plaque.

- ✔ **New therapies:** Some exciting treatments, such as cerebral angioplasty using a balloon-tipped catheter that expands inside an artery to open up the narrowed area and then uses stents and tiny coils (scaffold-like structures) to keep the arteries open, are now being used to treat strokes.

For hemorrhagic strokes caused by high blood pressure, *antihypertensive* (blood pressure-lowering) drugs may be given to slow blood flow and reduce the risk of bleeding. Surgery to repair a ruptured aneurysm or remove blood that's building up and causing pressure in the brain may also be done.

If you suffer a stroke, the doctors and nurses at the hospital will make sure that you are breathing properly and will assist your breathing if you need help, perhaps by administering oxygen or, if necessary, by putting you on a ventilator. They will also treat any swelling and pressure in your brain. Swelling, a cause of pressure on the brain, is generally treated with medications. In hemorrahagic stroke, pressure on the brain can also be the result of the leaking blood. Doctors can use a surgical procedure known as evaculation to drain the blood. This is generally done only in the case of an emergency.

People can and do survive strokes. A stroke rehabilitation program will help you restore the functions you may have lost. A team approach is used to provide you with speech, physical, occupational, vocational, and psychological therapies.

An ounce of prevention

As with coronary artery disease, the best way to prevent stroke is to reduce your risk factors. Here are some things you can do:

- **Stop smoking:** Contact the American Heart Association, American Cancer Society, or American Lung Association in your area for information on smoking cessation programs or to receive literature.

- **Monitor and control your blood pressure:** Get your blood pressure checked regularly and follow a low sodium diet. If you are on antihypertensive medication, take it even if you feel fine.

- **Drink in moderation:** Limit yourself to one alcoholic drink a day.

- **Be active:** Exercise for 30 minutes, three to four times a week.

- **Eat healthy:** Eat foods that are low in sodium, saturated fat, and cholesterol.

- **Look at your method of birth control:** Consider forms of contraceptives other than birth control pills, or discuss with your doctor switching to a low-estrogen product.

Hypertension

Blood pressure is the force exerted by the blood against the walls of your arteries as your heart beats. *Systolic blood pressure* (the top number) measures the pressure when your heart contracts, whereas *diastolic blood pressure* (the bottom number) is the pressure between beats when your heart is relaxed. So, with a blood pressure of 122/70 (read as "122 over 70"), 122 is your systolic pressure and 70 is your diastolic pressure. (In case you're interested, this pressure is measured in millimeters of mercury [mm Hg]).

A normal blood pressure for an adult is less than 140/90. You have hypertension if your systolic pressure is greater than or equal to 140 and/or your diastolic pressure is greater than or equal to 90. People with a systolic blood pressure between 130 and 139 and a diastolic blood pressure between 85 and 89 have high normal blood pressure and should have their blood pressure carefully monitored by their doctor. Isolated systolic hypertension (just the top number is high) is more likely to occur in women and increases the risk of heart disease and stroke.

In the majority of people, the exact cause of hypertension is not known. This type of hypertension is called *essential hypertension*. In other people, doctors can find a cause for their hypertension, such as kidney disease or adrenal gland tumors. In these instances, known as *secondary hypertension,* when the doctor finds the cause of the hypertension and corrects the problem, blood pressure usually drops back down to normal.

Although scientists don't know exactly why essential hypertension occurs, they have identified certain risk factors. Some risk factors can't be changed; others can be modified or eliminated. Risk factors for hypertension include the following:

- **Age, gender, and race:** You're more likely to see hypertension in Caucasian men under the age of 50 than in Caucasian women under the age of 50. But after age 50, this situation reverses. In African Americans, there's no difference between men and women.

  And African Americans develop hypertension at an earlier age than Caucasians, and it tends to be more severe.
- **Family history:** If your mom or dad has hypertension, you're more likely to develop it, too.
- **Overweight:** Being overweight increases the likelihood that you will have hypertension.
- **Smoking and excessive drinking of alcohol:** These can also raise your blood pressure.
- **Heart and kidney disease:** These diseases also increase risk.
- **Excess sodium:** Some people are sodium sensitive; for them, eating large amounts of sodium can cause hypertension.
- **Stress:** Stress increases you chances of having hypertension.
- **Physical inactivity:** Inactive men and women may have high blood pressure.

Some women develop pregnancy-induced hypertension or preeclampsia (a complication characterized by high blood pressure and fluid retention) during their last trimester. Blood pressure usually returns to normal after delivery, but be sure to tell your health care practitioner about any history of abnormal blood pressure, including that in a past pregnancy.

Why all the worry about hypertension? Because when your blood pressure is high, your heart has to work harder. Over time, this hard work causes your heart muscle to thicken abnormally so that it no longer pumps blood as efficiently. Unlike healthy blood vessels that stretch and contract like an elastic band, constant high blood pressure causes blood vessels to become hard, scarred, and less elastic. And hypertension also speeds the buildup of atherosclerotic plaque in your arteries. Eventually, high blood pressure can cause you to have a stroke, heart attack, and kidney problems and even go blind.

Recognizing the signs

Having high blood pressure doesn't make you feel any different. In fact, as many as 35 percent of people with hypertension don't even know they have it. Hypertension doesn't come with any obvious symptoms. The only way to know you have hypertension is to have your blood pressure checked. That's why it's called the "silent killer."

Knowing for sure

Checking your blood pressure is quick and easy by using a stethoscope and a *sphygmomanometer,* which consists of an inflatable cuff to wrap around your arm, a bulb that pumps air into or lets it out of the cuff, and a manometer, or gauge, from which the actual blood pressure numbers are read. You should have your blood pressure checked by your doctor at least every two years.

Don't be alarmed if your blood pressure is high on one blood pressure reading. Blood pressure can vary as much as 30 points on the same day, depending on the time, your stress level, recent salt intake, and other factors. To be diagnosed with hypertension, you need at least two elevated readings taken at two different visits.

Making it better

If you have high blood pressure, your doctor will first recommend lifestyle changes to try to lower your blood pressure. When these self-care measures aren't enough to control high blood pressure, your doctor will prescribe one or more medications for you to take.

Fortunately, you can do plenty to keep your blood pressure under control. To reduce your blood pressure

- ✔ **Halt the salt:** Cut back on sodium in your diet by avoiding salty foods and resisting the urge to reach for the salt shaker. And watch for hidden sodium in canned foods and bottled condiments.

- ✔ **Drop extra weight:** Lose those extra pounds.

- ✔ **Quit drinking:** Reduce the amount of alcohol you drink.

- ✔ **Work out:** Exercise regularly for at least 30 minutes, three to four times a week.

- ✔ **Avoid cigarettes:** Quit smoking and avoid secondhand smoke.

- ✔ **Relax:** Reduce stress.

- ✔ **Practice safe living:** Have your blood pressure checked at least once a year.

The most common classes of drugs that your doctor may prescribe to reduce your blood pressure include the following:

- ✔ **Diuretics:** These drugs help your kidneys flush excess water out of your body. Without this extra water load, your heart doesn't have to work as hard. Along with water, certain diuretics also cause you to lose potassium, and you may need to eat more potassium in your diet or take a potassium supplement. Other diuretics are potassium-sparing and do not carry this concern. Some common diuretics include furosemide (Lasix), chlorothiazide (Diuril), and chlorthalidone (Hygroton).

- ✔ **Sympathetic nerve inhibitors:** The sympathetic nerves carry messages from your brain to your arteries, telling them to narrow. Very simply, narrowed arteries raise your blood pressure. This class of drugs blocks these messages, allowing the arteries to relax and lower your blood pressure. Think of how you need a higher water pressure to get water to flow through a garden hose that you've narrowed by bending in half. When you release the hose, lower water pressure gets water to flow through it. The most common are beta-blockers, which include propranolol (Inderal), nadolol (Corgard), and metoprolol (Lopressor). Other sympathetic nerve inhibiting drugs are clonidine (Catapres), methyldopa (Aldomet), and prazosin (Minipress).

- ✔ **Vasodilators:** These drugs relax the blood vessels so that blood flows without resistance and include hydralazine (Apresoline) and minoxidil (Loniten).

- ✔ **Calcium channel blockers:** These drugs also reduce the heart rate, dilate the blood vessels, and reduce resistance to blood flow. Some examples are nifedipine (Procardia XL), diltiazem (Cardizem), and verapamil (Isoptin).

✔ **Angiotensin-converting enzyme (ACE) inhibitors:** ACE inhibitors block production of the active form of angiotensin, a substance in the body that makes arteries constrict and include captopril (Capoten), enalapril (Vasotec), and lisinopril (Prinivil). A diuretic may be added to enhance the potency of an ACE inhibitor.

Many blood pressure-lowering drugs may cause your blood pressure to drop when you suddenly sit or stand up from a lying position, making you feel dizzy or faint. So, sit or stand slowly, especially at night when you've been lying in bed. Dangle your feet over the side of the bed for a few minutes before standing up.

An ounce of prevention

You can reduce your risk of developing high blood pressure by reducing or modifying the risk factors over which you have some control. This means making the lifestyle changes recommended to help you keep your blood pressure under control.

For more information on heart disease, high blood pressure, and stroke, contact

✔ The American Heart Association, 7272 Greenville Ave., Dallas, TX 75231-4596; 800-AHA-USA1 (call 800-553-6321 for the American Heart Association's Stroke Connection); www.amhrt.org

✔ The National Stroke Association, 848 E. Orchard Rd., Suite 1000, Englewood, CO 80111; 303-771-1700; 800-787-6537; www.stroke.org

Chapter 16

Cancer

According to a 1997 report in the *Journal of the National Cancer Institute,* more than one-third of American women will develop cancer at some time in their lives.

But cancer is not necessarily a death sentence. The National Cancer Institute estimates that approximately 8 million Americans alive today have a history of cancer, many of whom can be considered "cured." In fact, an estimated 40 percent of the Americans who developed cancer in 1998 are expected to be alive in 2003. Experts reported the first ever drop in cancer death rates in 1996 and a drop in cancer incidence in 1998. And research has shown that you can take specific actions to significantly reduce your risk of becoming that one in three. This chapter looks at the origins and risk factors of many of the cancers that affect women, as well as diagnosis, treatment, and ways to reduce your risk.

Understanding Cancer Basics

Cancer — an uncontrolled growth and spread of abnormal cells — is actually a general name for about 100 different diseases characterized by the following traits:

✔ **Abnormal cell division:** Unlike normal, healthy cells, which grow, divide, and replace themselves to keep the body healthy, cancer cells don't have the control mechanism that turns off growth; they divide without restraint. When cancer cells divide over and over, they can become an abnormal growth called a *tumor*. Cancerous, or *malignant*, tumors can push aside or invade healthy tissue and cause organs to stop functioning.

✔ **Invasiveness:** Cancer cells often crowd out their neighboring cells and affect the function and growth of normal cells by competing with them for available nutrients. The cancerous growth takes over the organs so that they can no longer perform their usual duties.

✔ **Metastasis:** Cancer cells can spread from their original site to other organs, often via the blood or lymph system, a process known as *metastasis*.

✔ **Recurrence:** Cancer has a tendency to come back. After a period of remission, in which symptoms decrease or disappear, it may strike again, in the same part of the body or elsewhere.

Cancer can affect any body organ or tissue. In fact, we often refer to cancer in terms of the organ in which it originated (breast cancer or lung cancer, for example). Left untreated, cancer is usually fatal; its tendency to invade healthy tissue causes organs to cease functioning until the patient dies. However, sometimes cancer can go into spontaneous remission, which means that the symptoms either decrease or disappear entirely.

There is no one cause of cancer, and no one knows exactly why cancer develops in some people but not in others, but both external and internal factors play a role in cancer development. People who are exposed to environmental carcinogens (cancer-causing agents) such as high doses of ultraviolet light, radiation, tobacco smoke, asbestos, and toxic industrial substances, for example, are likely to get cancer. Poor dietary habits can also increase the risk of certain cancers, as can infection. Internal factors, such as hormones, immune and metabolic conditions, and heredity also contribute to cancer.

If cancer is caught early on, before it's destroyed much surrounding tissue or spread to other parts of body, the chances of a cure are much greater.

Detecting and Diagnosing Cancer

Because early detection increases the rate of cure, screening tests — periodic tests to discover the most common forms of cancers — have become a standard part of health care. Some screening tests, such as Pap tests and mammograms, are recommended for all women of a certain age, while others, such as screening tests for ovarian cancer, are recommended only for women who are at high risk.

In addition to undergoing the recommended screening tests, you need to be self-aware and look for any unusual changes. The American Cancer Society recommends that you see your doctor immediately if you notice any of the following warning signs of cancer:

✔ A change in bowel or bladder habits (frequency, consistency, pain)

✔ A sore that does not heal

✔ Unusual bleeding or discharge

✔ Thickening or a lump in a breast or elsewhere

✔ Indigestion or difficulty swallowing

✔ An obvious change in a wart or mole

✔ A nagging cough or hoarseness

If your doctor suspects cancer, she will likely perform tests, including x-rays, blood tests, and a *biopsy,* a laboratory study of a tissue sample, to confirm the diagnosis. Diagnosis involves analyzing a sample of cells under a microscope. Because each type of cancer has its own rate of growth and spreading pattern, your doctor or *oncologist* (a doctor who specializes in treating cancer) will perform tests to identify the type and location of the cancer, as well as the extent to which it has progressed.

Doctors and scientists have developed a staging system to help identify how far a type of cancer has progressed. Each type of cancer has its own specific staging system. But in general, the stages of cancer are

✔ **Carcinoma in situ:** This term, which means "in place," refers to a very early cancer that is limited to the surface of the organ involved.

✔ **Stage I – Stage IV:** Stages representing the progression from cancer that is localized to metastatic cancer (cancer that has spread to distant organs).

✔ **Recurrent stage:** Cancer that has reappeared.

Treating Cancer

Depending on the type of cancer and how far it's spread, cancer treatment may consist of a single treatment or a combination of treatments. The primary treatment (often surgery) is often followed by an adjuvant, or supplemental, therapy, such as chemotherapy. The three most common cancer therapies are surgery, radiation therapy, and chemotherapy.

Surgery

You can have surgery to determine whether a tumor is cancerous or not (called a biopsy); to stage the cancer; to remove a tumor; to remove most of a tumor (to make either chemotherapy or radiation therapy more effective); to relieve obstruction or pressures on nearby organs; or to check how far the cancerous cells have spread.

Surgery removes cancer cells from the body, thereby reducing the chances that the cancer will persist, metastasize, or recur. In this respect, surgery can actually cure a fair number of cancers. Surgery also increases the likelihood that further treatments will be successful. If the cancer is widespread, however, surgery is less likely to effect a cure.

Radiation therapy

Radiation therapy is the process of aiming radiation at the site of the cancerous tumor in order to kill the cancerous cells. This therapy has its greatest effects on the area of the body that it's aimed at.

Radiation is sometimes used as the sole treatment for cancer. It can also be used to shrink a tumor before surgery; to kill any remaining cancer cells after surgery; or in combination with chemotherapy. Radiation is also used to shrink tumors and prolong life when a total cure is unlikely.

Radiation can damage normal tissue as well as cancerous growths, and it does have side effects, such as diarrhea, dry mouth, hair loss, loss of energy, nausea, skin irritation, and difficulty swallowing. Depending on where the radiation is aimed (and how much radiation is used), these side effects can be intense or minimal.

Chemotherapy

Chemotherapy is the use of drugs to treat illness. Chemotherapy is *systemic,* which means that the drugs travel through your whole body and that healthy cells can also be affected. Any cell that divides rapidly (cancerous or not) is vulnerable. Normal cells usually recover shortly after treatment, however.

Chemotherapy can be administered orally (by mouth) or intravenously (through a vein). It can also be injected into a muscle or a body cavity. Depending on the drug, your state of health, and the potential side effects, you may be treated as an inpatient or outpatient in a hospital or as an outpatient in a clinic, your doctor's office, or at home. Regardless of the setting, chemotherapy is administered in cycles: a treatment period followed by a rest period, then another treatment period, and so on.

Because anticancer drugs affect cells that divide rapidly, they can also affect healthy cells such as the cells of your hair and stomach lining (which grow quickly), or the white blood cells that fight off infection, or the blood platelets that help the blood to clot, or the red blood cells that carry oxygen. For this reason, chemotherapy can have a wide variety of side effects, including hair loss, nausea/vomiting, mouth sores, susceptibility to infection, anemia, lowered white blood cell count, bone marrow depression (lowered ability to make red and white blood cells and platelets), changes in smell and taste, loss of appetite, tiredness and body aches, bloating and/or weight gain, and irregular menstrual periods or no period at all.

Most women experience a few side effects, but the majority of side effects disappear a few days after treatment. Some, such as hair loss, may take several weeks to disappear after the treatment ends.

Other treatments

Your doctor determines the appropriate combination of therapy based on your specific cancer stage and health situation. Depending on the type of cancer you have, other therapies that you may receive include the following:

- **Hormone therapy:** This therapy fights types of cancer that depend on hormones to grow (such as certain kinds of breast cancer). Drugs are used to stop hormone production or block the way hormones work, which prevents or inhibits cancer cells from growing. Side effects are usually mild but can include nausea, vomiting, swelling, weight gain, and, in some cases, hot flashes.

- **Immunotherapy:** This treatment introduces a synthetic form of a naturally occurring substance (such as the protein interferon) into your body to boost your body's natural defenses against cancer. Immunotherapy can also be used to protect the body from some of the side effects of other treatments. But it may have other effects of its own, including flulike symptoms.

- **Bone marrow transplant:** This treatment is useful for particularly aggressive or recurrent forms of cancer. High doses of chemotherapy and radiation can damage bone marrow (the inner active core of long bones), which produces new cells and helps maintain the body's immune system. In a bone marrow transplant, doctors remove, store, and then replace bone marrow after high-dose chemo treatment is complete. Alternatively, doctors may replace your marrow with that of a donor.

- **Monoclonal antibodies:** This treatment uses drugs that contain antibodies to deliver an anticancer effect directly to tumor cells.

- **Hyperthermia:** In this treatment, heat is used to stimulate white blood cells to attack cancer cells.

- **Laser treatment:** In this treatment, a laser beam is used to destroy cancer cells in a tumor by cauterizing them (burning them off).

Trying other avenues: Alternative cancer treatments

Most alternative cancer therapies (with the exception of experimental medical therapies) take the approach of helping the body heal itself, rather than attempting to kill off cancerous cells, and you can use many of them in conjunction with traditional cancer treatment. Be aware, however, that delaying traditional treatments to pursue alternatives can affect the success of traditional therapy.

Here are some alternatives that you may wish to investigate:

✔ **Psychological approach:** Counseling and focused imagery are used to enhance your quality of life, relieve pain and discomfort, reduce stress, and help you accept and deal with the physical crisis you are undergoing.

✔ **Diet:** Healthy diets stressing whole foods, fruits and vegetables, and nutritional or vitamin/mineral supplements are used to promote your overall health.

✔ **Health-promoting lifestyles:** Yoga, aerobic exercise, relaxation exercises, and detoxification (eliminating "chemicals" such as preservatives from your diet, avoiding car exhaust fumes, and so on) are used to develop a healthful way of life that supports the body in the process of healing damaged cells.

✔ **Spiritual approaches:** Faith healing and therapeutic touch are used to call on spiritual aids in support of healing.

✔ **Alternative immune stimulating therapies:** These therapies, including acupuncture, herbal remedies, and Chinese medicine are thought to bolster the body's immune system in some cases.

✔ **Clinical medical studies:** Participation in studies of the unconventional use of high-dose chemotherapy, radiation, and hyperthermia are a final option.

Pain relief

In addition to treatments designed to remove or kill cancer cells or stop them from growing, cancer treatment may involve treatment for pain.

Pain occurs in most cases of cancer, and it may be severe, especially in terminal stages. But not all people with cancer experience severe pain.

Cancer pain depends on the type of cancer and the stage of the disease. Pain may be caused by the growth of a tumor, which places pressure on a nerve, or poor circulation, which blocks the function of an organ. Pain can also result from side effects or complications of treatments, such as infection, and it can be dull or sharp, constant or intermittent, mild or severe.

Treatment for cancer pain, obviously, depends on its severity. For mild or moderate pain, your doctor may suggest or prescribe pain-relieving drugs, such as aspirin, and nonsteroidal anti-inflammatory drugs, such as acetaminophen (Tylenol) and ibuprofen (Advil). For severe pain, your doctor may prescribe narcotics, such as morphine and codeine. Other medications prescribed for cancer pain relief include antidepressants, anticonvulsants, steroids, and tranquilizers, which may help you tolerate discomfort.

Other types of pain relief, which can be used alone or in combination with medication to either reduce pain or reduce anxiety and help you cope with pain, include acupuncture, hypnosis, biofeedback, breathing and relaxation techniques, massage, and the application of hot or cold packs.

Breast Cancer

According to the *Journal of the National Cancer Institute,* a woman has a 12.6 percent chance of developing breast cancer in her lifetime — that's one in every eight women. Breast cancer is the second major cause of cancer death for women, but breast cancer itself is not lethal. The disease kills by spreading to other parts of the body.

Breast cancer comes in at least 15 different varieties; the type is defined based on where it develops, how far it has progressed, and the appearance of the cancer cells.

The risk of developing breast cancer goes up as you grow older. Factors that may put you at higher risk include the following:

- ✔ A personal or family history of breast cancer and/or ovarian cancer

- ✔ *Atypical hyperplasia* (abnormal cell growth that may lead to cancer) that has been confirmed by biopsy

- ✔ Early *menarche* (the onset of menstruation)

- ✔ Late menopause

- ✔ Recent use of oral contraceptives or postmenopausal estrogens

- ✔ Having no full-term pregnancies or having your first child after age 30

If you are wondering whether you should be tested for the breast cancer genes — known clinically as the BRCA genetic markers — you may find it helpful to know that experts do not believe that widespread screening of women is warranted because only a very small percentage of women carry the gene. However, you may want to consider being screened if you have a family history of breast and ovarian cancers, four or more close relatives with breast cancer, or are of Ashkenazi ancestry. Not all women who have breast cancer carry this gene, but those who have this gene are at increased risk.

Recognizing the signs

According to the American Cancer Society's screening guidelines, every woman should examine her breasts monthly once she reaches age 20 (see Chapter 2 for more information on the breast self-exam). If you are between the ages of 20 and 40, you should also ask your doctor to perform a physical breast examination (similar to the breast self-exam) every three years. Once you are over 40, you should have an exam once a year.

Be aware, however, that many symptoms don't appear in the earliest stages of breast cancer. Early breast cancer often shows up as an abnormality on a mammogram before the growth is big enough for you or your health care provider can feel it. Alternately, a lump or thickening doesn't mean that you necessarily have breast cancer. About 80 percent of biopsies performed on breast abnormalities show noncancerous conditions. (For more information about noncancerous breast conditions, see Chapter 19.)

Experts now recommend that you have a mammogram performed every year or two if you are between the ages of 40 and 49 and every year from age 50 on.

Knowing for sure

Your doctor can detect suspicious or abnormal areas of the breast by hand, mammogram, or ultrasound. But only a biopsy can determine whether a suspicious area is cancerous or benign.

Doctors can perform a breast biopsy using several different methods. The most common are as follows:

- ✔ **Fine-needle aspiration:** In this office procedure, your doctor inserts a thin needle into the lump to drain fluid, which can then be sent to a pathology laboratory to be analyzed for cancerous cells.

- ✔ **Needle-core biopsy:** This procedure, which is also done on an out-patient basis, involves a larger needle to obtain a better sample and requires a local anesthetic to numb the breast. Your doctor inserts the needle into the area thought to be suspicious to remove a small piece of tissue.

- ✔ **Open biopsy:** Open biopsy is a surgical procedure. Your doctor surgically removes either part or all of the lump through a skin incision in the operating room while you are under anesthesia.

Making it better

Breast cancer treatment is based on its type and stage and the woman's overall health. Surgery is the most common method of treatment, although radiation can be used as an alternative.

Surgical procedures, shown in Figure 16-1, include the following:

- ✓ **Lumpectomy:** Removal of the abnormal cancerous lump and a thin margin of surrounding tissue
- ✓ **Partial or total mastectomy:** Removal of part or all the breast
- ✓ **Radical mastectomy:** Removal of the entire breast, lymph nodes, and some chest muscles

Though mastectomy is still frequently chosen, lumpectomy in certain cases is equally effective. Studies have shown that for early stage cancer, women who have had a lumpectomy followed by radiation therapy live just about as long as women who have had a radical mastectomy.

Other therapies that may be used alone, or in combination with surgery, include chemotherapy; radiation therapy; tamoxifen (a drug that blocks the action of estrogen), which can theoretically increase the risk of recurrence of some breast cancers; paclitaxel (Taxol), a drug that reduces the risk of recurrence in patients with breast cancer that has spread to nearby lymph nodes; immunotherapy; and treatment with the drug 5-fluorouracil (5-FU), which can be delivered continuously by an intravenous pump, or the new oral drug capecitabine (Xeloda). Both drugs have been found to help shrink tumors in some advanced breast cancer patients whose cancer has already spread and whose other options have been exhausted.

For those women who must undergo a mastectomy, significant advances have been made in breast reconstruction techniques. Often, surgeons can perform breast reconstruction at the same time as the mastectomy.

Figure 16-1:
Surgical
options:
Lumpectomy,
total
mastectomy,
and radical
mastectomy.

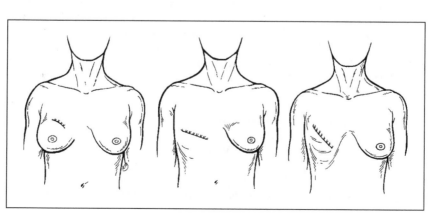

An ounce of prevention

You can do several things to reduce your risk of developing breast cancer:

- ✔ **Maintain a normal weight:** Weight gain, particularly after menopause, has been linked to an increase in breast cancer risk. Being overweight also makes breast exams more difficult.

- ✔ **Eat more fresh fruits, vegetables, and fiber:** Some evidence shows that fruits and vegetables, which contain antioxidant vitamins and other nutrients, offer protection against cancer.

- ✔ **Cut down on alcohol:** Studies show that the risk of breast cancer is significantly higher in women who have two to five drinks daily.

- ✔ **Re-evaluate hormone replacement therapy (HRT):** Be aware that some studies show that prolonged HRT may increase breast cancer risk. Chapter 20 discusses HRT.

- ✔ **Exercise:** Regular exercise has been linked to reduced breast cancer risk in several studies.

- ✔ **Don't smoke:** Researchers estimate that approximately half of all women are sensitive to the carcinogens in tobacco and, as a result, have a higher breast cancer risk.

- ✔ **Eat phytoestrogens:** Research has shown that women with a high intake of phytoestrogens, plant chemicals similar to estrogen, have a lower risk of breast cancer. Phytoestrogens are found in soybeans and soy products, flaxseed, whole grains, and some fruits and vegetables.

Cervical Cancer

Cervical cancer, or cancer of the *cervix* (the opening of the uterus that connects into the vagina), is one of the easiest cancers to prevent and detect. The majority of cases are closely associated with the human papilloma virus (HPV), a sexually transmitted virus whose spread can be prevented by practicing safe sex (see Chapter 22).

A routine Pap smear can detect cervical cancer in the early stages. When caught in its early stages, cervical cancer is one of the most effectively treated forms of cancer.

You are at increased risk of developing cervical cancer if

- ✔ You were sexually active before age 18.
- ✔ You've had multiple sex partners.
- ✔ You've had partners who have had multiple sex partners.

✔ You have genital herpes.

✔ You have genital warts. (Genital warts are caused by HPV.)

✔ You smoke.

✔ Your mother took diethylstilbestrol (DES) during pregnancy.

✔ You have a history of syphilis and gonorrhea.

Recognizing the signs

Cervical cancer is preceded by the development of abnormal cells known as cervical intraepithelial neoplasia (CIN), or dysplasia.

 Not all women with CIN develop cervical cancer, though cervical cancer develops from CIN. It is not possible to predict which women with CIN will go on to develop cervical cancer, so any suspicion of CIN needs to be worked up and treated.

You can have cervical cancer for as long as four to ten years without experiencing any symptoms. Symptoms don't appear until the cancer starts invading the deeper tissues. Consequently, the only way to detect cervical cancer in its early stages is with a Pap test.

As cervical cancer progresses, the most common symptoms are abnormal vaginal bleeding, bleeding after intercourse, unusually long menstrual periods, and abnormal vaginal discharge. Pain and general symptoms, such as fatigue, only develop after the disease is in its late stages.

Knowing for sure

Because the symptoms of cervical cancer take so long to develop, the first stage in diagnosis is usually the Pap test, a microscopic examination of a sample of cells taken from the cervix to screen for cervical cancer.

If an abnormal Pap test reveals potentially precancerous cells, your doctor can perform any of a number of tests to verify the diagnosis. She may start with an office procedure called a *colposcopy,* in which she looks at your cervix through a specially designed magnifying lens. She may then take tissue samples to analyze in the laboratory under the microscope.

Cervical biopsy methods include the following:

✔ **Punch biopsy:** In this procedure, the doctor uses an instrument resembling a long-handled paper punch to remove a sample of tissue about the size of half a grain of rice.

✔ **Endocervical curettage (ECC):** In this procedure, your doctor scrapes tissue from the cervical canal with a special instrument called a curette.

✔ **Loop electrosurgical excision procedure (LEEP):** This procedure uses low-voltage cautery attached to a stainless steel wire loop to shave off the surface of the cervix that contains the abnormal cells. The cautery attached to the loop seals blood vessels and lowers the risk of bleeding. A LEEP is an office procedure done under local anesthesia.

✔ **Conization:** Also known as cone biopsy, conization involves the surgical removal of a cone-shaped piece of tissue from the center of the cervix. It requires anesthesia in an operating room setting.

Regardless of how the tissue sample is taken, it is then examined under a microscope to look for cancerous cells.

Making it better

Treatment for cervical disease depends on the stage. Dysplasia, which is confined to the surface of the cervix, can be treated with conservative local therapies. Here are some other options:

✔ **Cryosurgery:** The cancerous cells are killed by freezing the surface of the cervix. This treatment is used for earlier stages of the disease.

✔ **Laser surgery:** A laser is used to cut away the cancerous part of the cervix.

✔ **Loop electrosurgical excision procedure (LEEP):** Low-voltage cautery is used to remove the cancerous section of the cervix.

✔ **Conization:** A cone-shaped section of tissue is removed.

Treatment of actual cervical cancer is different and is based on the level to which the malignant cells have invaded beyond the surface of the cervix:

✔ **Hysterectomy:** Surgery is reserved for early cases of invasive cancer confined to the cervix itself.

If the cancer is no longer just on the surface and has moved more deeply into the cervical tissue, your doctor may have to remove your cervix and uterus. If the cancer is farther along, she may have to perform a *radical hysterectomy,* which involves removal of the cervix, uterus, the upper third of the vagina, and the lymph nodes in your groin area. If necessary, she may also remove your ovaries and fallopian tubes, a procedure known as a *bilateral salpingo-oophorectomy.*

✔ **Radiation:** This therapy is used to treat cervical cancer that has spread locally within the pelvis.

Your doctor may use chemotherapy in an effort to make sure that all the cancerous cells have been eliminated.

An ounce of prevention

To reduce your risk of developing cervical cancer

> ✔ **Get regular Pap tests:** Pap tests can detect dysplasia at an early stage before invasive cancer develops.
>
> ✔ **Don't smoke:** Women who smoke are at least three times more likely to develop cervical cancer.
>
> ✔ **Practice safe sex:** Practicing safe sex (see Chapter 22) can reduce the risk of cervical cancer associated with HPV and other sexually transmitted diseases.

Colorectal Cancer

Colorectal cancer is cancer of the large intestine. Your large intestine includes the *cecum* (the pouch where the small intestine meets the large intestine), the *colon* (the main section of the intestine), and the *rectum* (the last 8 or 10 inches of the colon). Although either the colon or rectum can be affected, the disease is often called colorectal cancer.

Because the majority of cases of colorectal cancer occur in people over age 50, regular screening is recommended for all women beginning at age 50. You should begin screening earlier or undergo it more often if you have a personal or family history of colorectal cancer or *polyps* (little growths on the mucous membranes of the colon) or a history of inflammatory bowel disease.

Other risk factors include the following:

> ✔ A history of breast, endometrial, or ovarian cancer
>
> ✔ A low-fiber, high-fat diet
>
> ✔ An inactive lifestyle

Recognizing the signs

Some warning signs of colorectal cancer are diarrhea or increasing constipation; rectal bleeding or blood in your stool; skinny stool; frequent gas pains; a feeling like you aren't getting all the stool out; unexplained weight loss; constant fatigue; and anemia. Of course, many of these symptoms are also symptoms of other problems (some of them very common and ordinary). But don't hesitate to see your doctor if any of these symptoms persist for more than two weeks.

Knowing for sure

Your doctor has a variety of tests at her disposal to diagnose colorectal cancer:

- **Digital rectal exam (DRE):** In this test, your doctor inserts a gloved finger into your rectum and feels the rectal wall for lesions.

- **Sigmoidoscopy:** In this test, your doctor inserts a thin, lighted scope called a *sigmoidoscope* into your rectum to examine it. With a sigmoidoscope, your doctor can see the lower 10 or 12 inches of the rectum and colon. She can also take a tissue sample for biopsy.

- **Fecal occult blood test:** For this test, which you can also do at home (see Chapter 8), you collect stool samples. These samples are then examined under a microscope for blood.

- **Colonoscopy:** In this test, your doctor uses a flexible, thin, lighted scope called a *colonoscope* to view your colon. She can also take a tissue sample for a biopsy. This test is similar to a sigmoidoscopy but views a higher area of the large intestine.

- **Lower gastrointestinal series (GI):** For this two-part test, you are given a barium enema, which makes your intestinal tract stand out in contrast, and then are x-rayed.

- **CT scan or MRI:** Both the CT scan and MRI are used to create a detailed image of your colon and rectal area.

Making it better

Surgery is the most common treatment for colorectal cancer, though radiation therapy and chemotherapy may also be used, especially if the cancer has spread to the lymph nodes or beyond the bowel wall. Surgery options may include the following:

- **Polypectomy:** A cancerous polyp is removed. (If the cancer is localized to the polyp itself.)

- **Wedge resection:** A surrounding margin of tissue is also removed. (If it seems the cancer is beginning to spread.)

- **Bowel resection:** The cancerous tissue in the bowel is removed along with the nearby lymph nodes. If the cancer only occupies a small area of the bowel, the normal areas of the bowel on the margins can be sewn back together.

- **Colostomy:** An abdominal opening is made so that body wastes can be eliminated into a bag.

An ounce of prevention

To prevent colorectal cancer, do the following:

- **Cut down on fats:** Cutting down on fats (especially animal fats) reduces colorectal cancer risk.

- **Cut down on red meat:** Studies have shown that people who eat fish or chicken or no meat at all have a lower incidence of colorectal cancer than people who eat red meat.

- **Exercise:** Regular exercise is thought to reduce the risk of all cancers, including colorectal cancer.

- **Eat well:** Eat high-fiber foods, such as fruits, vegetables, and whole grains. These foods help digestion and cut down on the time that the lining of your intestines is exposed to carcinogens.

- **Cut down on alcohol:** Excessive alcohol intake has been linked over the long term to colorectal cancer and most cancers in general.

Endometrial Cancer

The *endometrium* is the lining of your uterus. Cancer of the uterus is called endometrial cancer because the vast majority start in the endometrium. This slow-growing cancer is one of the most curable and one of the most common. Endometrial cancer most often occurs after menopause, although it may occur earlier if you have risk factors.

Several risk factors are associated with endometrial cancer, and most of them have to do with prolonged exposure to estrogen. You're at higher risk for developing endometrial cancer if you

- Are over age 55

- Started your menstrual cycle early and/or entered menopause later than most women

- Are obese (fatty tissue converts some hormones into a form of estrogen)

- Have (or had) a problem with infertility

- Don't ovulate

- Have used estrogen therapy *without progesterone* over the long term

- Have a history of diabetes and high blood pressure

- Have used tamoxifen, which helps prevent recurrences of breast tumors

Recognizing the signs

The most common warning sign of endometrial cancer is abnormal vaginal bleeding, especially if it occurs *after* menopause. For women who have not gone through menopause, the warning signs include very irregular menstrual periods and/or bleeding between periods. As with other cancers of the reproductive tract, pain is *not* one of the first symptoms of endometrial cancer. Pain occurs much later as the cancer spreads (as does weight loss).

Some women may have no symptoms of endometrial cancer at all.

Knowing for sure

Your doctor can sometimes detect advanced endometrial cancer during a pelvic exam. Additional tests to confirm the diagnosis may include *endometrial aspiration* (in which a special vacuum is used to obtain a tissue sample for biopsy), *dilation and curettage* (in which a curette is used to scrape a tissue sample for biopsy), *ultrasound* (in which sound waves are used to create a picture of the inside of the uterus), and a *hysteroscopy* (in which a special microscope is used to examine the uterus).

Making it better

Doctors treat endometrial cancer in various ways, depending on the stage at which it is diagnosed. If your doctor diagnoses you with a precancerous condition such as *atypical hyperplasia*, you could be treated with the hormone progesterone for several weeks.

If endometrial cancer is diagnosed, your doctor usually recommends surgery, and you may need to have a hysterectomy and, possibly, a salpingo-oophorectomy. For more information on these procedures, see Chapter 20.

Lung Cancer

Since 1987, the leading cause of cancer deaths among women has been lung cancer (previously it was breast cancer). And the greatest risk factor for developing lung cancer is smoking. According to the American Lung Association, 87 percent of lung cancer deaths can be attributed to smoking.

You are at a greater risk of developing lung cancer if you smoke one or more packs of cigarettes a day for 20 years or more, started smoking before you were 20 years old, or have been exposed regularly to secondhand smoke. Exposure to radon, industrial materials such as asbestos, uranium, nickel, arsenic, coal dust, and chromates, radiation, and air pollution also increases your risk. You also may be at higher risk if you have (or had) diseases such as tuberculosis, emphysema, and other forms of chronic obstructive pulmonary disease, or even if you eat a diet that's low in vitamin A.

The two types of lung cancer, based on their cell type under the microscope, are small cell and nonsmall cell. Small cell lung cancer develops and spreads rapidly and accounts for about 20 percent of lung cancer cases.

About 80 percent of lung cancer cases are the result of nonsmall cell cancer. If caught in the early stages, nonsmall cell cancer is potentially curable — *if* the patient quits smoking.

Recognizing the signs

Lung cancer is very difficult to diagnose early because it doesn't have any symptoms until it has spread and is in its late stages. Once symptoms develop, they may include the following: a nagging cough (as a growing tumor blocks your airway), coughing up blood, persistent symptoms of pneumonia or bronchitis, chest pain or discomfort, shortness of breath, hoarseness, fever that doesn't have a definite cause, and weakness or fatigue for no other reason.

Knowing for sure

Most likely, your doctor will take a chest x-ray. He may test the mucous you cough up for abnormal cells. Your doctor may also select one of a variety of procedures to help in the diagnosis, including the following:

- **CAT scan or MRI:** Both are used to get a more detailed image of the lung.

- **Bronchoscopy:** A thin, flexible scope called a *bronchoscope* is threaded through your mouth or nose down into a lung to look at your lung tissue. A tissue sample can also be taken for biopsy.

- **Percutaneous needle biopsy:** A needle is inserted into your chest and used to remove a tissue sample for biopsy.

- **Mediastinoscopy:** A small scope called a mediastinoscope is inserted into an incision in the chest into the small area between your lungs, breastbone, and spine to look at the lymph nodes.

- **Thoracotomy:** An incision is made in the chest, cutting into the lung to remove a tissue sample for biopsy.

- **Video-assisted thoracoscopic surgery (VATS):** This method is used to determine how far the cancer has progressed (the stage of the disease). A few small incisions are made in the chest to remove small sections of lung cancer tissue. This process is less complicated than a thoracotomy and reduces the time the patient has to be in the hospital because smaller incisions are required.

✔ **LIFE Lung:** A flexible scope with a fluorescent light is used to locate possibly precancerous tissue. The precancerous tissue looks reddish brown in the light, while healthy tissue looks green.

Making it better

The two types of lung cancer are treated differently, but most treatment decisions are based on the stage at which the cancer is diagnosed:

✔ **Small cell:** This type, which spreads quickly, is usually treated with chemotherapy. About a third of small cell cases are *limited,* which means that the disease is confined to one side of the chest. These cases are treated with radiation therapy as well as chemotherapy.

✔ **Nonsmall cell:** This type is treated with surgery if caught in its early stages. Usually the surgeon removes either a lobe of the involved lung or the entire lung. If the cancer has progressed further, it may be treated with a combination of surgery and chemotherapy or radiation (which may be used to shrink the tumor before it's removed). If the cancer is not removable or has spread widely, chemotherapy and radiation are used.

An ounce of prevention

The best thing you can do to prevent lung cancer is not to smoke. In addition, avoid secondhand smoke and polluted air areas. Exercise in fresh air, and take vitamins.

Ovarian Cancer

Ovarian cancer is cancer of the *ovaries,* the two reproductive organs that produce female hormones and release eggs for fertilization. Sometimes called the "silent killer," ovarian cancer is very difficult to detect in its early stages because there are very few symptoms.

Though a woman can get ovarian cancer at any age, it's most often seen in women ages 55 and over.

Because ovarian cancer is so hard to detect, if you are in a high-risk group, you should be especially careful about getting yearly pelvic exams. Your doctor may also recommend that you be screened periodically by getting an ultrasound and a blood test that checks for the tumor marker CA 125. Although neither of these tests are considered very accurate by themselves (there are a lot of false positives), together they are currently the best tests available. You are considered at higher risk if you

- Are over 50 years old
- Have never been pregnant
- Have a personal or family history of breast or ovarian cancer (especially in a sister, mother, or daughter)
- Have a personal history of menstrual problems or infertility

A small percentage of familial, or genetically inherited, ovarian cancer is associated with two different genetic mutations. Though a very small percentage of women test positive for these genetic mutations, the BRCA1 and BRCA2 genetic markers are associated with increased risk of breast and ovarian cancer. If you think your family history implies that you may have inherited or could be a carrier for one of these genes, you may want to inquire about information on genetic testing.

Recognizing the signs

Most symptoms of ovarian cancer are very vague and nonspecific. The most common sign of ovarian cancer is a bloated abdomen, which is caused by the buildup of fluid in the pelvis. Another indication is vague abdominal discomfort, including gas that just doesn't go away and doesn't seem to be caused by anything in the diet. Abnormal bleeding is only rarely symptomatic of ovarian cancer.

Regular pelvic exams are important because a doctor may pick up ovarian cancer by feeling an enlarged ovary.

Knowing for sure

If your doctor suspects an ovarian growth or tumor, she may recommend an ultrasound of your pelvis. If anything abnormal shows up here, it can be followed by a *computerized axial tomography* scan (*CAT scan*) or MRI to get a visual image of your ovaries. If your doctor suspects that a tumor has spread beyond the ovaries, she may suggest a *lymphangiogram,* an *intravenous pyelogram,* or a *lower gastrointestinal (GI) series.* For these tests, you are injected with a material that shows up contrasts more clearly on an x-ray. Your doctor may also want to perform a *laparoscopy,* in which she makes a small incision in your abdomen under general anesthesia in the operating room in order to insert a viewing device so that she can take a closer look at your ovaries. At this point, she may also take a tissue sample for biopsy and analysis under a microscope in a laboratory.

Making it better

In order to determine the exact stage of ovarian cancer, surgery is first performed. This also allows the doctor to remove as much of the cancer as is surgically possible, including taking out other organs that the cancer has invaded. Often, one or both of the ovaries, the fallopian tubes, and the uterus are removed. If you are young and the disease is caught early, your doctor may remove only the affected ovary so that you can still get pregnant. If your cancer has progressed significantly, your doctor may suggest "debulking" surgery, which removes as much tumor as is surgically possible without endangering vital organs, and then chemotherapy or radiation therapy to destroy more cancerous cells.

You can receive chemotherapy by mouth in pill or capsule form, intravenously, intramuscularly (by deep injection into the muscle), or through a *catheter* (small tube) that is inserted through an incision directly into the abdomen. The catheter method is called *intraperitoneal chemotherapy*. Radiation therapy can also be given via catheter, a procedure called *intra-peritoneal irradiation*.

An ounce of prevention

To prevent ovarian cancer, consider taking oral contraceptives. Studies show that the Pill reduces the risk of ovarian cancer in high-risk women when used for as little as one year. The protection increases the longer you use the Pill — women who use the Pill for ten years have an 80 percent lowered risk of ovarian cancer.

Skin Cancer

The most common form of cancer in the United States is skin cancer. And according to a study by the American Cancer Society and government scientists, skin cancer is one form of cancer that is still on the rise.

The most common types of skin cancer are basal cell carcinoma and squamous cell carcinoma which, when caught early, are highly curable. The main difference between the two (other than how they look and the layer of skin in which they appear) is that basal cell carcinoma rarely spreads, while squamous cell carcinoma can spread. These two types of skin cancer are usually caused by too much exposure to the sun and other ultraviolet light.

The least common — yet most deadly — form of skin cancer is *melanoma*. Melanoma is related to sun exposure. There is no clear data on how many hours of exposure are required, because every person has a different susceptibility (genetic risk). Susceptibility is related in large part to skin type. Melanomas spread quickly.

Overall, you are at higher risk for developing skin cancer if any of the following apply to you:

✔ You are exposed to the sun often and for long periods of time.

✔ You vacation frequently in sunny places.

✔ You have many moles.

✔ You have light skin, light eyes, or fair skin.

✔ You have a tendency to burn or freckle.

✔ You have a history of painful or severe sunburns during childhood.

✔ You have a family history of skin cancer.

✔ You have *actinic keratoses* (precancerous skin patches that look dry and scaly).

Recognizing the signs

Because different kinds of skin cancer look different, you should be on the lookout for a variety of things:

✔ **Basal cell carcinoma:** This type most often looks like little pearly nodes that most often appear on your face around your eyes and nose (though they can be found anywhere on the body). The nodes can become open sores that bleed or crust over. These nodes grow deeper into the layers of your skin and can come back after they're removed.

✔ **Squamous cell carcinoma:** This type starts out as small lumps or flat red areas that slowly grow wart-like. Most often you'll find this type of cancer on areas of the body that are usually uncovered, such as hands, though they, too, can appear anywhere on the body. This kind of cancer can spread, but it develops slowly.

✔ **Melanoma:** This cancer usually develops from a pre-existing mole that gets bigger, changes color, and bleeds or itches. Melanomas also can appear as small brown, black, or multicolored irregular patches. Melanomas can spread quickly, invading all the layers of your skin.

For an easy way to remember the signs that a mole is developing into a melanoma, use the ABCD guide:

✔ **A:** Asymmetry (If the shape of one half of a mole doesn't match the other, talk to your doctor.)

✔ **B:** Borders that are irregular (If the edges of the mole are ragged, blurry, or notched, call your doctor.)

✔ **C:** Color that is variegated, varied within itself (Harmless moles are usually a uniform shade of brown.)

✔ **D:** Diameter bigger than a pencil eraser (Any change in size — sudden or over time — is cause for concern.)

The American Cancer Society recommends that you check your skin for changes in moles and the signs of skin cancer once a month.

Knowing for sure

If you think a mole or an area of your skin looks suspicious, see your doctor or dermatologist. Your doctor will examine the area and take a tissue sample to biopsy.

Making it better

Treatment for skin cancer depends on which type you have and how far its progressed. For basal cell and squamous cell carcinomas, you may be treated with the following:

✔ **Surgical excision:** This is a procedure in which the cancerous tissue is cut out. This may also be called a wide biopsy.

✔ **Radiation therapy:** This is a procedure in which radiation is aimed at the cancerous area.

✔ **Electrodessication/cauterization:** This is a procedure in which the cancerous node is burned off.

✔ **Cryosurgery:** This is a procedure in which the cancerous area of tissue is killed by freezing it off.

✔ **Laser therapy:** This is a procedure in which the cancerous tissue is vaporized with lasers.

✔ **Chemotherapy:** This is a procedure in which drugs are injected into the cancerous tissue to kill the cancer cells.

Melanomas are treated in various ways, depending on their location and depth of penetration of the skin layers. First, the cancerous growth is removed. It is necessary to also remove the nearby lymph nodes to know whether the cancer has begun spreading throughout the body. Depending on the stage of cancer, other therapies may be used as well.

An ounce of prevention

Exposure to the sun's ultraviolet rays is a major contributor to skin cancer. You can protect yourself by taking the following advice:

- Stay out of the sun when it's strongest — between 10 a.m. and 3 p.m.
- Wear sunscreen with a sun protection factor (SPF) of 15 or more daily.
- Cover up. Wear tightly woven clothes that cover your arms and legs.
- Wear a hat with a brim.
- Avoid tanning devices, such as tanning beds and ultraviolet lamps.

For more information on cancer in general or a particular type of cancer, contact one of the following organizations:

- The American Cancer Society, 111599 Clifton Rd., NE, Atlanta, GA 30329; 800-ACS-2345; 404-320-3333; www.cancer.org
- The National Cancer Institute, Cancer Information Service, 9000 Rockville Pike, Building 31, Room 10A31, Bethesda, MD 20892; 800-4-CANCER; 800-638-1234 (Alaska); 800-524-1234 (Hawaii); www.nic.nih.gov
- The National Alliance of Breast Cancer Organizations, 9 E. 37th St., 10th Floor, New York, NY 10016; 212-889-0606; www.nabco.org
- The National Breast Cancer Coalition, 1707 L St., NW, Suite 1060, Washington, DC 20036; 202-296-7477; www.natlbcc.org
- The Y-Me Breast Cancer Support Program, 212 W. Van Buren St., 4th Floor, Chicago, IL 60607; 800-221-2141; 312-986-8228; www.y-me.org
- The Society of Gynecologic Oncologists, 401 N. Michigan Ave., Chicago, IL 60611; 312-644-6610; www.sgo.org
- The American Lung Association, 1740 Broadway, New York, NY 10019; 800-LUNG-USA; 212-315-8700; www.lungusa.org

Chapter 17
Chronic Conditions

. . . .

. . . .

*Y*our new kitten is making you sneeze like crazy. When you finally get to your medicine cabinet, your fingers are so stiff from arthritis that you can't get your medicine bottle open. It's gonna be a bad day, or two, or three.

You have more than a little problem here. You have at least two. And they're *chronic*. That means if you don't fix them properly and keep after them on a daily basis, every day could be just like this one. Agony. This chapter tells you how to tackle chronic conditions, most of them quite serious, and some very debilitating.

Allergies

To survive in this pollen-, dust-, and bee-filled world, allergy sufferers must be tuned in to their surroundings, watching where they step, what they touch, and even what they eat.

About 50 million Americans have an allergy of some kind. Allergies are caused when the body's immune system, designed to attack bacteria, viruses, and other harmful invaders, instead reacts more aggressively than needed to a harmless substance. A sort of chemical reaction follows, causing swelling of body tissues and allergy symptoms such as sneezing, nasal congestion, or a rash.

In most cases, your first contact with an *allergen* — a substance that causes an allergic reaction — won't trigger a reaction. That's because your immune system has not yet developed its arsenal against the substance. Once exposed to a potentially harmful invader, such as a virus — or, in the case of allergy, a harmless invader, such as pollen — your immune system produces substances called *antibodies* to neutralize the invader. These antibodies stay in your body, ready to attack the invader the next time you encounter it.

The list of allergens is as varied as the reactions to them.

Recognizing the signs

Allergy reactions (and some of their common triggers) include the following:

- ✔ **Respiratory allergies:** The most common allergic response is *allergic rhinitis* (often called "hay fever"), which manifests itself in the nasal passages. Exposure to pollens, indoor or outdoor mold spores, *animal dander* (that's the sloughed-off skin of dogs and cats), dust, or a number of less-common triggers cause runny nose, congestion, postnasal drip, and itchy nose, throat, and eyes.

- ✔ **Skin allergies:** *Hives* (itchy, red welts) and eczema and allergic contact dermatitis (both rashes) are all types of skin allergies. Although the cause of hives is not always obvious, the most allergic common triggers are foods, drugs, and insect venom. The reaction can occur all over your body, may not show up until hours after exposure to the allergen, and may last for days on end.

  Eczema, or *atopic dermatitis*, is most common in children, and the majority of people with it have a family history of eczema and a personal history of allergy. Although the connection between eczema and allergy is not exactly clear, it is known that flare-ups of this rash (which Chapter 12 discusses in more detail) can be triggered by some of the same allergens that trigger respiratory allergic reactions — pollen, dust mites, and dander; however, the reaction manifests itself in the skin rather than the nose.

  Allergic contact dermatitis is caused only by direct contact with an allergen, such as the resin in poison ivy, nail polish, hair dye, underarm deodorant, metals, and latex. This type of reaction can occur on first exposure. (Chapter 12 discusses allergic contact dermatitis.)

- ✔ **Systemic reactions:** *Systemic reactions* are reactions that affect the entire body. These reactions range from gastrointestinal symptoms, such as cramping, vomiting, and diarrhea (which are common in food allergies), or a mild case of systemic hives, accompanied by itching, flushing, and swelling, to the more serious reaction known as *anaphylaxis,* which includes swelling of the *larynx* (voice box), difficulty breathing, reduced blood pressure, and, occasionally, shock, cardiac arrest, and death. Systemic reactions are triggered most often by allergies to food, drugs, and insect venom — all substances that are consumed or introduced directly into the body.

Knowing for sure

You may be able to figure out on your own whether you're allergic to something if the symptoms are minor and your contact with an allergen is obvious. If your lips swell and tingle shortly after you eat shrimp, for example, you may be allergic and may want to avoid eating shrimp.

When the trigger is not so obvious or when your symptoms are severe, you should see a doctor to pinpoint the exact cause, and learn how to handle your symptoms and avoid future contact with the allergen. Your family doctor may be helpful in this area or she may refer you to an *allergist,* a doctor who specializes in diagnosing and treating allergies.

Your doctor will take your medical history, likely going over the factors you've already reviewed in your own hunt for the cause of your symptoms. The doctor will also examine you, looking for those telltale hives, runny eyes, swollen nasal passages, and other symptoms. She'll also try to rule out any nonallergy causes for your symptoms.

After the doctor is pretty sure that you're suffering from allergies, you'll likely take one of four skin tests to pinpoint what it is that causes you to react:

- ✔ **Scratch test:** In this test, the doctor or her assistant makes a series of small scratches on your arm or back, rubs a different protein that may cause an allergic reaction into each scratch, and then waits to see whether you react with an itchy, red welt, or *wheal,* at a scratch site within the next 15 to 20 minutes.

- ✔ **Prick test:** This test works much the same way as the scratch test. The doctor or her assistant places small drops of allergens on your skin, and then uses a small needle to prick the skin under the drops. This is the most common allergy test.

- ✔ **Intradermal test:** In this test, the doctor or her assistant injects a solution containing the allergen into the skin, and then watches for your reaction.

- ✔ **Patch test:** This test is used to test for allergic contact dermatitis, which may take several days to manifest. Patches containing suspected allergens are placed on the skin and left there, usually for about 48 hours.

A positive skin test indicates the presence of antibodies. It does not prove that you are allergic to a substance, just that you have the potential to react to it.

The doctor may also suggest a blood test to diagnose the cause of your allergy symptoms. The *radioallergosorbent test,* or *RAST,* uses a single blood sample to measure the amounts of specific antibodies within your blood. If your blood contains a specific antibody, such as an antibody to ragweed pollen, chances are good that you may be allergic to the corresponding allergen.

If your doctor suspects a food allergy, she may ask you to keep a food diary to try to nail down the offending culprit. When your doctor suspects a specific food, she may ask you to avoid that food for a time, and then reintroduce it to see whether you react to it.

Making it better

Self-care for allergies is a two-pronged affair: You need to do what you can to avoid substances to which you're allergic, which may help you avoid allergy attacks. You also need to take steps to alleviate your symptoms when an attack occurs. Here are some tips for avoiding common allergens:

- **Don't stop to smell the roses:** Avoid outdoor allergens, such as pollen and mold, to reduce your chance of reaction. Keep your windows shut, and use your air-conditioning. Avoid mowing the lawn, cutting weeds, or raking leaves. Shower after outdoor activities. Avoid touching your eyes and nose. Wear a mask and gloves when gardening.

- **Ditch the dust:** Dust and damp-mop your home. Get rid of dust-collecting items, such as knickknacks and dried flowers. Keep closet doors closed. Regularly clean furnace and air-conditioning filters. Clean carpets regularly or remove them entirely. Wash your bed linens in hot water every seven to ten days.

- **Stick Fido and Fluffy into the tub:** If you can't bear to part with your pets, consider bathing them regularly to reduce allergens. Wash your hands after playing with your pet. Have someone else clean the litter box.

- **Stop indoor mold in its tracks:** Keep the humidity level of your home below 50 percent (a dehumidifier or air conditioner may help). Check your house for water leaks, repair any you find, and replace any carpeting that has gotten extensively wet or wood that has rotted as a result of water leakage.

When your prevention efforts fail, you can turn to over-the-counter medications for relief. Your choices include the following:

- ✔ **Antihistamines:** Histamine is a chemical mediator in the body that, when released during an allergy attack, produces swelling and itching. Antihistamines, medications that counteract those reactions, are used to control the nasal itching, runny nose, and eye irritation of hay fever as well as to relieve the itching of allergic skin rashes. Antihistamines come in both oral and topical forms, such as nasal sprays, eyedrops, and skin creams and sprays. They are often taken with decongestants. The oral medications can cause drowsiness.

- ✔ **Decongestants:** These are used to reduce swelling in the nasal passages, easing breathing. Like antihistamines, they come in both topical and oral forms. Topical decongestants, which you spray into the nose or drop directly into the eyes, provide quick, temporary relief from nasal congestion.

  Do not use topical decongestants for an extended period of time: Continued use can shorten the drug's effectiveness and lead to a *rebound reaction* — a more severe form of congestion.

- ✔ **Anti-inflammatory drugs:** These drugs, which counter the inflammation that occurs during an allergic reaction, include mast-cell stabilizers and corticosteroids. *Mast-cell stabilizers* keep the mast cells, or tissue cells, from releasing that nasty histamine. The most well-known mast-cell stabilizer is cromolyn sodium, which is available over the counter in a nasal spray. Corticosteroids, such as hydrocortisone, are available over the counter in cream and ointment form to relieve the inflammation of allergic rashes.

If you have allergies, you're stuck with them. With your doctor's help, though, you may be able to control your symptoms and lead a normal life.

Your doctor can prescribe stronger doses of the antihistamines and decongestants available over the counter as well as prescription-only antihistamines and antihistamine/decongestant combinations. Antihistamines available only with a prescription include nonsedating medications such as astimizole (Hismanal), loratadine (Claritin), cetirizine (Zyrtec), and fexofenadine hydrochloride (Allegra). Your doctor can also prescribe stronger versions of topical corticosteroids, as well as oral corticosteroids, which are used as a last resort as a short-term treatment for severe cases of hives and stubborn cases of allergic contact dermatitis.

Other prescription medications available to treat allergy symptoms include *epinephrine*, a synthetic hormone used to stimulate the heart and nervous system, and *leukotriene receptor antagonists*. Epinephrine constricts blood vessels, raises lowered blood pressure, and helps open closed breathing passages. It is most often used to relieve anaphylaxis, the most severe systemic allergic reaction.

Beyond treating symptoms, your doctor may suggest allergy shots. Known as *immunotherapy,* these shots desensitize a person to an allergen. Allergy shots, generally used only on people with allergic rhinitis and allergic asthma, gradually expose the body to small doses of an allergen. The theory is that in time, the allergen will no longer trigger an allergic reaction. The shots are given once or twice a week, and then are gradually decreased. After three to five years, the shots are stopped. New research suggests that the effect of the shots lasts well beyond that time.

An ounce of prevention

There's no surefire way to prevent developing allergies. You stand a pretty good shot — a 20 to 50 percent chance — of developing an allergy if one of your parents has any allergies. If both of your parents have an allergy, your risk shoots up to 40 to 75 percent.

Some research suggests that breast-fed babies have fewer allergy problems later in life. The American Academy of Pediatrics now recommends children be breast-fed for their first year of life to receive the full benefit of their mother's immune system.

For more information on allergies, contact

- ✔ The American College of Allergy, Asthma, and Immunology, 85 W. Algonquin, Suite 550, Arlington Heights, IL 60005; 800-842-7777; www.allergy.mcg.edu

- ✔ The National Institute of Allergy and Infectious Diseases, 31 Center Dr., MSC 2520, Building 31, Room 7A50, Bethesda, MD 20892; 301-496-5717; www.niaid.nig.gov

- ✔ The American Academy of Allergy, Asthma, and Immunology, 611 E. Wells St., Milwaukee, WI 53202; 800-822-2762; www.aaaai.org

Arthritis

You may have thought of arthritis as a condition of old age. Although it is true that almost half of everyone over age 65 has some type of *arthritis,* these diseases of the joints (arthritis literally means joint inflammation) know no age boundaries: Arthritis is the number one cause of disability among Americans over age 15. It afflicts nearly 1 in 6 Americans, about 285,000 of them children. And nearly two-thirds of arthritis sufferers are women.

Researchers have been unable to nail down a specific cause of arthritis, but risk factors for some types of arthritis include obesity, injury, and repetitive motions such as those experienced at work or in sports.

Many conditions fall into the arthritis family. Some of the most common are

- ✔ **Osteoarthritis:** This degenerative joint disease is caused by the deterioration of the cartilage that covers the ends of bones, which forces bones to rub against each other. The result is pain and loss of movement. It is the most common form of arthritis, affecting an estimated 20.7 million Americans, mostly over age 45.

- ✔ **Rheumatoid arthritis:** This condition is an autoimmune disease in which the body's malfunctioning immune system attacks healthy joints, causing swelling, joint damage, reduced movement, and pain. Rheumatoid arthritis afflicts approximately 2.1 million Americans, mostly women. In fact, women are three times more likely than men to develop rheumatoid arthritis. It may also occur at an earlier age than osteoarthritis, even in teenagers.

- ✔ **Gout:** This type of arthritis is caused by deposits of uric acid crystals in joints. It usually strikes a single joint — often the big toe — with sudden, severe pain. It is more common in men.

- ✔ **Infectious arthritis:** This type of arthritis is caused by an infection in a joint. The infections that can cause arthritis include Lyme disease, which is caused by a bacterium transmitted by ticks; gonorrhea, a sexually transmitted disease (see Chapter 22) that produces arthritis in approximately 1 out of 20 people who contract it; and viral infections such as hepatitis B, rubella, and mumps.

Recognizing the signs

Arthritis may not be easy to diagnose on your own when it first takes hold, particularly if you believe you are too young to suffer from it. Among the symptoms to look for are joint pain, stiffness that is worse in the morning, buckling or instability of a joint under stress, and loss of function. You should also look for bony enlargements at the joints, a limited range of motion, tenderness to the touch, and pain during motion of the affected joint.

Knowing for sure

Based on a physical exam and a history of symptoms, a physician can usually diagnose osteoarthritis. X-rays are generally only used to confirm the diagnosis. A lab test for the *rheumatoid factor,* an abnormal substance found in the blood of 80 percent of rheumatoid arthritis sufferers, may be used to detect that condition. And your doctor may take a sample of fluid from the infected joint to diagnose gout or infectious arthritis.

Making it better

No drug or treatment currently exists to cure arthritis (although treatments do exist for many of the infections that cause infectious arthritis). Doctors generally concentrate on controlling arthritis symptoms through physical therapy and pain medication. You can pursue many of these tactics on your own, but consulting a physician is imperative for an accurate diagnosis of the type of arthritis and to be certain you are doing everything possible — not mismanaging your care by unwittingly taking the wrong steps.

If you have arthritis, you may wish to try the following suggestions:

- ✔ **Watch your weight:** Extra pounds mean extra weight and pressure on joints and can make arthritis worse.

- ✔ **Exercise:** Range-of-motion and muscle strengthening exercises can reduce stiffness and help prevent some forms of arthritis from worsening. Check with your doctor or a physical therapist to see what type of exercise is right for you.

- ✔ **Rest:** Although exercise can be beneficial, you need to achieve a proper balance of exercise and rest. Rest is particularly important during flare-ups of rheumatoid arthritis, which put you at risk of damaging your joints.

- ✔ **Watch what you eat:** If you have gout, avoid foods high in *purines,* protein compounds found in rich foods, such as anchovies and organ meats. Purines can increase levels of uric acid in the body, aggravating the condition.

Finding a means to lessen the ache in your joints is your doctor's primary focus. With reduced pain comes greater mobility and a more active lifestyle. Your doctor may consider the following:

- ✔ **Anti-inflammatory medications:** Aspirin is one of the most commonly prescribed treatments for arthritis. It reduces the pain and inflammation of osteoarthritis and rheumatoid arthritis. Ibuprofen, acetaminophen, and prescription nonsteroidal anti-inflammatory drugs, such as diclofenac (Voltarol, Voltaren), indomethacin (Indocin), and ketoprofen (Orudis), also are frequently tried. A new class of anti-inflammatory drugs is expected to be approved. Known as cyclooxygenase inhibitors, or COX-2 inhibitors, they're as effective as aspirin, naproxen, and ibuprofen but don't have the same side effects (such as stomach upset).

Studies show that about one in five people who take aspirin and other nonsteroidal anti-inflammatory drugs (NSAIDS) in large doses or over a long period of time develops stomach or intestinal ulcers (see Chapter 10). If you are taking NSAIDS to control your arthritis symptoms, make sure that your doctor monitors you for signs of ulcers and ask about the possibility of taking misoprostal (Cytotec), a drug found in the arthritis drug Arthrotec. Misoprostol stimulates the growth of mucus-producing cells that form in the stomach and has been approved by the Food and Drug Administration (FDA) for use in preventing stomach ulcers in people taking NSAIDS.

✔ **Corticosteroids:** These potent, hormonelike drugs reduce swelling, inflammation, and pain. Oral steroids such as prednisone can be used for short-term relief of rheumatoid arthritis. Steroid injections, in which the drug is injected directly into inflamed joints, provide quick relief for both rheumatoid arthritis and osteoarthritis. A single injection can often provide permanent relief to an acute condition, but multiple injections can damage the bone and joint.

Your doctor may prescribe a variety of other medications, including slow-acting drugs thought to slow the progress of rheumatoid arthritis (gold salts; hydroxychloroquine (Plaquenil), a drug used to treat malaria; penicil-lamine, an antibiotic; and methotrexate, an immunosuppressive drug used to treat cancer, for example), sodium hyaluronate (Hyalgan), a newly approved drug that is injected into the knees of people with osteoarthritis to cushion the joint and relieve pain, and colchicine and indomethacin, which are used to treat gout.

In addition to medications, your doctor may recommend physical therapy, immobilization, rest, exercise, or surgery. Surgery can be performed to trim back tissue in a joint, to flush particles of debris out of a joint capsule, to immobilize painful, unstable joints, and to replace joints that have become painful and useless. As always, be sure to get a second opinion before opting for surgery.

An ounce of prevention

Even though a cause for arthritis has remained elusive, you may take certain steps to lessen or delay the blow of osteoarthritis.

✔ **Exercise regularly:** Low-impact activities such as swimming and yoga are best.

✔ **Maintain a healthy weight:** Avoiding being overweight reduces stress on your joints, and avoiding being too thin keeps your bone density in the normal range.

✔ **Watch your diet:** Research indicates that high doses of vitamins C and D slow the progression of osteoarthritis.

✔ **Don't repeat:** Avoid repetitive activities and injuries.

✔ **Protect yourself:** Wear a brace or use a foam resting pad for your wrists if you sit at a computer for many hours a day.

For more information on arthritis, contact

✔ The Arthritis Foundation, 1330 W. Peachtree St., Atlanta, GA 30309; 800-283-7800; www.arthritis.org

✔ The National Institute of Arthritis, Musculoskeletal, and Skin Diseases, NIH, 1 AMS Circle, Bethesda, MD 20892; 301-495-4484; www.nih.gov/niams

Asthma

The lungs are amazing, complex organs, supplying oxygen to the rest of the body, keeping it alive. But when someone having an asthma attack breathes in, air passages begin to close and that wonderfully functioning oxygen system falls flat, often to be revived only by medication.

About 14.6 million Americans have *asthma,* a disease in which the air passages in the lungs periodically become narrowed, obstructed, or even blocked. That number is growing by leaps and bounds, and researchers are scrambling for ways to keep it in check.

The stimuli that prompt an asthma attack are known as *triggers.* They include hundreds of substances, the most common of which are allergens such as pollen, dust, animal dander, and mold; cockroach fecal particles and decomposed body parts (sounds awful, but cockroach debris is quite common in cities); household chemicals; hair spray and other personal care products; pesticides; air pollution; tobacco smoke; foods; and some drugs. Even exercise can trigger asthma.

When someone with asthma is exposed to a trigger, the muscles surrounding their air passages squeeze the passages, reducing the flow of air. Then the cells along those passages produce loads of mucus, which clog the passages. The lining of the bronchial tubes become puffy and swollen, limiting how much air can get through.

Asthma attacks can last hours, days, or weeks, depending on how long it takes for the inflammation to subside.

Two primary types of asthma exist:

- ✓ **Extrinsic asthma:** External allergies trigger this asthma. An attack is clearly linked to the body's response to something inhaled or ingested. Because allergies (pollen, ragweed, and so on) play a role, extrinsic asthma tends to flare up more often during the peak allergy season of summer.

- ✓ **Intrinsic asthma:** This asthma is not related to allergy-causing molds or pollens. It is caused by a sensitivity to respiratory infections, exercise, stress, air pollution, and inhalation of chemical irritants.

When either of these types of asthma worsens in the night, the condition is known as *nocturnal asthma*.

Recognizing the signs

Not all asthma symptoms are present in every attack. The symptoms include shortness of breath, chest tightness, wheezing, excess mucus in the airway, coughing, and anxiety over shortness of breath.

Knowing for sure

Your doctor must determine whether your breathing difficulties are caused by asthma or by an infection, respiratory disease, or an adverse reaction to a drug. Doctors look for severe signs of asthma — two of which are that airway obstruction comes and goes and that it improves with medication. The doctor will talk about your medical history, ask you to describe your symptoms and try to pinpoint what triggers them. She may also ask whether an immediate family member has asthma as that increases your risk for the disease. Although most asthma develops in childhood, adults with no previous history of asthma can also develop the disease.

A physical exam will include checking for signs of allergies, wheezing, and a blue tint to the skin, which indicates a lack of oxygen. Several tests are likely to follow if asthma is suspected:

- ✓ **Pulmonary-function tests:** These examinations determine how well the lungs are performing. You put on nose clips, inhale fully, then exhale as hard as possible into a mouthpiece and tube attached to a computerized gizmo called a *spirometer*. The instrument measures the volume of air in the lungs when you exhale and the speed with which you expel that air.

✔ **Reversibility test:** This is a pulmonary-function test that is performed after you've taken some medication to open your airways. If the test shows your breathing is eased by the medication, you likely have asthma.

Your doctor may conduct skin tests to determine what substances you are sensitive to (for information on skin tests, see "Allergies"). She may also test you by exposing you to the very thing that is supposed to trigger your asthma — an allergen, food, or exercise, for example — just to observe your reaction and be sure that you truly have asthma.

Your doctor may refer you to an asthma specialist; you may also want to consider seeing one on your own.

Making it better

In all but the rarest of cases, asthma can be controlled. Sufferers can lead a normal life. And in some cases, asthma that is treated may seem to go away.

Asthma is one of those diseases that doesn't improve if you don't take an active role in your treatment. You must have a special relationship with your doctor, work to control or get rid of the substances that trigger your attacks, get into an exercise routine, manage your stress, and, most importantly, learn what medications work best for you and how to use them.

One task you likely will have is taking your *peak-flow measurements* (measurements of the maximum speed at which air can leave the lungs) with a meter every day, or less often if your condition is under control. These meters check your ability to exhale and can detect a potential attack, even before you're aware that your airways are narrowing.

If you have asthma, you're quite likely to be prescribed medication to control and prevent your asthma attacks. You may take a daily preventive medication and another when you have an attack. The key is that each person's asthma is different, and your doctor will work with you to create a management plan.

The most commonly prescribed types of asthma medications are:

✔ **Bronchodilators:** These drugs relax spasming muscles and open airways. They come in pills and liquids but work faster when inhaled with a small device called a *metered-dose inhaler*. Most people with asthma use one or more bronchodilators to keep their asthma in check. These drugs include beta-adrenergic agonists, or beta-agonists, such as albuterol (Proventil, Ventolin) and salmeterol (Serevent); xanthines, such as theophylline; and anticholinergic drugs, such as ipratropium bromide (Atrovent).

✔ **Anti-inflammatory drugs:** Anti-inflammatory drugs prevent or reduce swelling in the airways. Corticosteroids, or steroids, notably the inhaled variety, are among the most used anti-inflammatory drugs for treating asthma. Inhaled steroids such as beclomethasone (Beconase, Beclovent), flunisolide (AeroBid, Nasalide), and triamcinolone (Azmacort, Nasacort) are now the first line of defense in many asthma management programs. For severe asthma flare-ups that can't be controlled by inhaled steroids or for severe chronic asthma, your doctor may prescribe oral steroids, such as dexamethasone (Decadron) or prednisone (Deltasone). Other anti-inflammatory drugs in your doctor's asthma-fighting arsenal include cromolyn sodium (Intal) and nedocromil sodium (Tilade), which prevent cells from releasing inflammatory chemicals without using steroids.

✔ **Leukotriene modifiers:** This relatively new class of long-term asthma drugs attacks leukotrienes — substances that contract the airway, increase mucus secretions, and activate inflammatory cells. Available in pill form, they include zileuton (Zyflo), zafirlukast (Accolate), pranlukast (Ultair), and montelukast (Singulair).

Your doctor may also suggest you undergo allergy shots if you have extrinsic asthma. Known as immunotherapy, allergy shots gradually desensitize you to substances that trigger your asthma.

An ounce of prevention

Short of locking yourself in a sterile room, you can't really avoid developing asthma if you're predisposed to it. Once you have asthma, however, you can stick to your plan of medication, avoid triggers, exercise, and reduce stress to keep your attacks to a minimum.

For more information on asthma, contact

✔ The Allergy and Asthma Network, Mothers of Asthmatics, Inc., 3554 Chain Bridge Rd., Suite 200, Fairfax, VA 22030; 800-878-4403

✔ National Asthma Education and Prevention Program Information Center, National Heart, Lung, and Blood Institute, 4733 Bethesda Ave., Suite 530, Bethesda, MD 20814; 301-251-1222

Diabetes

You've probably heard of runners wolfing down a huge pasta dinner the night before a big race. That's because the body feeds on carbohydrates for energy. But what happens when the body can't absorb the sugar that is produced from the breakdown of carbohydrates — those sweet and starchy foods such as fruit, bread, pasta, and vegetables? The result is a condition known as *diabetes mellitus,* which is characterized by an abnormally elevated level of sugar in the bloodstream and urine.

The culprit in diabetes is the hormone *insulin.* Produced by the pancreas, insulin allows cells to absorb sugar for use as energy. When the pancreas produces no or inadequate insulin, diabetes results.

About 100 million people worldwide have been diagnosed with diabetes, about 16 million of them in the United States. Diabetes is the fourth leading cause of death by disease in the United States. Each day, an average of 1,700 people are diagnosed with diabetes; 1,000 die from its complications; 150 undergo amputations; 80 enter end-stage kidney disease treatment; and 70 become blind.

Over the long haul, diabetes increases the risk of stroke and heart disease and may damage the kidneys, nervous and circulatory systems, and the eyes.

According to the American Diabetes Association, more than 5 million people have it and don't know it. That's an alarming statistic, but one that if duly noted may prompt you to have your blood sugar checked if you show any symptoms or have a family history of the disease.

Left unchecked, diabetes can result in coma or even death because cells that are deprived of sugar begin to burn protein and body fat for energy. The breakdown of fats releases a toxic acid called *ketones,* which, in extreme cases can be fatal.

Several kinds of diabetes exist, all with some common symptoms:

✔ **Type 1 diabetes:** Also known as *insulin-dependent diabetes* because people with it usually require insulin injections to lower their blood sugar, type 1 diabetes is the most severe form. The majority of people are diagnosed under 20 years of age (which is why it once was called juvenile diabetes); however, people of any age can develop it.

This form of diabetes is an autoimmune disease, meaning the body's own immune system attacks the cells in the pancreas that produce that vital insulin. Although researchers have found no cause for the disease, they do know it can be inherited. Sufferers of type 1 diabetes face dangerous complications related to wide swings in blood sugar levels. If the blood sugar level is too high, it results in *hyperglycemia,* which can cause serious diabetic complications. If the blood sugar level is too low, it results in *hypoglycemia,* which can cause irritability, fainting, and even death.

✔ **Type 2 diabetes:** Formerly called adult-onset diabetes because it seldom develops in people under age 40, this form of diabetes accounts for 85 to 95 percent of all diabetes cases. This form of diabetes, known as *non-insulin-dependent diabetes,* because often diet regulation, alone or with oral medication, can keep the blood sugar within the normal range, also runs in families.

Four out of five people with type 2 diabetes are overweight, and scientists believe that the excess weight and age triggers the genetic predisposition to the disease.

✔ **Gestational diabetes:** Approximately 3 percent of pregnant women develop a form of diabetes known as gestational diabetes because of the hormonal and metabolic changes their bodies undergo.

Although gestational diabetes causes little harm to the mother, the unborn child can tend to be large and have oversized organs, making delivery more high-risk. Labor is more likely to be slow, difficult, or stall completely, with a higher rate of cesarean section. Such babies also tend to have less well-developed lungs at birth and can suffer from respiratory problems, low blood calcium, jaundice, stillbirth, and infection. For the vast majority of women (approximately 95 percent), gestational diabetes disappears after childbirth. But once a woman has had gestational diabetes, she's at risk for developing type 2 diabetes later in life.

Recognizing the signs

Symptoms of diabetes include frequent urination, extreme thirst, unexplained weight loss, fatigue, persistent hunger, blurred vision, itching genitals or skin, slow healing of cuts or bruises, and pain and/or numbness in hands and feet.

Knowing for sure

A blood test is used to determine whether the sugar level in the blood is elevated. Although a screening test can be done at a random time, a confirmatory test is usually conducted after a short period of fasting. The normal blood sugar range is between 60 and 100 milligrams per deciliter (mg/dl). A level higher than 126 mg/dl in two successive tests signals diabetes.

Another common test is the oral glucose-tolerance test, which begins with a fasting blood sample. Then, the patient drinks a sugar solution, after which blood tests are taken every 30 minutes for 2 hours to analyze how the body is handling the glucose. Normally, blood sugar levels rise after glucose is consumed, and then return to normal levels after the glucose has been metabolized. If the glucose readings are high to begin with or remain high more than one or two hours after the glucose was consumed, it signals the presence of diabetes.

Because the symptoms of type 1 and type 2 diabetes are similar, doctors often have difficulty distinguishing between the two in the early stages of the disease. Diagnosis often involves trying various treatments. Type 1 diabetes is the most severe form and requires the highest level of treatment.

Making it better

Regulation of blood sugar levels is key to the treatment of diabetes, so diet and exercise are recommended most often, sometimes in conjunction with insulin or other drugs.

The fact of the matter is, doctors can do only so much to control diabetes. The primary responsibility for coping with the disease rests with you, the patient:

- ✔ **Educate yourself:** Learn about the disease and how insulin, diet, and exercise affect your blood sugar.

- ✔ **Practice self-monitoring, if necessary:** If you're taking insulin or a hypoglycemic agent, you likely will use a self-monitoring blood glucose kit, which allows you, with a prick of your finger, to regularly test your blood sugar and adjust your medication doses and your diet as needed.

- ✔ **Eat a balanced diet:** The recommended diet for both type 1 and type 2 diabetes is the same as for the general population — balanced. The American Diabetes Association suggests a diet of 15 to 20 percent of calories from proteins, less than 30 percent from fats, and 55 to 60 percent from carbohydrates.

  People with diabetes may need to adjust the number of times they eat per day because high food intake can cause a big jump in blood sugar. The carbohydrates should be distributed throughout the day to avoid a large sugar load all at once. Additionally, people with type 2 diabetes generally need to lose weight and should work toward eating fewer calories each day. You should work closely with your doctor to develop a meal plan that will achieve your desired weight and blood sugar level.

- ✔ **Exercise:** Exercise is critical to diabetes management because it makes body tissues more sensitive to insulin. Check with your doctor about a safe level of exercise, and then make it part of your routine. Because exercise can reduce blood sugar levels, self-monitoring may be necessary to avoid a level that is too low.

- ✔ **Take care of your feet:** Foot care is important because the nerves of a person with diabetes don't sense when minor problems in this area are coming on and ignoring even a minor problem such as a cut or ingrown toenail can lead to a major infection. Foot care includes regular inspection and washing of feet, changing shoes twice daily, and avoiding wearing new shoes for long periods and going barefoot outside.

Treatment of type 1 diabetes generally involves regular, daily insulin injections along with a strict diet that helps keep blood sugar levels in the normal range. Exercise helps lower blood sugar and is highly recommended.

Type 2 diabetes often can be controlled with a strict diet and exercise plan. When that is not the case, drugs called oral hypoglycemic agents, which increase insulin secretions, are used to regulate blood sugar levels. If all else fails, a doctor may prescribe insulin injections.

Gestational diabetes most often is controlled with diet.

An ounce of prevention

At the moment, you can't prevent type 1 diabetes. If you have a history of type 2 diabetes in your family, you can get to work to stave off the disease's onset by keeping your weight down, exercising, and eating properly.

For more information on diabetes, contact the American Diabetes Association, 1660 Duke St., Alexandria, VA 22314; 800-232-3472; www.diabetes.org

Osteoporosis

Think of your bones as a framework of a house. When something in your house wears down, you replace it. Your bones are in a constantly evolving state as well. Some areas try to replace themselves, while other areas break down. Osteoporosis sets in when your body's "bony" house is breaking down faster than you can build it back up. This requires certain raw materials, the most important being calcium, vitamin D, and estrogen.

Osteoporosis literally means "porous bones." The disorder sets in when the bones gradually lose their mineral content (including calcium), which causes them to become less dense, as shown in Figure 17-1. Your body needs calcium to regulate blood pressure, maintain your heart rate, allow your muscles to contract, and build bones. When your body needs calcium, it borrows what it needs from your bones, thus weakening them and making the bones prone to fractures. Of the women who suffer hip fractures because of osteoporosis, 50 percent do not regain normal function, 15 percent die soon after the fracture, and 30 percent die within a year. The deaths usually are a result of blood clots, pneumonia, and other complications that result from confinement to a bed.

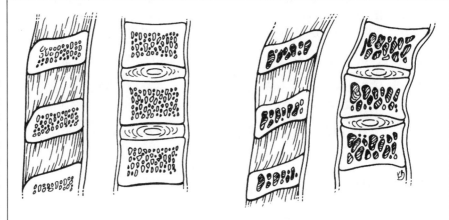

Figure 17-1:
Bones that
suffer from
osteoporosis
are less
dense than
healthy
bones.

More than 28 million Americans have osteoporosis. Women suffer more often from osteoporosis, largely because men start out with a larger bone mass and women lose theirs nine times more rapidly because of lack of exercise and a drop off in production of the hormone estrogen, which helps maintain bone mass.

Osteoporosis has no known cause; however, researchers believe it runs in families. Other risk factors include *bilateral oophorectomy* (the removal of both ovaries) without estrogen replacement therapy; natural menopause before age 40; a petite, small-boned frame; a sedentary lifestyle; a low calcium intake; fair hair and a fair complexion; too much alcohol or caffeine in the diet; smoking; a history of anorexia nervosa (which results in low estrogen levels); stomach disorders that cause poor calcium absorption; and the use of steroids, antiepileptic drugs, or anticoagulants.

Recognizing the signs

Symptoms of osteoporosis include gradual height loss, rounded shoulders, stooped posture, lower back pain, frequent bone fractures, and periodontal disease.

Knowing for sure

The key to diagnosing early osteoporosis is to scan bones for density. Bones that are less dense are at risk of fracture. The scan is generally done with one of several types of painless x-rays:

✔ **Single-photon absorptiometry:** This low-dose radiation x-ray is usually taken of the forearm and heel.

✔ **Dual-photon or dual-energy x-ray absorptiometry:** This more-precise, low-radiation x-ray is most often taken of the spine, femur, and hip. This is the preferred test because small bones such as those in the spine are most likely to fracture first and without major symptoms.

✔ **Quantitative computed tomography:** This high- or low-dose radiation scan is normally taken of the spine and forearm.

Bone density tests produce a figure that is compared with an average measurement of peak bone mass taken in adults around age 30. Osteoporosis is diagnosed if the figure is more than 2.5 times lower than peak bone mass, but the beginnings of osteoporosis are suspected if the number is less than 1.0 times that of young adults.

In addition to bone tests, your doctor may also perform blood and urine tests to measure the amount of calcium in the body and to help rule out other disorders.

Making it better

Once osteoporosis has wrought its damage, no medicine, vitamin, or exercise can make it disappear. Left alone, osteoporosis only gets worse. Treatment of the disorder involves keeping it from eating up any more bone mass.

If you have osteoporosis or may be at risk for developing osteoporosis in the future, you may need to change your lifestyle. Follow the preventive measures listed below. Aspirin, heat, massage, and orthopedic supports may ease physical discomfort.

The most widely prescribed treatments for osteoporosis are medications, including the following:

✔ **Hormone replacement therapy:** After menopause, this is the most-often prescribed course of treatment. Estrogen helps bones absorb calcium and maintain bone density and can cut bone fractures in half. Because therapy with estrogen alone increases the risk of endometrial cancer, it is usually prescribed in conjunction with progesterone to offset the risk unless you've had a hysterectomy.

✔ **Biphosphonates:** These drugs help increase bone density and prevent further bone loss. Only one of these drugs, alendronate (Fosamax), is approved as a treatment for osteoporosis, but etidronate (which is used to treat Paget's disease) has been shown to be helpful in some studies. Alendronate must be taken first thing in the morning on an empty stomach; some people get reflux (heartburn) if they lie down or bend over within one hour after taking it.

✔ **Sodium fluoride:** This treatment has been shown to stimulate bone formation, but is unclear whether it reduces fractures because the bone it helps form may not be as resistant to fracture as normal bone.

✔ **Calcitonin:** This hormone, which stimulates bone production, improves the cellular level of bones, slows the progression of osteoporosis, and in some cases, may even increase bone density. It is usually taken as a nasal spray twice a day.

✔ **Calcium and vitamin D:** These nutrients are often recommended for people with osteoporosis. Calcium, which helps the body build bones, may also help prevent bone loss. And calcitriol, the active form of vitamin D, increases calcium absorption.

✔ **Selective estrogen receptor modulators (SERMS), or designer estrogens:** These are the newest weapons in the osteoporosis-fighting arsenal. The first SERM, raloxifene (Evista) was approved in late 1997 for osteoporosis. It acts like estrogen on the bones but does not carry the same side benefits for the heart, brain, and colon.

An ounce of prevention

Researchers disagree as to whether osteoporosis can be completely prevented. But it appears you may be able to delay its onset and its severity, as well as slow its progression, by adhering to the following guidelines:

✔ **Make a milk mustache:** Eat calcium-rich foods and take a supplement if necessary.

✔ **Get your vitamins:** Eat a diet rich in vitamin D, magnesium, and vitamin C, which enhance calcium absorption.

✔ **Exercise:** Do weight-bearing exercise such as walking, tennis, bicycling, dancing, cross-country skiing, and weight training.

✔ **Limit yourself:** Avoid smoking and excessive caffeine and alcohol consumption.

✔ **Take hormones:** Consider beginning hormone replacement therapy at the onset of menopause, particularly if you are at risk for osteoporosis.

✔ **Try an alternative:** If you cannot take estrogen or choose not to do so, ask your doctor about alendronate (Fosamax). The drug, which has been used for several years as an osteoporosis treatment, was recently approved as an osteoporosis preventive.

For more information about osteoporosis, contact the Osteoporosis and Related Bone Diseases National Resource Center, 1150 17th St., NW, Suite 500, Washington, DC 20036; 800-624-BONE; www.osteo.org

Part IV
Your Reproductive Health

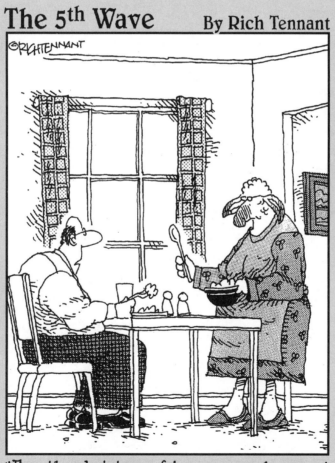

The 5th Wave   By Rich Tennant

"Exactly what type of hormone replacement therapy are you taking?"

In this part . . .

Your reproductive health includes more than just fertility. It also encompasses the health of your reproductive organs, the changes your reproductive system goes through during your life span, and your sexual health. This section addresses all these aspects of your reproductive health.

Chapter 18

Reproductive System Conditions

· ·

· ·

*T*he female reproductive system is as complex, high-tech, and delicate as a computer. When it's running well, you don't think about its complexity. You take it for granted and reap its many benefits. But when you have a systemic glitch — in either the hardware (the reproductive organs) or the software (the hormones that keep the whole system up and running) — you realize just how complex this system is. And because it is so complex, many things can go wrong — from the simple discomfort of menstrual cramps to life-threatening conditions, such as ectopic pregnancy. This chapter looks at common conditions that affect the reproductive system.

Amenorrhea

Amenorrhea is the complete absence of a menstrual period. In addition to such obvious causes as pregnancy and menopause, this condition can be caused by low estrogen levels, poorly or nonfunctioning reproductive organs, physical stress, and weight loss.

Female athletes, ballerinas, and most cover models have such extremely low body fat that their bodies can't produce reproductive hormones. They experience amenorrhea until their body fat is up to par. Yes, body fat is good for you — in moderation. If your body senses a starvation mode, it starts to shut down some systems to help you survive.

Over your life span, you are bound to miss a period or two because you didn't ovulate. But unless you're approaching menopause, you should report frequently missed periods to your doctor. Bringing back periods may be as simple as eating right or getting your body fat up to par. Just make sure that your doctor is involved in your treatment program so that neither one of you is missing anything serious.

Recognizing the signs

You won't notice amenorrhea until after the fact. A month will go by, and you won't have a period. If you skip two or more periods, make a doctor's appointment. Keep a menstrual calendar if you tend to be irregular, so you won't have to guess when your doctor asks you.

Knowing for sure

Your doctor will likely give you a pregnancy test to rule out pregnancy. After that, you can expect other blood tests to determine the hormone levels in your blood and to rule out other conditions such as premature menopause or thyroid disease.

Making it better

Eat a healthy diet with no more than 60 grams of fat per day. ***Remember:*** Too little or too much fat is not good. Make sure to get regular, but not overly strenuous, exercise. If you have been starving yourself to make the weight that society, your coach, or your instructor encourages, you're listening to the wrong people. Manipulating your eating to decrease your body weight can lead to bulimia and anorexia nervosa. For more information on these eating disorders, see Chapter 5.

Depending on the cause of amenorrhea, your doctor may recommend supervised weight gain. Or she may start hormone therapy, such as oral contraceptives, to replace your body's estrogen and bring back your periods.

An ounce of prevention

Keep a healthy body fat, watch your training, and keep your stress level to an absolute minimum.

Dysmenorrhea

The most striking thing about menstrual periods for some women is the unrelenting cramps. Cramps are caused by prostaglandins, which create contractions in your uterus. They also help push out menstrual flow. For some women, cramps may be debilitating. This painful condition is known as *dysmenorrhea*.

Recognizing the signs

The primary symptom is pain just before and during menstruation, which can occur in the lower abdomen, lower back, or thighs. Some women also experience nausea, vomiting, diarrhea, and body aches during their periods.

Knowing for sure

It's pretty easy to tell whether you have pain. But because other conditions, including endometriosis, uterine fibroids, and scarring caused by pelvic inflammatory disease, can also cause cramps, your doctor may want to perform a pelvic exam and other tests to rule out these more serious conditions.

Making it better

Many over-the-counter pain relievers can ease cramps. If your pain does not respond to these medications, your doctor may prescribe prescription pain killers.

Here are a few tips you can try on your own when you are experiencing cramps:

- **Walk around the neighborhood:** Certain exercises, such as walking, can alleviate pain by increasing *endorphins* (your body's feel-good chemicals).

- **Try yoga:** Certain stretches and positions may relieve the pain. Try the "cat cow." Get down on your hands and knees. Arch your back like a cat, and then relax your back to a flat, or cow, stance. Do this exercise a few times. Or flatten your back against a wall by bending your knees and sucking in your stomach. Then relax your back. These exercises help low-back pain by working your muscles. When muscles are busy, they don't have time for pain.

✓ **Exercise your innards:** Kegel exercises (see Chapter 23) work the bottom of your pelvis or pelvic floor and relieve pain in that area. Some experts have suggested having an orgasm. It relieves pain by relieving the congestion or buildup of pain-producing substances in the blood.

✓ **Try an over-the-counter (OTC) pain reliever:** You can choose from a number of reliable OTC pain relief medications. An estimated 80 percent of women who try them experience relief, especially if they take them in the day or two prior to menstruation, before the pain gets really bad.

Your doctor can prescribe pain medication and exercise and will carefully monitor your symptoms (if they get worse, tell your doctor). Oral contraceptives are another option. Because they prevent ovulation, they cause a lighter menstrual flow; they also reduce the production of prostaglandins, which reduces the severity of cramping.

An ounce of prevention

The same things you do to ease the pain during your period may help prevent your pain if you do them all month long. Take care of yourself: Eat a healthy diet, get regular exercise, and lower your stress level.

Ectopic Pregnancy

You can describe an ectopic pregnancy as a case of the wrong place at the right time. Normally, the egg and sperm unite in one of the fallopian tubes, and the fertilized egg travels through the tube into the uterus, where the embryo makes its home for the next nine months. Ectopic pregnancies start out fine: The egg and sperm unite and start to form an embryo, but the fertilized egg implants somewhere outside the uterus — usually in the fallopian tube. That's not fine. If you don't catch this condition in time, the growing pregnancy can rupture the fallopian tube, causing damage, infection, and hemorrhaging that may jeopardize your life.

It's hard to say exactly why the fertilized egg never completes its journey to the uterus. Scars from a previous infection, surgery, endometriosis, or tubal abnormalities may put up obstacles so that the fertilized egg gets waylaid on its journey and stays wherever it stops.

Recognizing the signs

You may not have any unusual symptoms during the first few weeks of pregnancy. Some women have the usual signs of pregnancy, such as morning sickness and tender breasts, and other women don't even know they are pregnant. In fact, the condition often goes undetected until the pregnancy breaks through the walls of the fallopian tube. But some women do experience symptoms, including

- Cramping and spotting early in pregnancy
- Vaginal bleeding (not your normal menstrual period)
- Severe lower abdominal pains on one side of the body
- Vomiting
- Nausea
- Dizziness
- Fainting

Pain can also radiate along the nerve pathways to another site, a process called *referred pain*. In ectopic pregnancies, pain is often referred to the shoulder. Shoulder pain in women who may be or are known to be pregnant may indicate a ruptured ectopic pregnancy.

Knowing for sure

Because ectopic pregnancies start out like normal pregnancies, it's sometimes hard to know whether they are occurring until after they rupture. Ultrasound tests, which use sound waves to create an image, can help determine whether a fetus can be seen inside the uterus or elsewhere. Blood tests for the hormone human chorionic gonadotropin (HCG) can also help. The placenta produces this hormone; levels increase in the first three months of pregnancy as the placenta grows. Lower than normal levels or levels that do not rise sufficiently when the test is repeated can indicate an ectopic pregnancy. Laparoscopy, in which a viewing scope is inserted into the abdomen at the belly button, can sometimes detect ectopic pregnancy before it ruptures.

Making it better

Ectopic pregnancy is an emergency situation. Get yourself to a doctor as soon as possible if you have the preceding symptoms or if you experience bleeding during pregnancy.

Sadly, ectopic pregnancy always results in the death of the fetus. The fallopian tubes weren't designed to care for a developing baby. And for women, this condition is the leading cause of pregnancy-related deaths during the first trimester (three months) in the United States. If the fallopian tube has not ruptured, your doctor will want to try to save your fallopian tube, so she may prescribe methotrexate (a chemotherapy medication that must be given in the office) to terminate an ectopic pregnancy. Or she may recommend surgery to remove the ectopic pregnancy or ease it out of one end of a tube that hasn't ruptured.

If the tube has ruptured and is hemorrhaging, your doctor will be concerned about saving you. Fallopian tubes are often removed in this situation: The surgery is called a *salpingectomy,* and it can be done via an incision in the abdomen or through a laparoscopic procedure, sparing the adjacent ovary, possible. Laparoscopic surgery is followed by a period of observation in the hospital or a quiet overnight stay, and the recovery period is shorter, so most doctors will try laparoscopy first if they think you need surgery.

An ounce of prevention

You cannot prevent an ectopic pregnancy, but you can reduce your risk by getting prompt treatment for any case of pelvic inflammatory disease (PID). If you have a sexually transmitted disease, you need to treat it as soon as possible and have your partner treated, too. Sexually transmitted diseases infect the reproductive organs and can cause scarring and blockage of the fallopian tubes, which can lead to ectopic pregnancy. (For more information on sexually transmitted diseases, see Chapter 22.) You are also at higher risk if you have had a previous ectopic pregnancy, pelvic surgery, or fallopian tube surgery.

A body parts primer

Following is a glossary for the reproductive organs talked about in this chapter:

- ✔ **Uterus:** A pear-sized hollow organ, also called the womb. It holds and maintains the developing fetus. The uterus contracts to expel its sloughed lining and blood during menstrual periods. These same contractions help expel the fetus.

- ✔ **Endometrium:** The lining of the uterus. During the reproductive years, the endometrium swells, sloughs, and repairs itself once a month.

- ✔ **Ovaries:** Two walnut-size organs that secret sex hormones, and the place where eggs originate, mature, and depart, located on either side of the abdomen just above the pubic hairline. The ovaries are connected to the uterus by the ovarian ligament and to the fallopian tubes by the infundibulopelvic ligament.

- ✔ **Fallopian tubes:** Two tubelike structures that connect to the uterus on one end, and curve downward and end in fringelike structures called the *infundibulum*. The infundibula sweeps the eggs into the uterus. Most fertilization (sperm uniting with egg) occurs in the fallopian tubes.

- ✔ **Cervix:** The opening from the uterus to the vagina. It produces mucus that cleanses the vagina and helps sperm move along into the uterus.

- ✔ **Vagina:** A muscular and flexible tubelike structure about 4 to 6 inches long, which receives the penis and sperm and acts as a pathway for menstrual blood and a baby to leave the body. The vagina, or birth canal, secretes mucus to help cleanse itself and protect against infections.

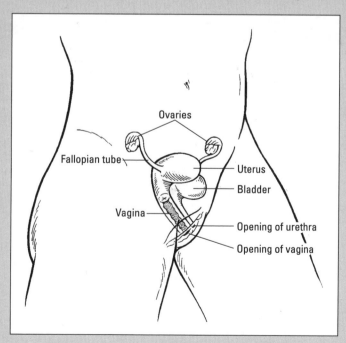

Endometriosis

For millions of women in the United States, each monthly cycle brings about more than just the typical menstrual cramps. The pain comes from sites — usually located in the pelvic cavity — where tissue from the lining of the uterus (or *endometrium*) has implanted itself (usually on the outside of the fallopian tubes, uterus, or ovaries). Because the endometrium responds to hormones such as estrogen and progesterone, this misplaced tissue imitates the menstrual cycle; it swells, bleeds, and sloughs each month. The misplaced blood and fluid may collect in pockets around the ovaries, forming painful sacs, or *cysts*. See Figure 18-1. The tissue may also form scars or *adhesions* (abnormal tissue that binds organs together), which can damage pelvic organs and cause infertility.

Endometriosis is most common in women during their reproductive years, particularly between the ages of 25 and 40. It is rare among women over the age of 50, which is about the time menopause occurs. The reason for this cut-off age is that *estrogen,* the hormone responsible for the swelling and sloughing of endometrium, is decreased during menopause, resulting in decreased endometriosis pain.

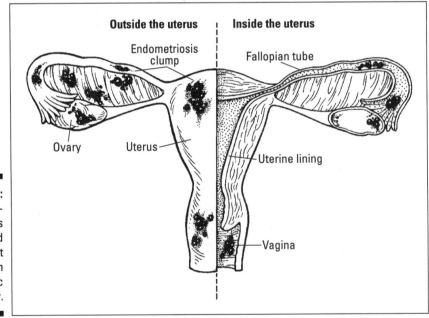

Figure 18-1: Endometriosis is misplaced tissue that ends up in the pelvic cavity.

Recognizing the signs

Although some minor cases of endometriosis may go unnoticed, for most women it hurts, plain and simple. You can have pain that is at its worst right before or during menstruation, lower back pain, painful intercourse, and painful urination or bowel movements. Symptoms also include heavy or irregular menstrual bleeding, low-grade fever, adhesions and scarring of the ovaries and fallopian tubes, infertility, and diarrhea or constipation.

Knowing for sure

Pelvic exams can sometimes help detect endometriosis: Certain areas in the pelvis may be painful to the touch. Tests may be done to determine or rule out other conditions such as pregnancy or infection, but a definitive diagnosis is generally made through *laparoscopy,* an outpatient surgical procedure in which a small camera attached to a viewing tool known as a *laparoscope* is inserted through the abdominal wall to look inside the pelvic cavity.

Making it better

Endometriosis has no cure. Most practitioners recommend approaching endometriosis treatment on a symptom-by-symptom basis. Mild pain can be eased with pain relief medications, heat applied to painful areas, and even acupuncture. Because endometriosis affects other reproductive organs and can result in infertility, if you are trying to conceive but haven't been successful, let your doctor know: She may want to rule out endometriosis as the cause.

You can do a few things on your own to help make the situation better:

- ✔ **Climb around your family tree:** You're seven times more likely to get endometriosis if you're related to a women who has it, so finding out how your relative was diagnosed and what she did to treat it may help.

- ✔ **Try over-the-counter pain relief:** Pain relievers such as aspirin, acetaminophen (Tylenol), and ibuprofen (Advil) may be enough to relieve mild pain.

- ✔ **Try an alternative:** Some women have found that complementary therapies such as acupuncture, acupressure, and massage ease pain.

If you're in your 40s, you may want to wait a bit to see what happens. Endometriosis decreases in severity during menopause in response to the decreasing levels of hormones. But if you are young and want to have children, you may want to consider your medical and surgical options.

If your condition doesn't respond to healthy lifestyle changes and pain medication and you don't want to have a baby right away, your doctor may prescribe oral contraceptives. These pills contain the hormones estrogen and progesterone in different forms and amounts higher than what's in your body. They help alleviate endometriosis symptoms by blocking ovulation, which blocks the swelling and bleeding of endometrial tissue.

A stronger drug option is danazol (Danocrine), an anabolic steroid (no, you won't be able to try out for the Olympics). This synthetic derivative of the male hormone *testosterone* is given to women with endometriosis. But its side effects include weight gain, bloating, depression, menopausal symptoms such as hot flashes and vaginal dryness, and masculinizing effects such as hairiness and voice deepening. Danazol also carries a high risk of birth defects, so it's recommended that you practice contraception in conjunction with this treatment. There's also a class of drugs called gonadotropin-releasing hormone antagonists (GnRH), which produce a sort of temporary menopause — the ovaries don't function at all or produce any hormones. As a result, the drugs reduce the pain and growth of endometriosis implants outside the uterus. These drugs, too, have side effects, notably menopausal symptoms, insomnia, and emotional changes. And prolonged treatment (more than six months) can cause bone loss, but this is reversible. With all medications, symptoms often gradually recur when treatment ends.

A more permanent treatment is surgery. With the aid of laparoscopy or laparotomy (which produces a larger incision), the doctor can take a look into your pelvic cavity at any endometrial tissue that's grown outside the uterus, and then surgically remove it by cauterizing it, burning it, or using laser surgery. Laser surgery can also be used to open cysts and release scar tissue. Be aware, however, that you may need to repeat these surgical procedures: Endometriosis can return.

For the most severe cases, *hysterectomy* (removal of the uterus) may be suggested, in conjunction with *oophorectomy* (removal of the ovaries). As a result of this surgery, the growth of the abnormally located endometriosis gradually is suppressed.

An ounce of prevention

Endometriosis is hard to prevent — especially if you have a previous family history. Using oral contraceptives for birth control may help reduce the risk of endometriosis developing or becoming worse.

Infertility

The happiest moment for a woman who wants a child is when that little test strip turns the right color. But for about 6.1 million American women and their partners, the test strip doesn't comply. Technically speaking, *infertility* is defined by time, as well as by success. If you fail to become pregnant after a whole year of trying, or you have not been able to carry a child to term, you're considered infertile. Infertility treatments can cost lots of money — tens of thousands of dollars — to do for you what Mother Nature seems unwilling to do.

A woman may not be able to become pregnant for many reasons. Sexually transmitted diseases, such as gonorrhea and chlamydia, can cause inflammation and scarring that block the fallopian tubes. Fibroids, benign tumors in the uterus, or other obstructions outside the uterus, such as endometriosis, can affect the fallopian tubes, or ovaries. Poorly functioning ovaries, or pituitary or adrenal glands may also be a problem: Hormonal imbalances can affect ovulation, as can thyroid disorders and chronic diseases such as diabetes. And that's only the half of it. It takes two to tango, so if you can't have kids, have your man checked out too.

Recognizing the signs

After a year of trying, noticing that you're going to have to help the stork get it into gear should be pretty easy.

Knowing for sure

Although infertility itself is obvious, the cause is not. Your doctor may perform a number of diagnostic tests to determine the cause of infertility, including

✔ Detailed history and physical exam

✔ Blood tests to measure hormone levels to determine whether you're ovulating

✔ Semen analysis, to see if your partner has sufficient number of normal sperm

Depending on the results of the initial work-up tests, further testing may be indicated, such as

✔ A hysterosalpingogram, in which dye is injected into the uterus as x-rays are taken to enable the doctor to see the shape of the inner cavity of the uterus and the inside of the fallopian tubes, along with any abnormalities or blockages.

✔ A laparoscopy, in which a viewing scope is inserted into a small incision in the abdomen to look for scar tissue or endometriosis or to examine whether the fallopian tubes are open; usually done in an operating room under general anesthesia.

✔ A hysteroscopy, in which a viewing scope is inserted through the vagina into the uterus to look for polyps, fibroids, or other causes of infertility. This may be done under local anesthesia, with sedation, or in an operating room under general anesthesia.

Making it better

The goal is to become pregnant — something you're often told how to prevent. Obviously, you want to make sure that you're having sexual intercourse on the appropriate days. You can chart your fertile periods by taking your temperature, using ovulation kits, and listening to your body. You can determine your most fertile time by checking your *cervical mucus,* the normal discharge that sometimes leaves a slight residue on your underwear. Mucus texture changes with your menstrual cycle to allow for maximum mobility or movement for sperm at the time of ovulation. These and other physical changes you can use to chart your fertile (and infertile) periods are discussed in detail in Chapter 21.

You may also want to look at other messages your body is sending you. Ovulation pain, or *mittelschmerz* (literally "middle pain"), occurs when the egg is released from the follicle in your ovary. Breast tenderness, cramping, or bloating may indicate that your menses will be arriving shortly.

Ovulation kits, too, can also help you to determine the right time to have intercourse. These over-the-counter kits are simple test strips that you hold under the stream of your urine when you go to the bathroom. A color change indicates you are about to ovulate. Kits differ with respect to which day and what time of the day you should check your urine, so read the instructions carefully. Some commonly used tests are ClearPlan, First Response, and Ovuquik.

Treatment for infertility often depends on its cause. If the problem is related to endometriosis, fibroids, or a specific infection, for example, treating the underlying condition may restore fertility. Surgery may remove scar tissue or adhesions or open a blocked fallopian tube, and fertility drugs may be given to stimulate ovulation or counteract hormonal problems.

Human menopausal gonadotropin (Pergonal) and clomiphene citrate (Clomid) are among the most common of many fertility drugs that increase ovulation and fertility. They are 40 to 80 percent effective, but they are not without possible side effects. Sometimes they can result in multiple pregnancies because they may cause several eggs to be released at once.

When conventional medical treatments fail, couples can turn to high-tech assisted fertility procedures, such as artificial insemination and in vitro fertilization. According to a report released in 1998 by the U.S. Centers for Disease Control and Prevention, these technologies deliver up to 20 to 30 percent of the time, depending on the expertise of the medical center and the condition being treated. Still, they offer many couples their last chance to have a biological child.

One of the easiest and least expensive of these high-tech treatments is *artificial insemination,* using either your partner's or a donor's sperm. This procedure involves placing sperm collected from a woman's partner or an anonymous donor near her cervix at the most fertile time of her menstrual cycle. This procedure is done when not enough sperm is present in the man's semen or when his sperm count is low enough that spontaneous conception would be unlikely otherwise.

In vitro fertilization (IVF) is used to conceive what are commonly known as "test-tube" babies. In this high-tech procedure, which is often used in women with blocked fallopian tubes or endometriosis, fertility drugs are used to stimulate the ovaries to ripen several eggs for ovulation. These eggs are then collected from the follicles of the ovaries with a hollow needle and a suction device in a minor office procedure. The eggs are fertilized in a glass dish with sperm collected from the woman's partner or donor. Several days after fertilization, the doctor inserts the fertilized eggs, or embryos, into the uterus using a long, thin tube inserted through the cervix. The more eggs transferred, the greater the chance of pregnancy — and the greater the chance of high-risk multiple births. IVF is quite costly (the average cost per monthly cycle was $7,800 in 1993, the latest year for which information is available), and it often takes three to five cycles to have a successful pregnancy.

A variation of IVF, *gamete intrafallopian tube transfer* (GIFT), allows fertilization to take place in the uterus. The eggs are collected during laparoscopic surgery, then mixed with sperm and transferred into the fallopian tubes. *Zygote intrafallopian transfer* (ZIFT) offers still another variation. In this procedure, the egg is collected and fertilized outside the body, and then the zygote (a fertilized egg that has not yet divided) is surgically placed into the fallopian tube.

Other options for women who are infertile include surrogate motherhood or adoption. *Surrogate motherhood,* in which the egg from the mother fertilized through IVF is implanted in another woman's (surrogate) uterus, is somewhat tricky. Contracts must be drawn up ahead of time to define the surrogate mother's role and what would happen if she were to change her mind about carrying the baby.

You may also want to consider adoption.

A study in contradictions

Trying to have a baby has to be one of the most contradictory experiences in life. You tell yourself to relax, but you become so tense that even your hair looks uptight. Well, here's some strange advice for conception — stop trying. *Note:* We do not mean avoid sexual intercourse, which is not a good way to become pregnant. The key here is to stop trying so hard. Babies have a habit of coming on their own terms, in their own good time (rather like your mother-in-law). All the charting, testing, and temperature taking won't make a baby. Even a healthy egg and a sperm at the right place at the right time have only a 30 percent chance of success. If you doctor has not diagnosed you as infertile, perhaps relaxing can increase your chance of getting pregnent.

An ounce of prevention

You can reduce your risk of infertility by taking care of yourself:

- ✔ **Call your doctor regarding any infections and pain or bleeding that is not normal:** That includes painful or prolonged periods (ones that lasts for more than seven days) and periods so heavy you have to change tampons or napkins frequently (see the section "Menorrhagia").

- ✔ **Reduce your stress:** Get lots of sleep (serious sleep), eat right, and take any prescribed or recommended medication or supplements.

- ✔ **Don't smoke:** If you do, quit as soon as you can. As few as ten cigarettes a day put you at risk for infertility.

- ✔ **Limit your alcohol intake to two drinks or less per day:** Save the bottle of champagne for the day when your baby is born (or when you are finished breast-feeding).

Menorrhagia

Menorrhagia, or heavy bleeding, often occurs when the uterine lining, which normally swells and sloughs off causing menstrual flow, is present in excessive amounts, causing excessive blood flow. Disturbances of the hormonal cycle, pelvic infections, or an enlarged uterus due to fibroids can cause this condition; other conditions, such as miscarriage, can mimic the symptoms.

Choosing a fertility clinic

According to the U.S. Centers for Disease Control and Prevention (CDC), the success rates for fertility clinics range from 7 percent to more than 35 percent, so if you're interested in high-tech help, it pays to shop around.

For each clinic you're considering, you need to know the qualifications and experience of the personnel, the types of patients they treat, the services they offer, and their rate of successful pregnancies, as well as the costs. The success of a fertility clinic cannot be determined by its rate of pregnancy alone. Many clinics limit the ages of their clients or the number of attempts they can make, which can increase their statistical success rate. And some clinics include the total number of conceptions in their rates, even if the pregnancies ended in miscarriage. What you really need is the clinic's "take-home baby" rate, the number of clients whose pregnancies end in live births. The national average was 19.6 percent in 1995, according to the CDC.

For more information on choosing a clinic or infertility procedures in general, contact the American Society for Reproductive Medicine, 1209 Montgomery Highway, Birmingham, AL 35216-2809; 205-978-5000; www.asrm.org.

Recognizing the signs

If your period is so heavy that you go through a sanitary napkin in two hours or less, you may have menorrhagia. Other symptoms include a feeling of weakness due to iron loss through the blood and pelvic cramping. Any change in the pattern of your bleeding, especially an increase in flow or the number of days you bleed, is something you should discuss with your doctor.

Heavy bleeding is not a condition that you should deal with on your own — especially if this is the first time it's occurred. Report any heavy bleeding or pain to your doctor immediately.

Knowing for sure

The normal amount of blood loss for a regularly menstruating woman varies from 1 ounce to $2^1/_2$ ounces. Any bleeding more than 3 ounces is considered abnormal. Physical examination and other tests can detect some conditions that cause prolonged or heavy bleeding. Other tests include ultrasound, pregnancy test, and blood count.

Making it better

Make yourself as comfortable as possible by taking care of yourself. You need plenty of fluids to make up for what you lose during your period. Also with your doctor's approval, you may need an iron supplement. To beef up your iron supply, you can add fortified cereals to your diet, along with high-iron foods, such as lean red meats and raisins. Use extra-absorbency tampons or napkins; a variety are made especially for heavy periods.

If your doctor determines that your heavy bleeding is not an emergency situation, you have several treatment options. Certain hormone therapies can reduce the growth of the lining of the uterus and prevent excess sloughing and bleeding.

As long as you don't want to have any more babies, a more aggressive treatment involves destruction of the endometrium using heat such as *endometrial ablation,* in which a laser is used to burn off the uterine lining, or the new ThermaChoice balloon. The latter technique delivers very hot water into the uterus via instruments inserted into the cervix. The hot water burns off the endometrium (the lining) but leaves the uterus intact. Some experts consider this procedure, which performed under local anesthesia, a safe alternative to hysterectomy.

Ovarian Cysts

Ovarian cysts are small, fluid-filled sacs on one or both ovaries that may or may not cause pain. These bumps are usually benign (harmless), but they can grow large and become very painful or rupture or can affect fertility.

The most common type of ovarian cyst is a *functional cyst* — a cyst that develops because of the normal functions of the ovary during the menstrual cycle. You can have two types of functional cysts. A *follicle cyst* forms when a follicle or groups of cells surrounding the egg in the ovary fail to release the egg. A *luteal cyst* forms when the follicle releases the eggs but doesn't shrink back down to its original size.

Dermoid cysts are not functional cysts; they are usually benign tumors that contain bits of hair, teeth, or bone and are thought to be remnants of abnormal embryo development. They usually need to be removed.

Recognizing the signs

Cysts often have no symptoms, but you may experience abdominal or pelvic swelling and pain, painful intercourse, or irregular or painful periods.

Knowing for sure

Ovarian cysts are usually detected during a pelvic exam. Your doctor may also use ultrasound, which creates an image using sound waves, x-rays, or laparoscopy, in which a viewing scope is inserted into a small incision in your abdomen, to confirm the diagnosis.

Making it better

Cysts often shrink or disappear on their own, so you may want to employ some patience to see whether they disappear. Always have regular exams so that your doctor can monitor the size of the cysts. Small benign cysts generally need no treatment if they are causing no symptoms.

If you experience pain or bleeding, inform your doctor.

If the cyst(s) is less than 5 centimeters (2 inches) in diameter, you have no pain, and you're premenopausal, your doctor may take a wait-and-see attitude to see whether the cyst will disappear on its own or prescribe oral contraceptives to reduce its growth. Before menopause, normally functioning ovaries often form small functional cysts, so the wait is worth it if you're not in too much pain.

If the cyst doesn't go away and you're postmenopausal, your doctor may perform a *biopsy* (a procedure in which a portion of the tissue is removed for diagnosis) to determine whether the cyst is benign or cancerous. Cancerous cysts are very rare. A doctor will be more likely to recommend surgery if you're in menopause.

Benign cysts need no treatment if they cause no pain or other symptoms. But if a benign cyst becomes large, causes pain, or ruptures, your surgeon will remove the cyst in procedure known as a *cystectomy*.

Pelvic Inflammatory Disease (PID)

Pelvic inflammatory disease, or *PID,* is really an umbrella term for different infections that affect the uterus (known as *endometritis*), the fallopian tubes (known as *salpingitis*), and the ovaries (known as *oophoritis*). The *-itis* endings means infection or inflammation of the affected organs. The infection can lead to the formation of scar tissue or *abscesses* (collections of pus surrounded by inflamed tissue).

A number of conditions can cause PID — sexually transmitted diseases, underlying infections you knew nothing about, urinary tract infections, or immune system or kidney problems. Organisms normally present in small amounts in the vagina and bowel can cause PID, or more dangerous bacteria can be introduced when a woman has unsafe sex without a condom; they enter through the vagina. Bacteria may also enter through the vagina when the cervix is dilated, such as after childbirth, abortion, a dilalation and curettage (D&C) procedure, or the insertion of an intrauterine device (IUD). PID is a rare complication of procedures such as D&C, abortion, or IUD insertion.

Recognizing the signs

PID can be hard to recognize because the symptoms are similar to those of other conditions. They include pain in the lower abdomen or pelvis, fever, abnormal vaginal discharge that is thick and foul-smelling, painful urination, painful intercourse, and menstrual periods that start early or are heavy.

Knowing for sure

Your doctor performs a pelvic exam in which she uses a cotton swab to take samples of your cervical discharge to determine which organism is causing the infection. She will also perform an internal pelvic examination to see if any of your pelvic organs feel tender. You may have a blood test taken to determine your white blood cell count to see how well your immune system is fighting the infection. You may have an ultrasound or laparoscopy to check for any inflammation, abscesses, or scar tissue.

Making it better

Early treatment of PID is essential to success: Left untreated, PID can result in infertility, chronic pelvic pain, secondary infections, and ectopic pregnancy. Take any infection seriously. If antibiotics or other medications are prescribed, follow your doctors orders and finish them. Don't assume that you're in the clear if your symptoms clear up. Call if your symptoms continue, especially if you've been directed to follow up due to test results.

If you've been diagnosed with PID, don't push yourself. Bed rest and medication help speed your healing. Do not have any sexual intercourse while you are being treated for an infection and check back with your doctor if your symptoms last longer than two to three weeks, sooner if your doctor has instructed you to do so. You may have what is classified as a chronic, or persistent, infection, and you may need a different course of action or perhaps stronger medication.

Your doctor will likely prescribe antibiotics to combat infection. If your PID is caused by a sexually transmitted disease, both you and your partner need to be treated or else you'll just keep reinfecting each other. If you're using an IUD, you should have it removed. If your infection is severe, you may require hospitalization, and the antibiotics may be given to you intravenously.

If the doctor detects an abscess, she may try antibiotics as a first course of action. If the abscess does not respond to medication, the doctor may suggest surgery to drain the area that is containing the pus. Any scar tissue that has formed as a result of the infection can sometimes be excised during laparoscopy.

As a last resort, a hysterectomy or *salpingo-oophorectomy* (removal of a fallopian tube and ovary) may be performed to relieve symptoms of severe, chronic PID. This is usually only done if prolonged courses of intravenous antibiotics do not relieve pain and fever, or if an abscess bursts and releases its contents inside the pelvic cavity.

An ounce of prevention

Preventing infections can help prevent PID. That means that you should do the following:

- **Practice safe sex:** Use a condom or vaginal pouch to prevent infected body fluids such as semen or cervical mucus from coming into contact with the vagina. The cervical cap and diaphragm also provide some protection. And oral contraceptives, which thicken cervical mucus, may prevent some organisms from reaching the uterus, reducing the risk of PID.

- **Don't douche:** Although douching does not cause PID, it may spread infection from the vagina into the uterus. *Note:* With the help of gravity and mucus, the vagina cleanses itself naturally. Also, douches strip away normal bacteria that wards off infection, changing the pH balance, or levels of acidity, and making the vagina and surrounding structures more vulnerable to infection.

- **Practice good hygiene:** Wipe from front to back after a bowel movement, and don't have vaginal intercourse immediately after anal intercourse.

Premenstrual Syndrome (PMS)

Lots of things in life aren't funny — IRS audits, traffic accidents, and PMS. Oh sure, everyone makes jokes about "that time of the month," but PMS is no laughing matter; it's a serious condition that affects an estimated 9 million to 12 million women in the United States. The medical establishment didn't take this syndrome seriously for some time. But over the past two decades, most doctors have stopped patting women on the hand and telling them it was all in their heads and started listening.

Premenstrual syndrome covers a wide range of symptoms — numbering more than 100 — that occur before menstruation. It's estimated that only 5 percent of women suffer from serious, life-altering symptoms, but many women experience the syndrome in a milder form. The characteristics and degrees of severity of PMS may differ from woman to woman, but the timing of the symptoms is predictable.

PMS is generally thought to be provoked by hormone levels rising and falling throughout a woman's cycle.

Falling levels of estrogen and progesterone and increased production of *aldosterone* (a masculine hormone naturally present in women's bodies) can set off a cascade of bodily changes. Other hormones may also play a role: Aldosterone leads to sodium retention and swelling. Low levels of estrogen increase levels of *monoamine oxidase*, a brain chemical that can cause depression, and reduce levels of *serotonin*, a brain chemical that affects mood and activity levels. The hormone levels return to normal at the start of menstruation.

Recognizing the signs

The trouble with PMS is that it covers such a wide range of symptoms that timing is more crucial to diagnosis than the symptoms themselves. Symptoms of PMS occur several days before menstruation and ease once menstruation starts. They include

- ✔ Acne
- ✔ Appetite changes and food cravings
- ✔ Breast tenderness or enlargement
- ✔ Constipation
- ✔ Diarrhea
- ✔ Difficulty concentrating
- ✔ Fatigue
- ✔ Fluid retention, which can result in abdominal bloating, swollen hands and feet, and weight gain
- ✔ Headaches
- ✔ Insomnia

- Lethargy

- Nausea and vomiting

- Premenstrual tension (depression, mood swings, irritability, anxiety)

Some women report a lower tolerance to alcohol, allergy flare-ups, and panic attacks. And women with PMS are more likely to get infections at this time. Experts believe that a women's immune system becomes slightly weaker before menses making her vulnerable to viral and bacterial infections.

Knowing for sure

A thorough medical history and careful recording of symptoms and days when symptoms occur are crucial. Symptoms include the bigger picture such as changes in activity levels, eating and sleeping patterns, and productivity levels at work. Your doctor will also look at *impaired social interaction.* (That's scientific talk for when you'd rather stay home and watch *Gilligan's Island* reruns than go out to that new Italian restaurant a few blocks away.)

Making it better

Don't diagnose this condition by yourself. Although PMS does not reflect any harmful underlying disorder, it can mimic more serious conditions, including cancer. So make sure that your doctor is aware of what your symptoms are. Follow her advice — she may suggest a trial month or two for you to record your symptoms before she puts you on any kind of treatment regimen. Also record any major life stresses — the death of a relative, for example — would give you a good reason to feel depressed and weepy.

Here are a few tips you can follow:

- **Keep a menstrual cycle diary:** Chart the symptoms and days when you experience anything that is not normal — that is, something that isn't experienced during the rest of your cycle. Doing so helps you know what to expect each month and for how long. If your symptoms are mild, knowing what to expect and when to expect it may be all you need to help you cope.

- **Lay off the java:** Caffeine increases irritability, anxiety, and mood swings. Unfortunately, caffeine shows up in some unexpected places: iced tea, soda, even over-the-counter preparations such as Midol, a menstrual pain reliever. Avoid excess caffeine while you are premenstrual, especially if you feel irritable or anxious. Once you get your period, you can take pain relievers that contain caffeine because they will help your body eliminate any excess fluid you retain.

✔ **Watch what you eat:** Your best bet is a high-complex carbohydrate, low-fat diet. Although you may crave sugar, you're better off eating raisin bran for breakfast than a candy bar. The carbohydrates in cereals can actually calm you down because carbohydrates have an effect on *serotonin* (a chemical that affects sleep) levels in the brain. Also avoid salt in the last few days before your period, which can help you reduce bloating and fluid retention.

✔ **Exercise:** Exercise can minimize and even eliminate some PMS symptoms. It reduces stress and depression and releases natural brain hormones known as endorphins, which make you feel good. Exercise also improves menstrual flow and may reduce menstrual cramps.

If your symptoms haven't decreased in severity or your condition gets worse, your health care practitioner may put you on hormone therapy, such as oral contraceptives. Birth control pills reduce pain because they suppress ovulation.

She may decide to treat your more irritating or severe symptoms with drugs that lower your prostaglandin levels and/or mild tranquilizers or antidepressants for mood disorders. Most of the medications have to be taken through your entire cycle, not just before or during your period, so make sure to discuss the pros and cons of this with your doctor.

Uterine Fibroids

The only lumps you should have in life are the kind that show in your mattress after a few years of use. Lumps and bumps in your body generally aren't good news, but uterine fibroids may not always be bad news. An estimated 25 percent of women between the ages of 30 to 50 years have these benign tumors, which are made of muscle cells. Fibroids can grow in the cavity of the uterus, within the wall, or outside the uterus. (See Figure 18-2.) They range in size from as small as a pea to as large as a grapefruit (though that size is rare). Most fibroids don't produce any kind of symptoms. And 99 percent of fibroids are not cancerous. Most shrink in size or disappear once menopause occurs.

Yet like bullies in a school yard, some fibroids make a lot of trouble. They may press hard on the bladder, spurring the need for repeat trips to the bathroom. They can trigger lower back pain or discomfort. And they can cause infertility because they can prevent fertilized eggs from implanting in the uterus. Fibroids can also wreak havoc on your menstrual cycle by causing bleeding between periods, making normal periods heavier, or prolonging the time you have your period. That kind of blood loss may be enough to cause anemia.

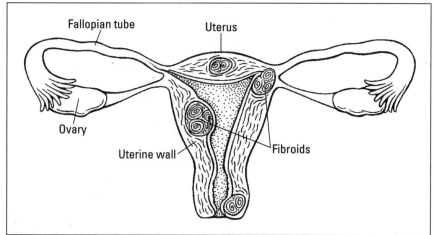

Fallopian tube

Uterus

Figure 18-2:
Fibroids,
little bumps
in or around
your uterus,
may not
produce
any
symptoms.

Ovary

Uterine wall

Fibroids

Recognizing the signs

Many women who have fibroids experience no symptoms, but some experience heavy or prolonged bleeding during menstrual periods; bleeding between periods; cramping; pelvic pain and pressure or low back pain; frequent urination; abdominal swelling; or pain during sex.

Knowing for sure

Fibroids are often discovered during a pelvic exam. If your doctor needs to confirm the presence of fibroids, she may use ultrasound to produce an image of the uterus, laparoscopy to view the uterus, or *hysteroscopy*, a procedure in which a viewing scope is inserted into the uterus through the cervix.

Making it better

Unless fibroids cause severe pain or pressure, are the cause of infertility, or grow to larger than 4 inches in diameter, they don't need to be treated.

If you're diagnosed with benign uterine fibroids, regular exams are critical. You'll want to keep track of their size, just in case. And you'll want to report any menstrual irregularities.

If fibroids are causing a problem, your doctor may consider the following:

✔ **Drug treatment:** Gonadotropin-releasing hormone antagonists (GnRH), estrogen-blocking drugs, may be used to cause the fibroids to shrink temporarily; however, these drugs have menopauselike side effects, such as hot flashes. For this reason, they are used only on a temporary basis before surgery to shrink the fibroids and decrease blood loss.

✔ **Myomectomy:** If you still wish to have children, your doctor may perform a myomectomy, a surgical procedure in which the fibroid is removed but the uterus is kept intact. This operation is not without risk, so you may have some side effects or complications, such as scarring or adhesion formation, that can cause chronic pelvic pain. Fibroids also have a nasty habit of returning, so if you doctor removes a fibroid and detects another in a follow-up a year or two later, it doesn't mean she missed one. Myomectomy can be performed through an abdominal incision if they are large, or a hysteroscope inserted through the cervix if they are small and located in the cavity of the uterus.

✔ **Endometrial ablation:** This technique allows the doctor to burn the uterine lining and any fibroids. It stops heavy menstrual flow and keeps the uterus intact, but it leaves the woman infertile.

✔ **Uterine artery embolation (UAE):** In this procedure, a chemical is injected into the uterine arteries nearest the fibroid. The chemical closes off the artery and shuts off the blood supply to the fibroid. The fibroid shrinks and eventually dies. You should not have this procedure if you plan to get pregnant because shutting off the blood supply to the fibroid may also disrupt the blood supply to part or all of the uterus.

✔ **Hysterectomy:** If your case is severe, your doctor may recommend a hysterectomy. Although fibroids were once the number one reason for hysterectomy, most doctors now believe that the surgery is necessary only when you have chronic pelvic pain, excessive bleeding, or severe symptoms that cannot be treated with myomectomy. Some doctors also recommend hysterectomy for large fibroids, while others believe that symptoms rather than size should dictate the surgery. If your doctor recommends hysterectomy, make sure that you get a second opinion.

Uterine Prolapse

It's no surprise that women over the age of 60 may experience the effects of gravity on their uterus. *Uterine prolapse,* a uterus that partially descends into the vagina, occurs as a result of diminished tone of the pelvic floor muscles and the stretching and weakening of the ligaments that support them.

Pregnancy and birth take a toll on your body. A tough labor and delivery may damage the supporting structures around your reproductive organs. Uterine prolapse can also be the result of a genetic weakness in the supporting structures because women who are childless may experience prolapse. Other causes include obesity, an enlarged uterus, and pelvic tumors.

Prolapse has different degrees of severity. Mild prolapse, with the cervix and uterus only slightly lower in the vagina, may cause no symptoms or only mild discomfort at certain times such as during intercourse. With severe prolapse, the uterus is escaping from the vagina to the outside of the body, and the symptoms of a bulge or something pushing out of the vagina are unmistakable.

Recognizing the signs

You may notice bleeding and discomfort or feel a pressure in the vaginal area. You may also have urine flow problems depending on whether the uterus is pressing on the bladder. You may also experience a constant backache or pressure, especially after straining your muscles, and pain during intercourse.

Knowing for sure

Your doctor can diagnose uterine prolapse during a pelvic exam.

Making it better

Depending on the degree of prolapse, you may want to consider all the treatment options.

Here are a few things you can do on your own:

- ✔ **Bulk up:** Constipation may be a symptom of or contribute to prolapse. Make sure that your diet includes adequate amounts of fiber (25 to 30 grams per day) and lots of water to keep your stools soft enough to have a bowel movement without excessive bearing down.

- ✔ **Lose weight:** If you're overweight, losing weight can help relieve pressure on your pelvic organs.

- ✔ **Exercise your pelvic muscles:** Kegel exercises (see Chapter 23) can help tighten the muscles around the vagina and rectum. These exercises may be helpful if you start them in the early stages of a prolapse.

Depending on the severity of your prolapsed uterus, your doctor may prescribe hormones to help improve ovulation to thicken the vaginal walls, fit you with a *pessary,* (a diaphragmlike device that is inserted into the vagina and helps support the uterus and hold it in place or suggest surgery. The surgeon may reposition the uterus and any other organs that have dropped, shorten stretched ligaments, and reinforce the muscles around the vagina, bladder, and rectum in a procedure known as anterior and/or posterior repair.

An ounce of prevention

To reduce your risk of uterine prolapse, follow the self-care tips in the "Making it better" section. You may also want to monitor your reproduction. Women with more than five children may be more at risk for prolapse.

Vaginitis

Burning and itching are pretty common in women of all ages, thanks to *vaginitis,* a catchall term for a whole host of conditions that inflame the vagina, including yeast infections and other fungal infections, bacterial infections, and infections caused by parasites. An estimated 75 percent of women experience a vaginal infection at least once in their lives.

The three most common types of vaginitis are

- ✔ **Yeast infections:** Also known as *candidiasis,* yeast infections are caused by the overgrowth of a yeastlike fungus known as *Candida*, which is normally present in the vagina in harmless quantities. This overgrowth may occur if your immunity is low, if you're taking antibiotics, or if you're a menopausal woman who does not take hormone replacement therapy. Some women experience yeast infections before their periods when their bodies are more susceptible to infection. And in menopause, the vaginal lining is thinner and more prone to infection. Yeast infections may be a recurrent problem for women who are exposed to warm, wet climates and warm, wet bathing suits or athletic clothes.

- ✔ **Bacterial vaginosis**: This type is a bacterial infection. Common causes include the bacteria *Gardnerella vaginalis* and group B streptococcus, which generally migrate to the vagina from the nearby skin around the bowel. Sexually active women may be predisposed to this infection; thrusting during intercourse can help more bacteria enter the vagina.

- ✔ **Trichomoniasis:** Also known as trich, this type is caused by the *Trichomonas vaginalis* parasite. This parasite is often transmitted via sexual intercourse (see Chapter 22 for more information).

Symptoms similar to those of vaginitis can also be caused by other sexually transmitted diseases, as well as the vaginal dryness of menopause, and the use of vaginal sprays, deodorant soaps, shampoos, spermicides, bubble baths, and douches.

Recognizing the signs

Symptoms of vaginitis include abnormal vaginal discharge (thick, white, and "cheesy;" off-colored, grayish-greenish with a fishy odor; or frothy yellow or greenish discharge with an unpleasant odor), itching, or burning.

Knowing for sure

Because vaginitis has many different causes, which necessitate different treatments, you need to see your doctor for an accurate diagnosis. Your doctor will take your medical history and perform a pelvic exam along with a microscopic examination or culture of your vaginal discharge.

Making it better

Treatment varies with the cause and severity of vaginosis. Vaginal infections are treated with various creams, ointments, suppositories, or pills.

Because many vaginal infections are treated by medications that are only available with a prescription, you need to see your doctor.

If you have a yeast infection that has already been diagnosed, you may wish to try an over-the-counter antifungal cream such as Monistat or Gyne-Lotrimin. You may also wish to eat some yogurt that contains "active cultures," the naturally occurring bacteria that helps your system ward off more severe infections. Women with recurrent infections sometimes report that eating yogurt with active cultures lessens the severity and occurrence of their infections.

If you have a yeast infection, your doctor may prescribe an antifungal cream, ointment, suppository, or pill. If your irritation is caused by vaginosis, you will generally be prescribed an antibiotic cream; the type of bacteria responsible for the infection dictates the antibiotic. If you have trich, treatment may consist of the oral antibiotic metronidazole (Flagyl) or another antibiotic in suppository, cream, or gel form.

An ounce of prevention

The moist, warm vagina is an ideal breeding ground for bacteria. You can reduce your risk of vaginitis by making the environment a little less hospitable to foreign bacteria.

To prevent all forms of vaginitis

- ✔ **Practice safe sex:** Doing so helps prevent infectious organisms from entering your body. And if you're being treated for vaginitis, a condom or female condom (vaginal pouch) can help stop the spread of the bacteria.

- ✔ **Wipe front to back:** Always wipe away from the vagina after bowel movements.

- ✔ **Air out:** Wear breathable underwear, panty hose with a cotton crotch, or loose-fitting pants. And make sure that your underwear, workout clothes, swimsuits, or anything that comes into contact with your vaginal area is washed in hot soapy water. Hot water may sound like murder on your delicates, but it will kill yeast. After a sweaty workout or a swim, shower and get into clean, dry, loose, cotton clothing.

To help prevent yeast infections

- ✔ **Eat Healthily:** A daily cup of yogurt containing live *Lactobacillus acidophilus* can help stop yeast from growing in the digestive tract and vagina. This healthy bacterium is available in capsule and tablet form.

- ✔ **Stay healthy:** Take antibiotics only if they're absolutely necessary. Ask your doctor if she can prescribe a prescription antiyeast treatment if you are prone to yeast infections after taking antibiotics.

Chapter 19

Breast Health

• •

In This Chapter

▶ Caring for inflamed breasts

▶ Understanding fibrocystic conditions

▶ Recognizing noncancerous lumps

▶ Discovering the pros and cons of cosmetic breast surgery

• •

*Y*our breasts are among your most distinctive features: They distinguish your profile from that of a man, enable you to provide sustenance to your young children, and contribute to your sense of fashion. This chapter looks at common breast conditions and helps you learn when and whether they should be treated. (See Chapter 16 for information about breast cancer.) This chapter also examines the pros and cons of cosmetic surgery to enlarge or reduce the breasts.

Mastitis (Breast Inflammation)

Mastitis, or inflammation of the breast, is the result of an infection in the breast. The condition is most common in breast-feeding women whose milk ducts have become blocked by bacteria that enter the breast through a cut, bite, or scratch.

Recognizing the signs

If you develop mastitis, you'll most likely notice some of the following symptoms: fever, swelling of the skin or nipple, redness, tenderness, and a tired, achy feeling.

Knowing for sure

If you're breast-feeding, these symptoms generally mean infection, and your doctor will probably not perform any diagnostic tests, although your doctor may want to rule out other causes of possible injury, such as trauma.

Making it better

Fortunately, mastitis can be successfully treated with a combination of medication and self-care. Using these treatments, the condition generally subsides in about 48 hours.

Early detection and treatment of breast infection is critical. If you don't treat the infection properly, it may develop into an *abscess* (a painfully infected area of tissue), which may have to be opened surgically to let the pus drain out. This can interfere with milk production.

You can help to treat mastitis and alleviate the discomfort associated with it by applying heat: take a hot bath or shower, or use a heating pad.

Because mastitis usually affects breast-feeding women, nursing mothers should keep the following in mind:

- ✔ **Continue to breast-feed:** Doing so helps drain the breast of milk, which eases the condition caused by the pressure of the built-up milk and discourages further growth of bacteria. The infection will not harm your baby.

- ✔ **Keep emptying your breasts on a regular basis:** If you can't continue nursing, drain the breast milk manually or with a breast pump. You can freeze the milk and give it to your baby later. (For more information on breast-feeding, see Chapter 26.)

In addition to the self-care regimen mentioned in the preceding section, mastitis is treated with antibiotics that are safe for breast-feeding women. Consult your doctor for a proper diagnosis and the most appropriate medication for you. Antibiotics are especially important early in the condition to avoid abscess formation.

An ounce of prevention

Although there's no definitive way to prevent breast infection, you can reduce your risk if you are breast-feeding by keeping your nipples clean and dry between feedings and wearing nonirritating clothing, such as cotton nursing bras.

Fibrocystic Conditions

If you're a woman of childbearing age, the odds are that you will develop a fibrocystic breast condition at some point — if you haven't already. Fibrocystic condition, which also includes other terms such as fibrocystic changes, cystic disease, chronic cystic mastitis, and mammary dysplasia, is simply a fancy (and anxiety-provoking) way of describing benign, lumpy breasts. Fortunately, the key word here is benign. Fibrocystic conditions are characterized by benign, or noncancerous, fluid-filled cysts in the breast, and the prescribed treatment is oftentimes to do nothing.

Sometimes, nonmalignant lumps are referred to as cysts. They're not. Many forms of "noncystic" benign lumps exist. (See "Benign Breast Lumps" later in this chapter.) For information about distinguishing between cysts and cancerous lumps, see the sidebar "Do fibrocystic conditions increase your risk of developing breast cancer?"

Fibrocystic conditions are extremely common. In fact, fibrocystic conditions are the most common cause of lumps in women of childbearing age: It is estimated that one-third to one-fourth of all women will experience fibrocystic breast symptoms at some point in their lives. Because this condition is so common, doctors no longer refer to it as fibrocystic disease. Simply put, lumpiness is just normal breast tissue in which one or more long, threadlike fibers divide into cysts (sacs that contain fluid).

If your breasts swell and feel tender and lumpy just prior to your period, chances are good that you have fibrocystic breasts. The symptoms are thought to occur in response to high or low levels of the hormones estrogen and progesterone and are affected by fluctuations of the menstrual cycle. Lumpiness tends to manifest itself seven to ten days before a woman's period begins and then subsides after menstruation begins. The lumps often disappear or shrink after menopause.

Recognizing the signs

Symptoms associated with fibrocystic condition may vary from mild to severe. You will, however, typically notice the following patterns:

- Lumps that feel fluid-filled, like clusters of peas or grapes (although they may become as large as golf balls). Cysts are usually movable, soft, and tender to the touch (sometimes painful). They can be present in both breasts, and the lumpiness is often located in the upper-outer quadrants of each breast.

- Tenderness (perhaps even pain) in one or both breasts, especially under your armpits.

✔ Breast fullness and swelling, often cyclical in nature and worse right before your period.

✔ Lumps that develop or multiply just before the menstrual period and then subside or disappear a few days after it begins. Some women may experience discomfort throughout the menstrual cycle.

A breast cyst may stretch in size when filled with fluid, which is why the size varies throughout the menstrual cycle. Some cysts are so small that they're hardly detectable, while others can easily be felt by palpating the breast.

Knowing for sure

The only way your doctor can know for sure that a lump in your breast is a cyst is to rule out cancer.

Your doctor will probably start by discussing your medical history and performing a complete physical examination of your breasts. The exam, which includes a visual inspection for asymmetry, puckering, and changes in the nipple and skin texture and palpation of your breasts, armpits, and collarbone to feel for lumps, enables her to better determine the lump's location and size as well as assess your own individual risk of breast cancer.

Monthly breast self-exams are crucial for all women, particularly if you have fibrocystic breasts. You should "memorize" your breasts and regularly examine them for any lumps or thickening that don't fit your usual pattern of fibrocystic changes. Be sure to notify your doctor immediately if you notice any changes that are out of the norm. (For more information on breast self-exams, see Chapter 2.)

Other diagnostic tools that your doctor may use include the following:

✔ **Mammogram:** This test produces an x-ray of the breast and can tell whether some lumps are benign or cancerous. To ensure the greatest accuracy, mammography and ultrasound are often used together.

✔ **Ultrasound:** This test uses sound waves to create an image of the breast and may be used to determine whether a lump is solid or fluid-filled. Fluid-filled masses are usually benign; solid masses require biopsy. Ultrasound is especially helpful for examining dense breasts.

✔ **Fine-needle aspiration:** In this nonsurgical *biopsy* (a test in which tissue or fluid is removed and analyzed), a hollow needle is inserted into the lump. If the lump is a benign cyst, the fluid is drained and analyzed. This procedure, which collapses the lump if it's a cyst, is normally performed in your doctor's office or in the mammography unit. Aspirating a cyst simultaneously diagnoses and treats the condition.

✔ **Needle-directed biopsy:** A needle is directed into the area thought to be abnormal on your mammogram, while you are still in the mammography department. An additional x-ray can be taken to make sure the needle is taking a sample from the part of the breast that is of greatest concern. The tissue sample is then analyzed.

✔ **Open biopsy:** In this test, a larger sample of breast tissue is removed through a surgical incision and examined under a microscope. This option is the most thorough for diagnosing a lump.

Keep in mind that a biopsy is surgery (although minor) and should be avoided whenever possible. For this reason, most lumps should be aspirated before they are biopsied.

A biopsy is certainly warranted, however, under select circumstances, such as the following:

✔ If the lump doesn't go away after fine-needle aspiration

✔ If the cyst has recurred after multiple aspirations

✔ If the fluid drained from aspiration is bloody

✔ If analysis of any fluid or cells from the other procedure reveals the possible presence of abnormal cells

Making it better

If your fibrocystic lumps cause minimal discomfort, no specific treatment may be required. In fact, the cysts may actually disappear on their own with time. In many cases, however, some form of treatment is required, be it self-care or medical.

There are many things you can do to reduce and/or eliminate lumps as well as to minimize the discomfort associated with them. Here are a few examples:

✔ **Try an over-the-counter pain reliever:** Over-the-counter pain relievers such as aspirin, acetaminophen (Tylenol), or ibuprofen (Advil) may relieve some discomfort.

✔ **Wear a support bra:** A well-fitting bra that provides adequate support may reduce discomfort in some women. A good exercise bra is especially important if you do any high-impact activities such as jogging.

✔ **Cut the caffeine:** Some women have reported a decrease in symptoms, mainly breast pain and tenderness, when they decreased their caffeine consumption.

✔ **Get on the vitamins:** Increase your intake of vitamins E, A, and B₆. Several studies have found a daily dose of vitamin E (600 international units, or I.U.) effective in reducing breast discomfort as well as the size and number of lumps.

✔ **Go low on salt:** Restrict your diet of any excess salt, which can contribute to fluid retention. When you retain water, all your body tissues swell up, including your breasts.

Research is mixed on the effectiveness of some of these self-care methods, although most appear to be effective, healthful steps to follow.

Your doctor may have a few suggestions as well, including the following:

✔ **Oral contraceptives:** Your doctor may prescribe oral contraceptives to create a consistent low level of the hormones estrogen and progesterone, which may deter the growth of more lumps and help to relieve symptoms that fluctuate with your menstrual cycle.

✔ **Medication:** A drug called danazol (Danocrine) is sometimes used to reduce swelling, relieve breast pain, and in some cases, eliminate severe breast lumpiness. Danazol is a synthetic form of a male hormone. Although it may eliminate severe breast lumpiness and pain, it is associated with several possible side effects, including the loss of menstrual periods; weight gain; acne or oily skin; facial hair; and rarely, voice deepening. It should not be used by women trying to get pregnant. You should consult with your doctor about possible options.

Do fibrocystic conditions increase your risk of developing breast cancer?

Just because you have a fibrocystic lump doesn't mean that you're at increased risk of contracting breast cancer. Although some earlier studies indicated that women with fibrocystic breasts were at slightly increased risk of developing breast cancer, newer studies indicate that is not the case. But that doesn't mean you're completely out of the woods. You need to be aware that precancerous lesions occasionally accompany breast cysts. These lesions, notably *atypical lobular hyperplasia* and *ductal hyperplasia,* are characterized by excessive growth of abnormal cells and do carry an increased risk of breast cancer developing in the future. Only a biopsy can determine whether hyperplasia is present. In addition, your benign condition may make it more difficult for you or your doctor to detect a cancerous tumor if one should develop because cysts that are assumed to be benign may be right next to or on top of a malignant lump. So, if you have a fibrocystic condition, make sure that you perform a breast self-exam each month and make sure that your doctor examines your breasts regularly.

An ounce of prevention

When it comes to fibrocystic conditions, most of the preventive measures you should take are those listed in the earlier self-care treatment section. In addition, regular breast exams are critical.

If you have lumpy breasts, in addition to performing monthly breast self-exams, you should be examined more frequently than just once a year by a doctor or gynecologist who has extensive clinical experience in breast disease. How often you need to be seen will depend on your individual condition. A baseline mammogram before the age of 35 may also be a good idea, particularly if you have a family history of breast cancer.

Benign Breast Lumps

What exactly are benign lumps? Well, they usually form within the breast's milk-secreting glands, nestled within fatty breast tissue. Lumps come in a variety of sizes, shapes, and textures. They're usually, although not always, tender, movable, and affected by the menstrual cycle. Besides fibrocystic condition, other common benign breast lumps include fibroadenomas, lipomas, intraductal papillomas, breast calcifications, and traumatic fat necrosis. The following is a brief description of each.

Fibroadenomas

Fibroadenomas typically occur in very young women, usually those in their teens or early 20s. These lumps, which are composed of fibrous and glandular tissue, generally feel round, rubbery, and movable. Fibroadenomas are normally painless and unaffected by the menstrual cycle. And unlike cysts, which feel soft and fluid-filled, fibroadenomas are solid lumps. Doctors usually recommend a mammogram, often with an ultrasound, to diagnose fibroadenomas because the lumps have a characteristic appearance. If there is any doubt, however, the lump should be biopsied.

Some doctors recommend surgical removal of the lumps; others will operate only if the lumps grow large enough to change breast shape or if there is any suspicion they are masking cancer. In either instance, fibroadenomas do not increase a woman's risk of breast cancer. Nevertheless, the exact cause of these lumps remains a mystery, and they cannot be prevented.

Intraductal papillomas

These tiny, wartlike lumps grow in the lining of the milk ducts, usually near the nipple. They sometimes cause dark and/or bloody nipple discharge and may even produce infection and inflammation by blocking the milk ducts. Intraductal papillomas are usually removed to confirm that they are not cancerous lumps.

Breast calcifications

Breast calcifications are tiny deposits of calcium in the breast, detectable only through mammograms. Two distinct types exist — macro- and microcalcifications.

Macrocalcifications are benign lumps that reflect degenerative changes in the breast. A biopsy is usually not required. Macrocalcifications typically occur in women ages 50 and over. In fact, the National Cancer Institute reports that they are found in 50 percent of women over age 50 and in 10 percent of younger women.

Microcalcifications are tiny deposits of calcium in the breast as seen on mammograms. A certain type of grouped microcalcifications in one area may appear suspicious for cancer, and a biopsy is recommended.

Traumatic fat necrosis

These are round, painless lumps comprised of dead fat cells that form after injury (trauma) to the breast or after a breast biopsy or surgery. The skin surrounding the lump may appear red. Traumatic fat necrosis appears most commonly in older women and women with large breasts. Fortunately, these lumps are not tied to cancer, and removal is usually not necessary. The body generally absorbs them.

Cosmetic Breast Surgery

Cosmetic breast surgery to reduce or augment breast size has become increasingly popular in recent years. Although risks are associated with both breast reduction and augmentation surgery, modern medicine has indeed achieved many state-of-the-art advances in cosmetic procedures. In the end, only you can make the decision of whether to pursue breast surgery. The following sections will shed new light on these controversial procedures and better assist you in making an educated, rational decision that's right for you.

Breast reduction surgery

Breast reduction, or _reduction mammoplasty,_ is performed for medical or cosmetic reasons. Typically, it's a combination of the two. This procedure, which is illustrated in Figure 19-1, reduces the size of large breasts.

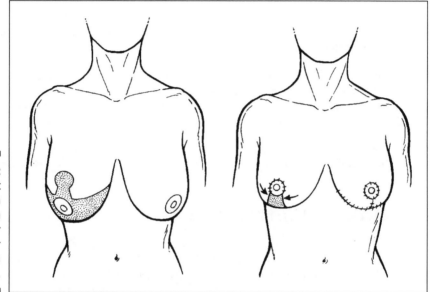

Figure 19-1:
Breast
reduction
surgery can
be done for
medical or
cosmetic
reasons.

If you have extremely large breasts, you probably endure various uncomfortable and even painful ailments, including chronic back pain; skin irritations and shoulder grooves from "digging" bra straps; difficulty breathing; and painful breasts.

There's no denying the tremendous emotional impact that very large breasts can have on a woman, causing many "healthy" women to seek refuge through breast reduction.

If you have extremely large breasts and are contemplating breast reduction for medical and/or cosmetic purposes, consider the following before deciding whether breast reduction is right for you:

✔ **Timing is everything:** Experts stress not to have reduction surgery if your breasts are still growing (your bra size has changed over the past year). By doing so, you only risk the possibility of having to repeat the surgery once your breasts regrow.

✔ **It's all in the weight:** Remember that weight loss and, more significantly, weight gain will affect the outcome of reduction surgery by causing your breasts to change size accordingly. For best, long-lasting results, be sure that you're prepared to maintain your current weight.

Breast reduction surgery is usually performed under general anesthesia and assumes the same risks as other major surgeries; namely, infection.

The surgery consists of two parts (performed under a single surgical session): reducing the actual breast size and moving the nipples back to their original places.

The nipple and areola are cut but not completely removed, remaining attached to the breast by a stalklike piece of tissue in order to keep their blood supply; excess breast tissue is extracted; the nipple and areola are sewn back to the breast.

In some instances, however, you do have a risk of scarring. Depending upon how well you heal, the scar may be barely visible or rather prominent.

Breast augmentation surgery

Breast augmentation surgery has been the source of much controversy in recent years. That's because in 1992, the Food and Drug Administration, citing the dangers of silicone gel-filled implants, banned these implants for any use other than breast reconstruction after cancer surgery. This left only saline-filled (salt water) implants available for breast augmentation. And that's how it stands today.

Saline-filled breast implants are deemed safer than silicone gel-filled implants because salt water is naturally present in the body. Should a saline implant leak or rupture, the body will absorb the solution rather than treat it as a foreign matter. However, saline implants are enclosed in a casing made of a silicone product. Experts believe that the amount of silicone within the casing is so small that a leakage shouldn't pose a threat. Studies are still being conducted.

Breast augmentation, or *augmentation mammoplasty,* (see Figure 19-2) increases breast size by surgically placing pouches of saline under the existing breast skin or, in some cases, under the chest muscle. Of course, these implants don't last forever and may have to be replaced years later. And additional surgery and/or medical procedures may be needed after implantation due to problems or complications. Nevertheless, millions of women have found the procedure to be beneficial, and it remains a popular, though highly controversial surgery.

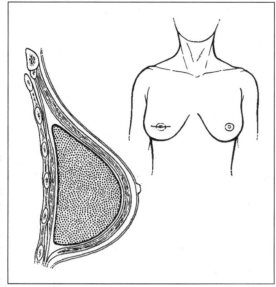

Figure 19-2:
Breast
enlargement
surgery
involves the
placement
of implants.

Following are the leading potential problems associated with breast augmentation:

✔ **Capsular contracture:** This is a tightening of the scar tissue surrounding the implant. It may cause pain, hardening of the breast, or a change in breast appearance. It is corrected surgically.

✔ **Additional surgery:** You may need additional surgery to treat a serious problem with the implants or to remove a ruptured implant.

✔ **Calcium deposits:** These may also form around the surrounding tissue, causing pain and hardening of the scar tissue.

✔ **Changes in nipple or breast sensation:** Sensation may gradually return later.

✔ **Possible inability to breast-feed:** Changes in nipple or breast sensation may affect the response of the nipple during breast-feeding.

Currently, it's not known whether leakage from an implant may be passed to a child during breast-feeding.

✔ **Interference with mammogram readings:** This is a potentially dangerous situation because implants can delay the early detection of breast cancer by "hiding" lumps. Women with implants should inform the radiologist and mammography technician about the implants before mammography is performed.

✔ **Shifting of the implants:** This can result in an unnatural breast shape and, possibly, pain.

✔ **Appearance problems:** These include incorrect implant size, uneven breasts, and wrinkling of the implant.

✔ **Breast pain:** Changes in the breast as a result of augmentation may cause pain.

✔ **Scarring:** Typically, any scarring you develop from augmentation surgery should fade over time to thin lines, although the darker your skin the more prominent the scars.

If you're contemplating breast augmentation, you should have realistic expectations of the surgical outcome in order to base your decision. The following points will help you to decide whether breast enlargement will produce the outcome you desire:

✔ Ask your doctor for "before" and "after" pictures of patients she has operated on.

✔ Talk to other women who have had the same surgery performed by your surgeon at least a year before. Keep in mind, however, that no one can guarantee that the same results will occur.

✔ Know the individual factors that have an effect on surgery outcomes, including your overall health; chest structure and body shape; healing ability; bleeding tendencies; prior breast surgery; infection; skill of surgical team; type of surgical procedure; type and size of implants.

Breast augmentation can be performed on an outpatient or inpatient basis, using either local or general anesthesia. Surgery may last from one to two hours, depending upon whether the implant is inserted in front of or behind the chest muscle and whether one or both breasts are involved. Following surgery, you'll experience temporary side effects, including pain, swelling, bruising, and tenderness.

Chapter 20

Menbopause

● ●

In This Chapter

▶ Understanding the mechanics of menopause

▶ Recognizing the menopausal symptoms

▶ Learning about health risks in menopause

▶ Deciding on hormone replacement therapy

▶ Understanding the hows and whys of hysterectomy and surgical menopause

● ●

lthough the term *menopause* actually refers to the point when your body stops menstruating, people tend to use it to encompass the whole process that your body goes through as your ovaries gradually shut down hormone production. If you want to get technical about it, the process leading up to the point when your menstrual periods stop is called *perimenopause*. Menopause is only considered official once you haven't had a period for 12 months. After that point, you're considered *postmenopausal*.

You may experience a variety of symptoms when you are in perimenopause, from hot flashes to mood swings. But the hallmark of perimenopause is changes in your menstrual pattern. This chapter looks at the reasons behind these and other symptoms, examines how menopause (what we call both menopause and perimenopause) affects your overall health, and looks at the various treatments available to help you cope with these changes.

What's Going On?

To get a clear understanding of what's going on during menopause, you need to understand what happens as your body goes through its menstrual cycle.

Your ovaries are filled with egg cells, or *oocytes*. Oocytes are kind of like dormant seeds. An oocyte and its surrounding support cells have the capacity to develop into a follicle that ultimately releases an egg. But like seeds, not all oocytes mature and develop. They need the right conditions, and they compete with one another for survival. As you age, your oocytes die off and become depleted so that while you start out life with a million or two, by the time you reach menopause, you have only a few thousand left.

Your menstrual cycle is regulated by the estrogen and progesterone hormones that are produced by the ovary when a follicle releases an egg. The presence (or lack) of these hormones triggers the different responses in your body. See Figure 20-1.

When your estrogen and progesterone levels are low, the hypothalamus in your brain produces a hormone that kick-starts your pituitary gland into producing follicle stimulating hormone (FSH) and luteinizing hormone (LH). The presence of FSH and LH encourages some of the oocytes to develop and mature into follicles. One (or occasionally two or more) follicle beats out the others and matures further. As the follicle develops, it releases estrogen into your body. The estrogen feeds the lining of the uterus, which grows and thickens. When the follicle finally matures, it releases an egg (ovulation). The follicle is transformed into the *corpus luteum,* a small yellow cyst on the surface of the ovary that secretes progesterone.

Progesterone causes the lining of the inner uterine walls to thicken and form blood vessels and stockpile nutrients to support a potential fertilized egg, or fetus. The release of estrogen and progesterone continues for about 14 days. If the egg isn't fertilized, the high levels of estrogen and progesterone cause a decrease in the production of FSH and LH, which causes the corpus luteum to stop producing hormones and feeding the lining. The lack of progesterone then causes the lining of the uterus, or endometrium, to break down, causing you to menstruate. At that point, your low estrogen and progesterone levels trigger your hypothalamus to start the process all over again.

You go through this cycle month after month — until you approach menopause. At that point, at least for most women, the process becomes much less predictable. Your periods may come closer together, late, or you may skip them entirely. You may have light intermittent bleeding, called *spotting,* or you may have very heavy bleeding. Here's why these changes take place.

As you approach menopause, your ovaries produce less estrogen and have trouble producing viable follicles. Your pituitary may crank out the FSH, but the oocytes just don't respond. When ovulation becomes irregular, it affects the production of progesterone, which is needed for cyclic menstruation to take place. So your uterine lining may build up, but not shed, throwing your cycle out of kilter. Your period may be delayed, or it may start on time but continue longer than normal or be heavier or lighter than normal.

Eventually, you stop ovulating altogether, gradually your ovaries stop producing estrogen, and your periods cease.

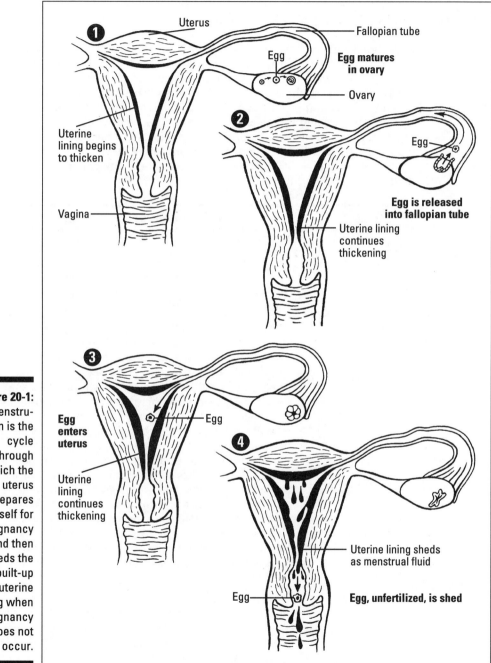

Figure 20-1: Menstrutation is the cycle through which the uterus prepares itself for pregnancy and then sheds the built-up uterine lining when pregnancy does not occur.

Menopausal Symptoms

In addition to changes in your period, menopause produces changes that affect your entire body. Due to a lack of estrogen, estrogen-sensitive organs, such as your uterus, ovaries, and breasts, shrink, while other estrogen-sensitive tissues, such as the vaginal walls and the tissue of the urethra, become thinner and less elastic. Bone mass begins to decrease, and skin becomes thinner and less elastic. These changes may or may not produce symptoms, but if they do, they're likely to take some time to appear. Other symptoms, such as hot flashes, may occur immediately after estrogen production goes down. Table 20-1 runs down the some common menopausal symptoms.

Table 20-1	Common Menopausal Symptoms
Symptom	*Description*
Frequent urination	Some women find that they urinate more frequently after menopause. This condition occurs when the tissues lining the urethra become more fragile and shrink after estrogen levels fall. The bladder can't hold as much urine.
Hot flashes	Hot flashes, sensations of intense warmth, are the most common complaint of menopausal women. These personal heat waves, which are accompanied by a pink flush in the head, neck, and upper body, heavy perspiration, and a rapid pulse, and are followed by chills and shivering, can last anywhere from a few seconds to two minutes. Experts believe they are caused by both the sudden drop in estrogen that occurs when you enter menopause and by a hormonal disruption of the body's thermostat, which is part of your hypothalamus. As a result of this disrup-tion, your heart races, and your blood vessels open to push more blood to your skin's surface quickly, where it can be cooled by the outside air. You sweat to cool the skin further. But then your thermostat senses that you are too cold, so your blood vessels constrict, the blood drains away from the skin's surface, and you shiver.
Mood swings	As your estrogen level fluctuates, you may become irritable, moody, and anxious and have trouble concen-trating. And although depression is not caused directly by lower estrogen levels, you may become depressed as a result of the changes in your life. Although irritability and some anxiety during menopause are normal, prolonged depression is not. If you have trouble with depression, get help. (For more information on depression, see Chapter 14.)

Symptom	Description
Sleep disturbances and fatigue	Sleep disturbances, such as insomnia and the resulting fatigue, are not actually side effects of low estrogen. They're side effects of your hot flashes. Women with frequent hot flashes may be awakened hourly because they feel so warm and/or sweaty. Over the course of days and months, such disrupted sleep can cause memory lapses, anxiety, and fatigue. If you're feeling fatigued but don't recall awaking, you may be having frequent hot flashes that are keeping you right at the edge of consciousness.
Urinary incontinence	You may have had more trouble holding in your urine after you had children. Pregnancy and vaginal delivery stretch your pelvic muscles, which causes you to lose support to your urethra and bladder. Aging can have the same effect or compound it. As you go through menopause, the loss of estrogen also diminishes this muscle tone. As a result, some women experience incontinence, particularly when they cough, sneeze, laugh, lift, or jump. (Chapter 11 discusses possible solutions for this problem.)
Vaginal dryness	As your estrogen level goes down, *vaginal atrophy* occurs, meaning the tissue that lines your vagina thins and dries out. When you don't have much natural lubrication, intercourse can become really uncomfortable. Over time, your vagina becomes shorter, more narrow, and less elastic.

Dealing with hot flashes

Here are some ways to deal with hot flashes:

✔ **Avoid spicy foods, hot drinks, caffeine, and alcohol:** All these can trigger hot flashes.

✔ **Change your blankets:** Use a light blanket and sheet at night.

✔ **Dress lightly:** Wear layers that you can take off when you get too hot.

✔ **Keep cool:** Turn room temperatures to a low setting.

✔ **Exercise:** Women who exercise regularly report fewer hot flashes.

✔ **Reduce stress:** Practice stress reduction techniques, such as meditation and yoga.

✔ **Keep a journal:** Track your flashes to see what your triggers are.

Fighting vaginal dryness

Here are some ways to combat vaginal dryness.

✔ **Have more sex:** Frequent sex or masturbation helps maintain lubrication and vaginal elasticity.

✔ **Use lubrication:** Try water-based lubricants, such as K-Y Jelly.

✔ **Talk to your doc:** Your doctor can prescribe estrogen. Oral or patch forms of estrogen have benefits for your entire body, including the genital area, but estrogen creams inserted directly into the vagina will work faster to produce the desired local effect.

Menopause Health Risks

In addition to producing physical symptoms, your body's lack of estrogen during menopause can put you at increased risk for certain conditions, notably heart disease, stroke, and osteoporosis. Table 20-2 outlines.

Table 20-2	Health Risks Associated with Menopause
Risk	*Description*
Heart disease and stroke	As your estrogen level changes, so does your health profile. Estrogen has played several roles over the years separate from governing your female organs and reproductive system. It has helped keep your blood pressure low by keeping the blood vessels supple and flexible, and it has helped keep your cholesterol levels down, which prevents your arteries from becoming clogged. Estrogen's beneficial effects on blood pressure and cholesterol reduced your risk of having a heart attack or stroke (discussed in Chapter 15). As you grow older and your estrogen level decreases, your risk of heart attack and stroke increases. Heart disease is the number one killer of women. And it appears most often after menopause. You can fight back by exercising more, eating well, and keeping your weight down. You can also ask your doctor about hormone replacement therapy (HRT).
Osteoporosis	Your bones are living tissue. *Osteoclasts* (bone-eating cells) are constantly breaking down your bones, and *osteoblasts* (bone-building cells) are rebuilding them with calcium. Estrogen plays a role in the maintenance

Risk	Description
	of healthy bones by preventing the bone-eating cells from becoming too aggressive. As your estrogen level goes down, the delicate balance of bone health starts to get out of whack and you start to lose bone density. Loss of bone density, called *osteoporosis*, is considered by the National Institutes of Health to be one of the four deadliest diseases among women in the United States. Osteoporosis, which makes your bones very brittle, leads to compression of the vertebrae (the small bones in your spinal column and neck), causing what's called *dowager's hump,* and fractures in larger bones — especially hip fractures. As Chapter 17 details, you can fight osteoporosis by taking calcium and vitamin D supplements (vitamin D helps your body to absorb the calcium); exercising; and doing weight-bearing exercises regularly. HRT can also help.

Hormone Replacement Therapy (HRT)

With all the symptoms and health risks associated with decreasing estrogen levels during menopause, you'd think that taking estrogen would be a no-brainer. But replacement hormones have risks and benefits of their own. Hormone replacement therapy (HRT) is a decision you really need to think through and work out with your doctor.

Hormone replacement therapy is just what its name implies — a therapy in which you take hormones to supplement or replace those you lose during menopause. Replenishing these hormones alleviates many of the effects of menopause. HRT is used to relieve menopausal symptoms, to treat and prevent osteoporosis, and to prevent heart disease. HRT comes in many forms. The main ingredient, not surprisingly, is estrogen. In fact, you may hear some people refer to HRT as estrogen replacement therapy, or ERT.

Estrogen: The main event

More than half a dozen types of estrogen are on the market. Those used in HRT can be either natural, which means they occur naturally and are similar to the estrogens made in the human body, or synthetic, which means they are made from chemicals or a combination of the above. Most estrogen used in HRT is natural.

Estrogen comes in several forms:

- **Pills and patches:** Pills and patches provide estrogen systemically, which means that these forms are processed through your whole body and provide many of the health benefits we detail later in the chapter.

- **Creams:** Estrogen cream is applied directly to, and affects only, the vagina and genital area. It's prescribed for women who have trouble with the drying and irritation of vaginal atrophy.

- **Implants:** Still in development, the vaginal ring is inserted deep in the vagina where it continuously releases low amounts of estrogen. The vaginal ring is designed for women whose major complaints are vaginal atrophy and urinary problems.

Progesterone: The complement to estrogen

Estrogen isn't usually prescribed alone. Without progesterone to balance estrogen, your uterine lining (endometrium) builds up and thickens. Over the long term, this buildup can lead to an increased risk of abnormal cell growth or even endometrial cancer. However, if you've had your uterus removed, you may be prescribed estrogen alone, or *unopposed.* You may also receive estrogen alone in cream form. In most cases, estrogen is prescribed in combination with progesterone.

The addition of progesterone reduces the risk of endometrial cancer. However, progesterone may also add water retention and PMS-like symptoms temporarily to the equation. Your doctor can make adjustments in the type of progesterone or the dosage if you experience these side effects.

You can take progesterone in one of two ways. You may either take it in a low-dose form every day along with your estrogen, or you may take it at a higher dose for 10 to 14 days each month to mimic your menstrual cycle's ebb and flow. If you take it cyclically, you may have regular periods, usually at the end of the progesterone days.

Male hormones: Additional help

In some cases, your doctor may recommend that you also take *androgens.* Before menopause, your ovaries not only produce estrogen, they also produce male hormones. Once you reach menopause, both types of hormone production fall. At this point, experts don't know exactly how the loss of male hormones affects women, though it's thought that loss of sexual urge (libido), low energy, moodiness, nervousness, inability to sleep, and discontent may be due at least in some cases to a low level of male hormones. If estrogen replacement doesn't help offset these particular symptoms for you, your doctor may recommend the addition of male hormones.

Male hormones come in pill form and you can get estrogen/male hormone combinations as well (to cut down on the number of pills you need to take). Male hormones also come in a long-acting shot that you get once a month.

The pros and cons of HRT

There is no question that taking hormone replacement therapy (HRT) relieves the symptoms of menopause, and for many women who take it, that's the issue. Over time, studies have been done on the long-term effects of taking HRT, and benefits and drawbacks have come to light.

On the plus side, HRT relieves symptoms such as hot flashes and vaginal atrophy, helps cut your risk of developing heart disease, and prevents osteoporosis. Estrogen may also delay the onset and lower your risk of developing Alzheimer's disease, reduce tooth loss and macular degeneration (a leading cause of blindness among the elderly), and lower the risk of colon cancer.

On the minus side, when estrogen is taken alone (without the counteraction of progesterone), it can cause your uterine lining to thicken and grow, which can ultimately lead to endometrial cancer. Taking progesterone along with estrogen reduces this risk.

HRT may also increase gallbladder problems. Women on HRT are more likely to have their gallbladder removed than women who are not.

The more controversial issue is HRT's impact on breast cancer. Although some studies have shown that HRT slightly increases the risk of breast cancer, others have shown no increase or even a reduced risk. The difficulty in establishing an HRT/breast cancer connection lies in the fact that no one yet knows what causes breast cancer and that some, but not all, forms of breast cancer depend on estrogen for growth. For this reason, women with breast cancer should not take HRT.

HRT can pose problems for certain women, such as those with a history blood clots, particularly if these clots occurred during pregnancy or during birth control use. Women with active liver disease and women with undiagnosed vaginal bleeding should also have a thorough workup before going on HRT.

As scientists learn more about the specific effects of HRT on different parts of a woman's body, they will be able to develop therapy approaches that bypass the risks and still provide the benefits. This process has already begun. Products that are targeted specifically toward the prevention of osteoporosis and prevention of heart disease are already on the market.

Alternatives to HRT

If you cannot take HRT or you decide against it, you can still do plenty of things to relieve menopausal symptoms and cut your health risks. A proper diet and exercise plan can help reduce your risk of both heart disease and osteoporosis. A healthy sex life can help reduce symptoms of vaginal atrophy. But that's only the beginning. Table 20-3 outlines some other non-HRT options for dealing with the risks and symptoms of menopause.

Table 20-3	Alternatives to HRT
Alternative	*Description*
Medications	If you opt against HRT, you can still opt for medical treatment. A large number of medications are available to treat heart disease. (Chapter 15 discusses these medications, along with other preventive and treatment measures.) And in recent years, a number of medications have come on the market to prevent or slow the progression of osteoporosis. These medications, which we discuss in Chapter 17, are targeted primarily at postmenopausal women. Medications are also available to treat symptoms such as hot flashes and vaginal dryness. For hot flashes, your doctor may prescribe anti-hypertensives, or blood pressure-lowering medications, which may provide relief to women with high blood pressure; and sedatives and tranquilizers, which relieve anxiety and have a calming effect. For vaginal dryness, your doctor may recommend vaginal lubricants.
Phytoestrogens	Some plant foods, such as soybeans, flax seed, and whole grains, contain chemicals that your body can convert to estrogen. These chemicals, known as phytoestrogens, or plant estrogens, offer only about $1/400$ the dose of a pharmaceutically prepared estrogen; however, in women who eat a diet high in the foods that contain them, they may reduce mild hot flashes. Bear in mind, though, that although phytoestrogens are natural, they are still a form of estrogen and determining what dose you are getting is difficult. If you're considering phytoestrogens as an option, talk with your practitioner.
Herbs	Herbs have been used for years to treat a variety of conditions, including menopausal symptoms. Just because they are natural doesn't mean that they are always safe, however. Some can cause unexpected allergic or toxic reactions if they are taken in too large or

Alternative	*Description*
	too frequent a dose, and some can interact with other medications. You're wise to consult your doctor for recommendations of formulas and dosages. That said, the herbs sometimes used to relieve menopausal symptoms include the following:
	Dong quai: A phytoestrogen that is used to relieve hot flashes, breast tenderness, sore joints, insomnia, and anxiety.
	Ginseng: A phytoestrogen used to treat menopausal discomforts, stimulate the immune system, normalize blood pressure, and reduce cholesterol levels.
	Black cohosh: A phytoestrogenic herb whose root is used to relieve hot flashes, night sweats, vaginal dryness, incontinence, irritability, anxiety, headaches, and depression.
	Licorice root: This herb may relieve vaginal dryness and hot flashes, possibly by balancing the estrogen-progesterone ratio, although scientific data doesn't exist.
Biofeedback	This psychological therapy uses the conscious mind to control involuntary body functions, such as respiration, heartbeat, and body temperatures. After training in the therapy, some women are able to reduce the frequency and severity of their hot flashes.
Alternative therapies	Other alternative therapies are also used to treat menopausal symptoms. These include *homeopathy, naturopathy, acupuncture,* and *acupressure.* (See Chapter 2 for more information.)
Attitude	Finally, remember that your attitude has a lot to do with your menopausal experience. If you approach menopause as an exciting new phase in your life rather than as an end to your youth, you may find the adjustment easier to make, regardless of what, if any, treatments you choose.

Diet and Exercise

A low-fat, high-fiber diet featuring a variety of fruits and vegetables has been found to help reduce the risk of heart disease. Fruits and vegetables are rich in heart-protective antioxidant nutrients, while fiber helps lower cholesterol. For further heart protection, make sure that you're getting enough vitamin E, vitamin B6, and folate. To guard against osteoporosis, you need adequate calcium, magnesium, vitamin D, and vitamin K. (For Recommended Dietary Allowances, see Chapter 1.)

Exercise, too, offers protection. Numerous studies have shown that aerobic exercise lowers your weight, improves your cholesterol levels, and reduces stress, all of which benefit the heart. And weight-bearing exercise also stops or slows bone loss and stimulates the formation of new bone.

Hysterectomy and Surgical Menopause

For some women, menopause doesn't start at age 45 or 50, it starts when they undergo surgery to have their ovaries removed. Surgical removal of the ovaries, known as *oophorectomy,* is a frequent cause of early menopause.

If your ovaries are removed, you develop instant menopause with symptoms occurring within days. In this case, estrogen replacement therapy is a necessity for normal bodily sexual functioning.

You may need to have your ovaries removed if you have ovarian cancer, severe pelvic inflammatory disease (PID), endometriosis that has developed in your ovaries, or a severe case of ovarian cysts. If you need a *hysterectomy,* surgical removal of the uterus for another reason, discuss with your doctor whether removal of the ovaries is necessary.

By the age of 60, approximately one-third of American women have undergone hysterectomy, and approximately 40 percent of them have also had their ovaries removed.

Coming to terms with hysterectomy and oophorectomy

You may know that surgical removal of the uterus is known as hysterectomy and that surgical removal of the ovaries is known as oophorectomy, but it's not always as simple as that. Depending on a woman's condition, her doctor may perform any of several types of hysterectomy, often along with oophorectomy. These procedures are

✔ **Subtotal hysterectomy:** Surgical removal of the uterus.

✔ **Total hysterectomy:** Surgical removal of the uterus and cervix. (See Chapter 18 for more information.)

✔ **Oophorectomy:** Surgical removal of the ovaries.

✔ **Total hysterectomy with bilateral salpingo-oophorectomy**: Surgical removal of the uterus, cervix, fallopian tubes, and both ovaries.

✔ **Radical hysterectomy:** Surgical removal of the uterus, cervix, fallopian tubes, both ovaries, the upper part of the vagina, and some lymph nodes. (See Chapter 18 for more information about radical hysterectomy.)

The top three reasons physicians perform hysterectomies are uterine fibroids, prolapsed uterus, and endometriosis.

But although hysterectomies are often recommended for these conditions, which Chapter 18 discusses in detail, they are not the only treatments available. If your doctor recommends a hysterectomy for one of these conditions, get a second opinion.

Hysterectomies are necessary for cancer of the uterus, vagina, fallopian tubes, or ovaries, however. They are usually necessary for invasive cervical cancer, for severe, uncontrollable infection, for severe, uncontrollable bleeding, for life-threatening blockages of the bladder or bowels by the uterus or growths on the uterus, and for rare complications of childbirth, such as uterine rupture.

Avoiding an unnecessary hysterectomy or surgical menopause

You can avoid having an unnecessary hysterectomy or undergoing an early menopause by being a savvy consumer:

🖙 **Ask questions:** If your doctor recommends a hysterectomy or oophorectomy, ask why you need it, what will happen if you don't have the surgery, and whether you have other alternatives.

🖙 **Get a second opinion:** Not all doctors treat all conditions in the same way, and your doctor may have overlooked an alternative treatment that may be more agreeable to you.

🖙 **Don't make a hasty decision:** If your condition is not life-threatening, take some time to consider whether the surgery is for you. After all, the decision will affect you for the rest of your life.

🖙 **If you must have a hysterectomy, ask your doctor to leave your ovaries intact:** If your ovaries are healthy and you do not have a family history of ovarian cancer, you have every right to request that your ovaries stay in place. Tell your doctor of your decision and write it on the hospital's consent form.

Chapter 21

Contraception and Postconception Alternatives

*A*lthough you may love children, you may not want them to be a potential consequence of every sexual encounter. That's where contraception comes in.

Also known as birth control or family planning, *contraception* is the deliberate prevention of conception or pregnancy.

A number of contraceptive options are available, and each has pros and cons — some protect you against sexually transmitted diseases, and some don't; some involve health risks, while others are risk-free; some are permanent, and some are not; some are available at the drugstore, and some are available only by prescription; some can be self-administered, while some require surgery. You need to educate yourself before you make your choice. And you need to make your decision *before* you have sex. This chapter discusses the various contraceptive options available to you, as well as your options if you become pregnant and don't wish to be.

Some General Words of Wisdom

It's still true that celibacy is the only *foolproof* method of avoiding pregnancy. None of the contraceptive forms and methods here are 100 percent effective — especially if you don't use them properly. But some come pretty close. Don't be naïve enough to think that you can't get pregnant if you have unprotected sex just one time. The risk can be high: Approximately 85 percent of sexually active women who don't use contraception in the course of a year become pregnant.

Just because a certain form of contraception prevents pregnancy well doesn't mean that it prevents you from getting sexually transmitted diseases. If you are having sex with multiple partners — or even with one partner whose sexual history, drug habits, or health status is unknown to you — you are at risk of contracting AIDS and other sexually transmitted diseases. Spermicides are known to provide *some* protection against *some* sexually transmitted diseases. But the only contraceptive device known to protect against the transmission of the AIDS virus is the latex condom. (For more information on preventing sexually transmitted diseases, see Chapter 22.)

Reversible Contraception for Your Lifestyle

Finding the right contraceptive is generally not a one-time deal. As your lifestyle changes, you may want — or need — to change your form of contraception. A young, single woman has different needs than a married woman who is taking a break between having her first and second child. And a woman who is nursing has different concerns than one who is not. This section talks about the reversible options available to you.

Over-the-counter solutions

If you are having sex with more than one partner, you need to protect yourself against sexually transmitted diseases. The condom is an obvious choice.

The condom

Condoms, sometimes called *rubbers* or *prophylactics,* are thin sheaths made of latex rubber, plastic, polyurethane, or animal tissue that are worn over a man's penis. They prevent pregnancy by preventing your partner's semen from coming in contact with your vagina. They come in a variety of sizes, styles, and colors and are either dry or lubricated. Each condom comes in a small, flat packet made of foil or plastic and is small enough to slip into a purse or even a wallet. They are readily available and can be purchased at just about any drugstore or grocery store. Condoms are dated with either an expiration date or the date they were manufactured and have a shelf life of about five years. After that, they should be disposed of because packages can dry out and crack open, and the condom material can weaken and disintegrate.

What you don't know about condoms could hurt you

Your choice of condom and the way you use it can affect your health:

- Only latex condoms are proven to provide protection against sexually transmitted diseases, such as HIV.

- One to 3 percent of people are allergic to latex. If you or your partner has a latex allergy, polyurethane condoms with spermicide also provide some protection against HIV and other STDs. Not enough comparative scientific data is available yet to know whether polyurethane condom protection is as good as latex, however.

- If you want to use a lubricant and you are using a latex condom, don't use mineral oil or petroleum jelly: Oil-based lubricants can cause latex to deteriorate. Use K-Y Jelly or another water-based lubricant instead.

Some men say that condoms reduce the sensations they feel during sex. And putting on a condom just when you are both getting passionate can interrupt the spontaneous mood. You can adjust for this problem by putting the condom on your partner and including it as part of foreplay.

A condom can fail if it is put on incorrectly, if it comes off or breaks during vigorous sex, or if it has defects. You or your partner must also hold on to the rim of the condom during withdrawal to prevent leakage. You can reduce the risk of pregnancy further by using another form of contraceptive, such as a spermicide, in combination with a condom.

Condoms are typically 86 percent effective in preventing pregnancy.

Spermicides

A *spermicide* is a form of contraceptive that is inserted into your vagina before intercourse. Spermicides come as foams, jellies, creams, films, and suppositories. Regardless of its form, once in your vagina, a spermicide melts into a liquid that coats your vagina. The liquid kills off sperm before they come in contact with your cervix.

How to use a condom

A condom should be put on your partner's erect penis before it comes in contact with your vagina:

1. Take the condom out of the package and unroll it about ¹/₂ inch to create a reservoir for the semen.

2. Pull back the foreskin, and center the condom on the tip of the penis.

3. Pinch the air out of the tip of the condom.

4. Unroll the condom over the penis.

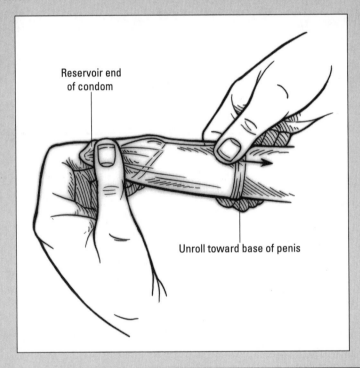

Reservoir end of condom

Unroll toward base of penis

Like condoms, spermicides are readily available and can be found in just about any drugstore or grocery store. On the minus side, they need to be used about ten minutes before intercourse (to give enough time for the spermicide to melt and spread in your vagina), which can interrupt spontaneity. They can be messy and leak. They may irritate your vagina and the skin of the man's penis (if you're using a spermicide in combination with a condom, this shouldn't be a problem). And spermicides are less effective than some other contraceptives when used alone.

Spermicides are typically 74 percent effective in preventing pregnancy.

Applying a spermicide — the right way

To get the most effectiveness, here are some guidelines for using a spermicide:

✔ Different types of spermicides are used differently, so always follow the instructions on the package.

✔ Spermicides must be reapplied every time you have intercourse.

✔ Most spermicides must be inserted ten minutes before intercourse if you're using them as your sole method of contraception.

✔ Lie on your back or squat on your heels to inject the spermicide deep into the vagina.

✔ Avoid douching for six to eight hours after intercourse.

The female condom

If you want to be in control, you may want to consider the female condom.

The female condom, or vaginal pouch, is a pouch made of soft polyurethane with two rings at either end — one open, the other closed. It looks kind of like a big, loose condom. You put the closed-ringed end of the pouch high up in your vagina against your cervix. The open-ringed end stays on the outside of your vagina, covering the lips a little. When you have sexual intercourse, your partner inserts his penis into the open-ringed end. The semen is collected in the pouch, which like the male condom, is removed and thrown away after one use.

The female condom will protect you against some sexually transmitted diseases, possibly even AIDS. But if you think you can get twice as much protection by using both a male condom and a female condom, think again. The two rubbing together can stick and pull or tear both off, providing you with no protection at all.

The vaginal pouch can come off during sexual intercourse, and the rings can be irritating. And like the male condom, some people find that the female condom reduces spontaneity and sensation during sex. On the other hand, the female condom is available over the counter at drugstores.

The female condom is typically 79 percent effective in preventing pregnancy.

Doctor-prescribed contraception

If you can't find an over-the-counter contraceptive method to suit you, your doctor can prescribe one of three nonhormonal options — the diaphragm, the cervical cap, and the intrauterine device, or IUD.

Using a diaphragm or cervical cap the right way

Here are some guidelines for proper use of diaphragms and cervical caps:

✔ Check to see that your diaphragm or cervical cap is still in place after sexual intercourse (either can come loose with vigorous sexual activity).

✔ Make sure that your diaphragm or cervical cap stays in place for six hours after sexual intercourse.

✔ Check your diaphragm or cervical cap frequently for weak spots or holes by holding it up to the light. (A pinhole to you is the Holland Tunnel to a sperm!)

✔ Have your diaphragm or cervical cap size checked yearly and after each pregnancy.

The diaphragm and cervical cap

Diaphragms and cervical caps are both barrier methods of contraception like the condom (they prevent the sperm from connecting with the egg), but they aren't available over-the-counter because your gynecologist or health care provider has to custom fit them to you.

A *diaphragm* is a rubber cup with a flexible rim that fits snugly into your vagina to block the path to your cervix. (See Figure 21-1.) Because sperm are tiny and can conceivably wiggle their way around the diaphragm, you use a diaphragm along with spermicidal jelly or cream applied to the rim to form a seal and immobilize the sperm.

Figure 21-1:
Ask your doctor about pre-scribing a diaphragm.

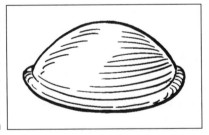

A *cervical cap* works on the same principle with one difference. Although a diaphragm blocks the path to the cervix, the cervical cap fits right over the cervix like a little hat. The cervical cap is also made of rubber, but it's smaller than a diaphragm — about the size of a large thimble. The cervical cap is also used with spermicidal jelly or cream.

One advantage of using a diaphragm or cervical cap is that the spermicide you use with them provides some (but not the best) protection against some sexually transmitted diseases, including gonorrhea and chlamydia. They are also pretty easy to insert and, like a condom, insertion can be made a part of foreplay. After the diaphragm or cervical cap is in place, (assuming they are inserted properly) neither you nor your partner can feel them.

If you have an irregularly shaped cervix or a sagging uterus or if your pelvic or vaginal muscles are weak, you may not be able to use a diaphragm or cervical cap. Your gynecologist or health care provider will let you know.

Diaphragms and cervical caps are typically 80 percent effective in preventing pregnancy.

Intrauterine devices

Intrauterine devices (or IUDs as they are commonly called) offer long-term, reversible contraception. These T-shaped devices, made of polyetheylene, are placed into the uterus and work by preventing egg fertilization, although experts are not exactly sure why. They do not prevent STDs. To insert an IUD, your health care practitioner will hold your vagina open with a speculum (a duckbill-shaped instrument with handles), attach an instrument known as a tenaculum to your cervix to steady your uterus, and insert a tube containing the IUD (with its T-bar wings bent back) into your uterus through your cervix. She then pushes the device into place by using a plunger in the tube. She then removes the tube, plunger, tenaculum and speculum, leaving the IUD in place. (The wings spring into place when the device is in the uterus.) The procedure may cause cramplike pain that can be relieved with rest or an over-the-counter pain reliever.

IUDs enable you to be perfectly spontaneous. Neither you nor your partner feels the IUD, and you don't have to remember to do anything (such as take a pill) or interrupt coitus.

Currently, two types of IUD are on the market:

- **Paragard:** This plastic device contains a little copper, which has a spermicidal effect. Paragard is extremely effective and can be left in place for up to 12 years.

- **Progestasert:** This IUD contains progesterone, a natural hormone. If you're worried about using an IUD because you've heard that it will give you heavier, more painful periods, you may want to try Progestasert.

Note: Progestasert is slightly less effective than Paragard and has to be replaced about once a year. If you are considering having another child (but want to space them a couple of years apart), Progestasert may be an option for you.

The drawbacks of IUDs are that they can cause cramps and heavy menstrual flow — especially right after insertion — and spotting between periods. In rare cases, the IUD can perforate the wall of the uterus when it's inserted. Although the risk of infection is highest in the first three weeks after the IUD is first inserted, multiple sex partners (or infected sex partners) can raise the risk of fallopian tube infection, which increases your risk of ectopic pregnancy, can cause sterility, and could ultimately require hospitalization and surgery, possibly even hysterectomy.

On the other hand, both the American Medical Association and the World Health Organization consider IUDs to be one of the safest and most effective reversible forms of contraceptive for women.

The Paragard IUD is typically more than 99 percent effective in preventing pregnancy. The Progestasert IUD is typically 98 percent effective. If you do become pregnant while wearing an IUD, you should have the device removed as soon as possible. The presence of an IUD increases the risk of miscarriage, infection, and premature birth.

Hormonal methods

If you're in a stable, monogamous relationship (unless you need to prevent the transmission of a known case of herpes or HIV), you may want a contraceptive method that doesn't interrupt the flow of passion, is reliable, and is easy to use. At this point, you may wish to consider hormonally based contraceptives, such as oral contraceptives, Norplant, or Depo-Provera.

Oral contraceptives

Oral contraceptives (sometimes referred to as "the Pill") are pills made from synthetic hormones that are taken daily to prevent pregnancy. Oral contraceptives are available only by prescription.

Two different types of oral contraceptives are available. You need to talk with your doctor to figure out which is best for you.

  ✔ **Combination pills:** This type of pill combines two hormones — estrogen and progestin — which stop your ovaries' production of hormones. They prevent your eggs from ripening, and they stop ovulation.

  Combination pills come packaged either in a 21-day pack or a 28-day pack. If you choose the 21-day pack, you take one pill daily for 21 days. Then you take nothing for the next seven days while you menstruate.

  The 28-day pack actually has the same 21 combination pills along with an extra seven placebo (inactive) pills that you take while you menstruate. The 28-day pack is useful for people who find it easier to remember to take a pill every day without a break to stay on track.

✔ **Minipill:** This pill contains only progestin. It works by thickening the mucus made by your cervix, which prevents sperm from passing through and joining an egg. The minipill is taken every day; it has no on-and-off cycle.

Oral contraceptives have several advantages. Both the combination pill and the minipill can make your menstrual cycle more regular and reduce menstrual flow and cramps. They can also cut your risk of ovarian cancer, endometrial cancer, pelvic inflammatory disease, and iron-deficiency anemia. The combination pill may also reduce the risk of acne, ectopic pregnancy, noncancerous breast tumors, and ovarian cysts.

On the other hand, you could have spotting between periods (small amounts of blood flow), tenderness in your breasts, and you could put on (or lose) weight, experience nausea, vomit, and/or become depressed. These side effects usually decrease after you are on the Pill or minipill for two or three months, however.

Once on the combination pill, you *may* have a slightly higher risk of developing blood clots, stroke, a heart attack, or a liver tumor. These risks become greater as you grow older and are also more closely associated with people who smoke, have diabetes, or have high blood pressure or high cholesterol. Although it was once feared that the combination pill greatly increases the risk of breast cancer, a large study published in 1996 found that it confers no long-term risk and only a small short-term risk. Your doctor will ask you questions about your health history and take your answers into consideration before prescribing oral contraceptives.

One more point about the combination pill: If you are breast-feeding and thought you'd just start up on your old pill again, don't. You should not take the combination pill if you are breast-feeding (unless you are supplementing with formula) because the milk will contain traces of the hormones. You should not take the combination pill or minipill if think you may be pregnant.

Oral contraceptive cautions

If you are on the Pill or minipill and you experience any of the following symptoms, talk with your doctor:

✔ Sudden pain in your chest

✔ Swelling or pain in your legs

✔ Shortness of breath

✔ Severe headache

✔ Loss of vision, or blurred or double vision

The Pill and minipill are 99 percent effective in preventing pregnancy if taken exactly as prescribed every day. The minipill is 97 percent effective if you are taking it while breast-feeding. Both pills are 95 percent effective with typical use.

Norplant

If you're not very good at remembering to take a pill every day, you may want to consider Norplant.

Norplant is another hormone-based contraceptive that is only available by prescription. But you don't swallow it, you sort of . . . wear it. Norplant consists of six cardboard matchstick-size rods of a synthetic form of progestin that are implanted just under the skin of your upper arm. Your doctor numbs a small area of your arm with a topical anesthetic, makes a small incision (usually less than 1/4 inch in length), inserts the rods under the skin, and bandages the skin. The procedure, which takes about ten minutes, is not exceptionally painful, although you may experience some itching, swelling, and tenderness for a few days after the insertion. The progestin is released gradually and continually into your body, both preventing ovulation (like combination pills) and thickening cervical mucus (like minipills) to prevent the sperm from connecting with the egg.

Norplant is effective for five years. And though it lasts a long time, once the rods are removed, you can get pregnant again immediately. Unlike the combination pill, Norplant can be used by breast-feeding mothers, though not during the first six weeks of the newborn's life.

A common side effect of Norplant is irregular bleeding. Once Norplant has been implanted, your periods could become irregular, you may have spotting between periods, your menstrual flow could become heavier, or you could have no period whatsoever for months at a time.

Norplant cautions

If you are using Norplant and you experience any of the following, talk with your doctor:

✔ Pain, bleeding, or pus (abnormal discharge) at the site where the doctor implanted the Norplant rods

✔ Norplant rods that seem to be coming out

✔ Bleeding that lasts much longer and seems to be much heavier than a normal period

✔ Regular menstrual cycles for a long period of time, followed by a late period

Slightly less common side effects are headaches, nausea, appetite changes, weight fluctuation, tenderness in your breasts, acne, hair loss, depression, vaginal dryness, an increase in face and body hair, and changes in skin color over the spot where the Norplant rods were inserted.

One more caveat: Your doctor may have trouble removing the Norplant rods and removal may take repeated tries. Even perfectly inserted rods may become surrounded by scar tissue. As with any prescription contraceptive, your doctor is going to take a health history and will rule out Norplant if you have serious liver disease, blood clots, or vein inflammation, if you are pregnant, if you have unexplained vaginal bleeding, or if you can't tolerate irregular bleeding.

On the other hand, you may be able to use Norplant under medical supervision even if you have diabetes, high blood pressure, high cholesterol, heart disease, migraine headaches, seizures, or clotting or bleeding disorders.

Norplant is more than 99 percent effective in preventing pregnancy.

Depo-Provera

Depo-Provera is a synthetic progestin that is given in the form of an injection (in your arm or buttocks) every 12 weeks. Depo-Provera both prevents ovulation and thickens cervical mucus to prevent the sperm from connecting with the egg.

The difference between Depo-Provera and the other hormonally based contraceptives is that once you stop using it, it takes an average of ten months to get pregnant again (and it can take up to a year and a half). So, even though it's convenient, you shouldn't use this method if you are planning to get pregnant reasonably soon.

Depo-Provera can cut down on menstrual cramps and provide protection against some cancers. And it can be used if you are breast-feeding (six weeks after delivery) because it doesn't contain any estrogen.

Depo-Provera cautions

If you are using Depo-Provera and experience very heavy menstrual flow (much heavier and longer than your regular period) or severe abdominal pain, headaches, or depression, call your doctor.

But Depo-Provera can cause irregular bleeding. Your periods may become erratic, you could have spotting between periods, your period could last longer, or it could disappear for months at a time. And side effects can last up to eight months after you stop getting the injections.

You could also have side effects such as headaches, dizziness, nausea, appetite loss (or gain), weight gain, sore breasts, nervousness, hair loss, increased hair growth, acne, skin rashes, depression, vaginal dryness, and increased or decreased sex drive.

Your doctor will review your medical history before prescribing Depo-Provera. Several factors, including serious liver disease, breast cancer, allergy to the synthetic hormone depotmedroxprogesterone acetate, or the inability to tolerate irregular bleeding, can rule it out.

Depo-Provera is 99 percent effective in preventing pregnancy.

Natural family planning

You have a few different approaches to avoiding pregnancy if you don't want to use a contraceptive. These methods are usually referred to as *natural family planning*. In order to practice natural family planning, which takes commitment from both partners, you must become familiar with your own body's cycle of fertility and menstruation.

Your *menstrual cycle* starts on the first day of menstrual flow of one period and ends on the first day of menstrual flow or your next period. The average menstrual cycle is 28 days long, though it's perfectly normal to have a menstrual cycle that is anywhere from 23 to 35 days long. Fourteen days before your next menstrual period your body *ovulates* (releases an egg). If you have a 28-day cycle, this is around day 14. However, if you have a 30-day cycle, ovulation will occur around day 16. If your cycles vary from month to month, it is not possible to predict ovulation exactly by the calendar, and you will have to watch for other signs as well. Generally, you are fertile (and can become pregnant) during the three to four days before you ovulate, on the day you ovulate, and three days after. When you practice natural family planning, you avoid sexual intercourse during this fertile period.

Note: The key to natural family planning is predicting accurately when you will ovulate. You can do so in a few ways: You may practice the basal body temperature method, the mucus inspection method, the rhythm (or calendar) method, or a combination of all of them (which is called the symptothermal method). Or you may attempt to prevent contact between the sperm and the egg by practicing withdrawal. (Some doctors, clinics, and churches offer instruction on these methods.)

Bear in mind that your period can be affected by so many things — stress, diet, illness — that it's likely that your calculations are going to be off now and then, which increases your risk of getting pregnant.

One last point about natural family planning. *None* of the natural family planning methods protects you against sexually transmitted diseases.

The Basal Body Temperature method

The *Basal Body Temperature method (BBT)* involves taking your temperature every morning upon waking. (You'll need an accurate thermometer — one of the digital ones is probably best.) Your temperature will go up around 0.4 to 0.8 degrees F the day you start ovulating and will stay that way until you start your next period. For the next three days, in order to avoid getting pregnant, you should avoid sexual intercourse.

The temperature method has one big drawback. Sperm can survive anywhere from three to eight days during your fertile period. So, if you have sexual intercourse a couple of days before you ovulate, you can still become pregnant. You can avoid this problem by combining the temperature method with the mucus inspection method and/or the rhythm method.

The temperature method is typically about 75 percent effective in preventing pregnancy.

The mucus inspection method

The *mucus inspection method* is a way of detecting your most fertile period by checking your vaginal secretions. Your cervical mucus is usually cloudy, or creamy white and somewhat thick. But during the fertile period before ovulation, the amount of your cervical mucus increases and changes, becoming clearer and more runny — kind of like egg white. You may feel this as a damp sensation on your underwear or notice it on toilet paper. About a day or so after ovulation, your cervical mucus dries up, once again becoming thick and opaque.

When you use the mucus inspection method, you avoid sexual intercourse during the period of time when your mucus is clear and runny and for three days after it dries up. And during your "nonfertile" period, experts recommend that you have sexual intercourse only every other day because you may confuse the dampness of seminal fluid with a change in your cervical mucus.

The major drawback of using the mucus inspection method is that figuring out whether your mucus is changing or not can be difficult. And figuring out exactly when you are ovulating can be hard, too. You can deal with this problem by combining the mucus inspection method with the temperature and rhythm methods for more accuracy.

The mucus inspection method is typically about 75 percent effective in preventing pregnancy, especially when combined with awareness of the calendar and your cycle.

The rhythm method

Using the *rhythm method* doesn't mean you have to be able to dance well, but you do have to know how to count! You may choose to use the rhythm, or calendar (as it's sometimes called), method if you have a very regular and predictable menstrual cycle.

Before you use the rhythm method, you need to become very familiar with your menstrual cycle Start by charting your cycle for six months to a year. Use either the temperature method or one of the ovulation predictor kits available at your local drugstore to determine when ovulation occurs within each cycle. Then, use this information to predict your future cycles and avoid sex during your fertile periods.

The rhythm method is typically about 75 percent effective in preventing pregnancy.

The symptothermal method

With the *symptothermal method,* you chart your periods and ovulation each month, noting changes in cervical mucus and temperature. By becoming very familiar with your body's cycles, you can accurately predict your fertile period and avoid sexual intercourse during that time.

The symptothermal method is typically about 75 percent effective in preventing pregnancy.

Withdrawal

Withdrawal means that when you have sexual intercourse, your partner removes his penis from your vagina just before he ejaculates, which prevents the sperm from coming in contact with your egg.

Although you can practice this method any time you have no other options, it has some drawbacks. First, it's very hard for a man to pull out just when he is about to ejaculate (every instinct is telling him to go on). Consequently, you have no control because you can't be sure when he is about to ejaculate. Second, a man releases a small amount of seminal fluid *before* he ejaculates, so pulling out doesn't prevent all the sperm from making their journey.

Withdrawal is typically 81 percent effective in preventing pregnancy.

Emergency Contraception

So, you had sexual intercourse, but you didn't use a contraceptive. Maybe you were caught up in the passion of the moment, or maybe your partner's condom broke. Believe it or not, you still have contraception options.

Two methods of emergency contraception are available: emergency IUD insertion and emergency hormonal contraception. You can get these forms of contraception only from your health care provider.

Emergency hormonal contraception

Emergency hormonal contraception is simply a high dose of oral contraceptives (usually the Pill) taken at a prescribed interval. You can take emergency hormonal contraception up to 72 hours after you've had unprotected sex and still cut your chance of getting pregnant by 75 percent or more.

Hormonal contraceptives such as the Pill usually work by preventing ovulation or thickening cervical mucus. But at high doses, hormonal contraceptives also seem to block implantation of the fertilized egg in the wall of the uterus. Using emergency hormonal contraception has no serious side effects, and if you are already pregnant, the hormones won't hurt the fetus. An emergency contraceptive kit called Preven is now available.

About half the women who use the Pill as emergency hormonal contraception become nauseated by it, and a good number throw up. Taking an antinausea drug such as Dramamine at the same time is a good idea. Nausea, vomiting, and a 75 percent effectiveness rate don't exactly make this a good *long-term* choice of contraception, but then again, it's not meant to be. However, you may want to ask your health care practitioner to advise you. Emergency hormonal contraception can be kept on hand in case you need it.

Emergency hormonal contraception is typically 75 percent effective at preventing pregnancy.

Emergency IUD insertion

With *emergency IUD insertion,* you can have the Paragard (copper) IUD inserted by your health care practitioner within five to seven days of having unprotected sexual intercourse and still significantly reduce your risk of pregnancy. Inserting the IUD causes an inflammatory reaction in your uterus that blocks sperm and prevents implantation.

Emergency IUD insertion is the most effective form of emergency contraception, but it, too, isn't for everyone. If you are already at risk for contracting a sexually transmitted infection, inserting an IUD puts you at greater risk for getting pelvic inflammatory disease. Your health care practitioner will need to examine you and perform tests for sexually transmitted disease.

Emergency IUD insertion is 99 percent effective in preventing pregnancy.

Permanent Contraception

Permanent contraception (or sterilization) is just that — permanent. It's meant only for people who don't want to ever have children again. It's considered permanent because no one can guarantee that surgery to reverse it will be successful. Believe it or not, sterilization is the most commonly used method of family planning in the United States.

Two types of permanent contraception are available — one for men and one for women:

✔ **For men:** The surgical procedure to sterilize a man is called a *vasectomy,* and it involves sealing off, tying, or cutting the man's vas deferens, which carries the sperm from the testicles to the penis. Vasectomy is quick (it only takes about half an hour) and less expensive than female sterilization; the man recovers more rapidly, too.

Male sterilization is more than 99 percent effective in preventing pregnancy.

✔ **For women:** Female sterilization blocks the fallopian tubes so that the egg cannot travel down to the uterus. Female sterilization is a surgical procedure that can take anywhere from 10 to 45 minutes and can be done either under general or regional anesthesia and sometimes even under local anesthesia.

First, the surgeon, or ob/gyn needs to get to your fallopian tubes. She most often makes an abdominal incision to use laparoscopy or minilaparoscopy (see Table 21-1). The surgeon may then clamp the fallopian tubes, tie them shut, clip them, or cut them. Or she can block them by cauterizing (burning) them. If another surgical procedure is being done, such as a cesarean section, tubal ligation is often performed at the same time.

Women who undergo hysterectomy are also permanently sterilized. But hysterectomy isn't done just as a sterilization procedure because of the potential complications. (For more information on hysterectomy, see Chapter 20.)

Procedure	Explanation
Laparoscopy	The doctor makes a small incision at the bottom edge of the naval and inserts a long, thin, telescopelike instrument through the incision to view and access the fallopian tubes.
Minilaparotomy	The doctor makes a small incision in the lower abdomen near the top of the pelvic bone so the fallopian tubes can be lifted out to be tied or cut.
Laparotomy	The doctor makes a long incision through the muscle layers of the abdomen to view and access the fallopian tubes.

Table 21-1 Surgical Procedures Used for Female Sterilization

The risks and side effects of female sterilization, which range from bloating and mild pain to possible cardiac arrest, vary depending on which procedure is done. Your health care practitioner will explain your options, along with their risks and benefits.

Female sterilization can be reversed *in some cases*, though surgery is necessary. Basically, the surgeon sews the ends of the fallopian tubes back together. But success depends on which sterilization procedure was used and how long ago it was done.

Female sterilization is 97 to 99 percent effective in preventing pregnancy, depending on the technique used and how long ago it was done. Sometimes tubes do grow back together, but scarring can occur in the area, putting the woman at an increased risk of ectopic pregnancy.

For more information about your contraceptive options, contact any of the following:

- The National Family Planning and Reproductive Health Association, 122 C St., N.W., Suite 380, Washington, DC 20001-2109; 202-628-3535
- The Access to Voluntary and Safe Contraception International, 79 Madison Ave., 7th Floor, New York, NY 10016; 212-561-8000; www.avsc.org
- The Planned Parenthood Federation of America, Inc., 810 7th Ave., New York, NY 10019; 800-230-PLAN; www.ppfa.org/ppfa

Abortion and Adoption Options

So, you discover that you are pregnant — and you don't want to be. At this stage in the game, you have a lot of thinking to do. You basically have two options: You can terminate the pregnancy, or you can carry the baby to term and put it up for adoption.

Abortion

Abortion, quite simply, is the termination of a pregnancy. But although the definition may be simple, the procedure, which has been around in some form or another for centuries, is a source of complex, heated debate. On one side are those who believe a woman should have the right to choose abortion; on the other side are those who believe a woman should not have that right. The U.S. Supreme Court in 1973 ruled that a woman's right to choose abortion is constitutionally protected, but individual state laws and practitioners' views on abortion can affect a woman's access to abortion.

Although most states do not require women to tell their partners before they have an abortion, the majority do require women under the age of 18 to notify or get the permission of at least one parent before they undergo this procedure. In addition, a number of states have passed laws that require women to wait for a certain amount of time (usually 24 hours) after they have been counseled about their pregnancy options before they can actually have an abortion.

Counseling is only one of the preliminary steps you will undergo if you opt for an abortion. You will be asked to complete paperwork that indicates that you have been informed about your options, understand the risks and benefits of the abortion procedure, and that you have made the decision to have an abortion of your own free will. You will also undergo a series of blood tests and a physical exam. You may also be given a sonogram (a test in which sound waves are used to view the pregnancy inside the uterus) to determine how long you've been pregnant because that will help your doctor determine which type of procedure to use. The various procedures are categorized into two types: surgical and medical.

Surgical abortion

Surgical abortion terminates pregnancy by surgically removing the embryo or fetus from the uterus. This procedure can be done two ways: by opening the cervix and removing the contents of the uterus or by inducing labor so that the fetus is expelled as it would be in childbirth.

Up to 14 weeks of pregnancy, most surgical abortions are done by a procedure called *suction curettage,* or *vacuum aspiration.* This procedure, which takes only about 10 to 15 minutes to perform, is usually done on an outpatient basis in a doctor's office or clinic. In this procedure, you lie on your back on an examining table with your legs in stirrups, just as you would for a gynecologic exam. Your vagina is washed with an antiseptic, and a local anesthetic is injected in or near your cervix. Next, the opening of your cervix is stretched by inserting progressively wider dilating instruments to allow a tube attached to a suction machine to be inserted. Your uterus is then emptied out with a suction. Then, a metal loop, called a *curette,* is used to gently scrape the walls of the uterus to make sure that it's been emptied.

Between 14 and 24 weeks of pregnancy, surgical abortions are generally done by using a procedure called *dilation and evacuation (D&E).* This procedure, which is basically an expansion of the suction curettage method, is also usually done on an outpatient basis. Again, you lie on your back on an examining table, and your vagina is washed with an antiseptic. Then, absorbent dilators are put into your cervix. The dilators stay in for several hours to absorb fluids from your cervical area. Often, they are left in overnight. As they absorb fluids, they gradually thicken, opening the cervix wider, which can result in cramping or a feeling of pressure. You may be given antibiotics to prevent infection.

The second step takes about 10 to 20 minutes. For this part, you may be given drugs intravenously to dull the pain and prevent infection. A local anesthetic is injected either in or near your cervix, and the absorbent dilators are removed. Finally, a suction machine and instruments are used to remove the fetus and tissues.

After you have an abortion, you rest under medical supervision for about an hour or so to check for complications such as fever, bleeding, or unexpected pain. Some clinics require you to have somebody with you to take you home and check up on you. Often, you'll have a dark, menstrual-like flow on and off for a couple of weeks afterwards.

Medical abortion

In a *medical abortion,* pregnancy is terminated by a drug, herb, or chemical agent, rather than by a surgical procedure. These substances, which are known as *abortifacients,* dilate your cervix or cause your uterus to contract, inducing early labor.

Although at the present time the Food and Drug Administration (FDA) has not approved any drugs specifically to terminate pregnancy, medical abortions are available in some clinics as part of a clinical trial and from some physicians who prescribe an approved drug for an unapproved, or *off-label,* use.

Two drugs can be used for medical abortions: *methotrexate*, an approved cancer drug, and *mifepristone*, or RU-486, a drug that was developed specifically to induce abortion. (Mifepristone has not yet been approved by the FDA, although an FDA committee in early 1998 recommended its approval.) Because these drugs do not work well later in pregnancy, they are generally used only in the first six weeks of pregnancy.

Medical abortions are done in two steps. On the first visit, you receive an injection of methotrexate, which stops fetal cells from dividing, or a pill containing mifeprestone, which blocks the hormone progesterone, causing the uterine lining to break down. Several days later, you return and are given vaginal suppositories of a second drug, misoprostol, which causes the uterus to contract. The embryo and tissues that developed during the pregnancy pass through the vagina like your period. If the drugs fail to induce the abortion, surgical techniques are used to end the pregnancy.

Induction method (after 24 weeks)

Because abortion is generally safer when done early in a pregnancy, abortions done in the third trimester of pregnancy are extremely rare. They are generally done only if there is a serious threat to the woman's life or health or if the fetus is severely deformed or already dead. The procedure most often used in these instances is called the *induction method*. The induction method has to be done in the hospital, and you have to stay overnight. In these cases, labor is induced by injecting urea (a solution that causes urination), salt solution, prostaglandin (a hormone), or a combination of these substances into the uterus, resulting in the delivery of stillbirth.

Postabortion care

For the first two weeks after an abortion, you should avoid douches, tub baths, tampons, and sexual intercourse.

Adoption

If you're pregnant and don't wish to end your pregnancy, you may consider giving your baby up for adoption. In adoption, a child born to one woman becomes the legal responsibility and child of someone else — often someone who can't have children of her own. In many cases, adoption can be a win-win-win situation, benefiting the birth mother, the adoptive parents, and the child.

Once you decide to give up your baby for adoption, you then need to decide which route to take. You can arrange for the adoption either through an agency or independently through a lawyer. Even if one of your family members adopts your child, a judge in family, or surrogate, court must approve the adoption. In most states, either the biological father has to sign the papers to put the baby up for adoption or a court has to terminate his right to custody of the baby.

If you place your baby with an agency, the agency provides you with counseling, may provide you with (or refer you to) medical care and housing, handles all the legal paperwork, makes arrangements for the birth of the baby, and chooses the new adoptive family for the child.

If you choose to place the baby through a lawyer, she will handle all the legal matters and locate the adoptive parents. In many cases, the adoptive parents will pay all the medical bills (and sometimes the housing costs) associated with your pregnancy and the birth of the baby as well as counseling costs. (Some states don't allow independent adoptions because of the risk that one side is out to exploit the other.)

Once you decide whether to go through a lawyer or an agency, you must then decide whether you want the adoption closed or open:

- **Closed adoption:** Identifying information about the adoptive and birth parents is kept confidential. Alias names may be used if there is communication between the adoptive and birth parents, for example. In some cases, there is a clean break from the very beginning, while in other cases, adoptive parents and birth parents may choose to communicate with each other during a transition period. After such a transition period, a break is made, which is thought to help make a separation between you, the baby, and his or her new, adoptive parents.

- **Open adoption:** You and the adoptive parents have some degree of contact and your real names are used. You and the adoptive parents can decide how much contact you want there to be. The terms of any ongoing relationship vary from one family to the next; each family works out an agreement that suits their needs. For example, you can participate in choosing the adoptive parents, you can maintain limited contact with them, or you can simply make sure that the adoptive parents always have full access to your health history and genetic background.

Although both open and closed adoptions are legally binding, state laws can vary, so getting good information from the agency or lawyer you use is important. Finally, you need to know your options for revoking your consent to the adoption if you were to change your mind.

Questions to ask yourself if you're considering adoption

Here are some questions you want to ask yourself if you're considering adoption:

✔ Does the father agree with the adoption decision?

✔ Do I want to go through an agency or through a lawyer?

✔ Who will pay for prenatal medical care?

✔ Do I need living assistance? Who will pay for it?

✔ Who will select the adoptive parents?

✔ How much contact do I want with the adoptive parents?

✔ Who will pay for the birth costs?

✔ What are my options if I change my mind?

For more information about adoption, contact the following:

✔ The Independent Adoption Center, 391 Taylor Blvd., Suite 100, Pleasant Hill, CA 94523; 510-827-2229; www.adoptionhelp.org/nfediac

✔ The National Adoption Information Clearinghouse, P.O. Box 1187, Washington, DC 20013-1182; 703-352-3488; 888-251-0075; www.calib.com/naic

✔ The National Council for Adoption, 1930 17th St., N.W., Washington, DC 20009; 202-328-1200; info@ncfa-usa.org

Chapter 22

Sexually Transmitted Diseases and You

· ·

· ·

*W*hat makes sexually transmitted infections so dangerous is that they are so often silent and invisible, giving no signs or symptoms of their presence until years later, when the damage is done and cannot be undone.

Pelvic inflammatory disease, infertility, ectopic pregnancies, arthritis, cancer, as well as liver and kidney damage, heart and brain damage, and blindness are the tolls that sexually transmitted diseases take. But you may never have a clue that you're infected unless you begin looking at your lifestyle instead of your symptoms. This chapter looks at how sexually transmitted diseases are spread, diagnosed, and treated, as well as what you can do to reduce your risks.

How Sexually Transmitted Diseases Are Transmitted

Sexually transmitted diseases (*STDs*), also known as sexually transmitted infections, or STIs, and once called venereal diseases, or VD, are quite simply invasions of the sexual regions or organs of your body by tiny living organisms that cause uncomfortable, painful, or damaging changes in your body when they set up housekeeping there.

Sexually transmitted diseases are, by definition, infectious diseases — diseases that are transmitted, or spread, from one person to another by the movement of a particular organism from person to person. That organism may be a bacterium, which a full course of antibiotics can usually eliminate, or it may be a virus, which stays in your body for life. But unlike most other common infections, which are spread by drinking infected water or breathing infected dust or moisture particles suspended in the air, STDs require direct physical contact — usually (but not always) intimate, sexual contact — in order for the organisms that cause them to move from one person to another.

STD organisms can only survive in a living body or within the fluids of a living body. Consequently, an infected part of one person's body must directly touch someone else's body, or an infected fluid must be spread from the infected person to someone else — including by way of a contaminated needle or other contaminated object — in order for these organisms to travel from one person to another. This central fact determines what is safe and what is not safe during sexual activity with a partner who has (or who may have) an STD.

Among the body fluids known to carry or transmit the organisms responsible for various STDs are

- ✔ Fluids of the body's sexual regions, including
  - • Penile secretions (any liquid that flows from the penis during sexual play or at any other times)
  - • Semen (the sperm-containing liquid that may drip from the penis prior to orgasm and is ejected during orgasm)
  - • Vaginal secretions (the lubricating fluid that flows from the vagina during sexual play, intercourse, orgasm, or at any other times)
  - • Breast milk
- ✔ Saliva and oral secretions
- ✔ Blood and blood-related fluids, such as pus or fluids from a scab or sore
- ✔ Nasal and throat secretions or mucus
- ✔ Tears and urine

Not all STDs can be transmitted by way of all the fluids listed above. You will need to look up specific STDs (see the section "Now Presenting...The Top STDs" later in this chapter) to find out which of these fluids can spread a particular organism.

Further, not all parts of the body are equally vulnerable to contact with an infected fluid. The skin is usually a good protective barrier to infection — unless it has cuts or sores, which act like open windows and doors to STD organisms.

What make very weak barriers are the *mucous membranes* throughout your body — the porous tissue that lines the inside of the mouth, nose, and throat; the inner surfaces of the vagina, urethra, and rectum; as well as the tissue under the eyelids that lie against the eye. All these areas are particularly susceptible to invasion by organisms of every kind, including STD organisms.

Knowing When You Are at Risk

You are at risk and may be infected with one (or more than one) STD organism, if

✔ You have anal, oral, or vaginal intercourse without using a condom each and every time.

✔ You have sex with multiple partners.

✔ You use IV drugs and share needles.

✔ You are monogamous (that is, you have sex with only one partner), but your partner has sex with others, is bisexual, or uses IV drugs and shares needles.

✔ You kiss and touch intimately with a partner who is not monogamous, is bisexual, or uses IV drugs and shares needles.

✔ You have been raped or sexually abused.

✔ You are under 20 years old or became sexually active when you were under 20. (Teens' cervical and vaginal cells — as well as their immune systems — generally are more vulnerable to infection, especially by viruses.)

If you are at risk, either because you have practiced, or because you have been subjected to, one of these risks through a partner, you need a complete physical examination to determine what infections you may have. Do not be led by your symptoms or by the absence of symptoms. More often than not, STDs exhibit no symptoms at all in women, so symptoms are no indication of whether you are infected.

Knowing Where to Go for Care

The next critical step, after recognizing whether you are at risk, is to find yourself a competent and caring health care provider. Ideally, all primary care practitioners should ask all their patients about sexual health and risk status, but unfortunately, many do not. Publicly funded clinics try to make this kind of care more accessible, but many are overbooked and do not always provide the high-quality, sensitive care that all women deserve. You may prefer to see your own gynecologist. Certified nurse-midwives are becoming a common alternative to the traditional ob/gyn. They are highly qualified to give reproductive health care and counsel and are often less expensive.

Your practitioner will need to ask you a variety of questions about your lifestyle, sexual practices, and any symptoms. She will examine you, paying particular attention to your vulva and the surrounding perineal tissue, as well as to your vagina and *cervix* (the entrance to your uterus). Finally, she will obtain some tissue scrapings and/or fluid samples for laboratory examination (and may also order blood work), in order to identify any specific organism that may be present.

Usually, your practitioner will call you within about a week to report the results of these tests and to recommend the best course of treatment if an STD has been identified. Take a few moments at this point to ask your health care provider more pressing questions. Be sure that your practitioner explains the treatment to you thoroughly and has you schedule a follow-up appointment. Also important is that your partner be treated — or at least tested — for the STD(s) right along with you. Only by mutual testing, treatment, and follow-up can you be sure that the STD(s) has been eradicated and that you and your partner are no longer at risk of further long-term effects.

If you have an infection that is not curable, that is, one of the STD viruses, find out all you can about ways of minimizing its effects, avoiding recurrences of active episodes of infection, and protecting your current or future sexual partners from its spread.

Protecting Yourself

Figuring out how to use a condom so that its level of protection is worth the bother may be enough in itself to make you think twice about the risks of casual sex. No matter how dull and unpopular the other options for avoiding infection may be, STDs themselves are not at all fun or cool. If you've been through one already, you may be willing to try options you never thought you would consider. The following "safe sex" practices will definitely protect you from an STD, though you may fear you won't have a life:

✔ Abstain from all deep kissing, genital contact, and any form of intercourse.

✔ Abstain until you find a partner willing to make you his only partner and who you are convinced has had no other sexual partners before you.

What's not "safe" sex ?

In the growing landscape of STDs and their many ways of spreading, life is getting more and more treacherous for women who have multiple or casual intimate partners. Yet little is said about "safe sex" beyond the advice to use condoms and avoid "unprotected" sex.

That's decent advice, but it's just a start. Depending on the organism, you may not be safe kissing or sharing intimate touch with a partner. Here are some lesser known dangers — plus what's required to avoid them!

✔ **Deep kissing and genital kissing are not safe with a partner who's infected with hepatitis B, herpes, and cytomegalovirus (CMV) — all of which can be spread by oral contact.** The only way to protect yourself with certainty from a partner infected with one of these three viruses is to avoid all contact between body parts where any mucous membrane or body fluid is accessible. That means avoiding: oral kissing with inner lip, cheek, and/or tongue; contact between the tongue and eyes; unprotected genital kissing or licking; as well as contact by the hand with body fluids (because your hands touch so many areas of your body, thus spreading the viruses).

✔ **All forms of sexual contact are unsafe if you have unhealed skin lesions due to STDs such as chancroid, syphilis, or herpes.** These lesions make you three to five times more vulnerable to infection by HIV (the virus that causes AIDS). Staying safe under these conditions means avoiding contact not just between an HIV-infected partner's blood or semen and your vaginal or anal membranes but also between his blood or semen and any body areas where you have a cut, lesion, or sore.

✔ **Deep tongue penetration during kissing, even without oral sex, can expose you to the gonorrhea bacterium, which is occasionally harbored in the throat of a person with no other obvious symptoms.**

✔ **Deep kissing and unprotected oral sex are not safe if either partner has chlamydia, which can be harbored or spread to the respiratory tract, where it can cause pneumonia or become a trigger in chronic conditions such as asthma, particularly in children and adolescents.**

Pregnancy, birth, and STDs

Several STDs can cause serious problems for mother or baby when an infected woman becomes pregnant and gives birth. If you think you could be pregnant and have been exposed to any risk factors discussed in this chapter, make an appointment as soon as possible to be tested for STDs (including HIV), as well as for pregnancy so that you can begin treatment immediately.

The good news is that babies of women who do obtain treatment during pregnancy are frequently free of infection and healthy. The following list covers the STDs known to cause problems, their specific risks for unborn and newborn babies, and how to protect against these risks whenever possible:

- **Cytomegalovirus (CMV) is transmitted from mother to fetus in 10 to 20 percent of cases:** No known treatment exists to prevent transmission nor to cure fetal infection once it spreads. CMV can cause permanent disabilities such as hearing loss and mental retardation in babies.

- **Chlamydia and gonorrhea both can infect the fetus during its descent through the vagina just before birth and can often cause blindness if the baby is not treated for the infection during the first day of life:** Chlamydia can also cause pneumonia in the newborn, but this, too, can be treated with antibiotic therapy. In a pregnant woman, however, untreated gonorrhea can sometimes cause premature labor or stillbirth of the baby.

- **Herpes can result in a serious infection in a newborn if the infant is exposed to the** virus from an active lesion in or near the birth canal during labor and vaginal delivery: Long-term conditions resulting from the infection may include brain damage, developmental delays, disability, and, occasionally, death. Your doctor may recommend a cesarean section if you have an active herpes outbreak when in labor if it seems that it will avoid exposing your unborn baby to the virus.

- **HIV can be transmitted from HIV-infected mothers to their children, and babies who become infected eventually die:** Prior to AZT and the newer, related drugs, HIV was transmitted from mother to fetus in 20 to 30 percent of pregnancies involving an HIV-infected mother. Today, studies show that this rate can be reduced below 10 percent through treatment beginning in mid-pregnancy and extending into the newborn period. Even infants born without prior treatment can benefit from drug therapy during the first six weeks of life, and these therapies appear to be relatively safe for mother and baby. HIV is also transmitted through breast milk, so HIV-positive mothers must not breast-feed, and their partners must be careful to avoid taking in any breast milk during love-making, until the woman's milk supply has stopped.

- **Syphilis can also spread from mother to fetus during pregnancy, but antibiotic treatment early in pregnancy can prevent permanent damage to the fetus:** Untreated syphilis infection in the mother may result in stillbirth or birth defects such as heart defects, brain damage, and blindness.

A tall order. Now, for reality. If you don't think you can live within those confines (and more power to you, if you can!), try the next group of options, ordered from the most protective, to the least protective:

- ✔ Have only one sexual partner at a time — one who, likewise, has no other current sexual partners than you — and both get yourselves checked for STDs (and get treatment and follow-up, if needed) at the start.

- ✔ Have only one sexual partner at a time, use a condom and nonoxynol-9 spermicide each and every time you have vaginal or anal intercourse, and avoid oral sex. Nonoxynol-9 spermicide has been found in some studies to destroy STD organisms, including human immunodeficiency virus (HIV), the virus that causes AIDS, on contact.

- ✔ Have only one partner at a time, use a male condom and spermicide each time you have intercourse, including oral sex.

- ✔ If you have multiple partners, use a condom with spermicide each and every time you have intercourse, including oral sex.

- ✔ Use a male condom or a dental dam whenever you have oral sex.

- ✔ Use a diaphragm, sponge, or cervical cap and spermicide every time you have vaginal intercourse, and avoid anal or oral sex. (These limited barrier methods can help protect you from a few STDs but are no protection against open lesions or HIV; also, unprotected anal sex is especially risky because anal mucous membranes are thinner than vaginal ones and can tear more easily, creating an easy entrance for STD organisms.)

Now Presenting . . . The Top STDs

Here are the top STDs, in alphabetic order. For each, we list prevalence, transmission, symptoms, diagnosis, treatment, complications, and how to protect yourself.

Chlamydia

This infection, caused by a parasitic bacterium, is the most common STD in the United States.

Prevalence: Chlamydia is the fastest spreading STD in the world, with 4 million new cases reported each year in the United States alone, and 50 million new cases per year worldwide.

Transmission: Chlamydia can be spread by vaginal, oral, or anal intercourse, although there are occasional reports of transmission apart from intercourse, such as from the hand to mucous membranes of the eye. Chlamydia can be contracted from a person with no symptoms.

Symptoms: Up to 75 percent of women and 25 percent of men exhibit no symptoms. If symptoms do appear, they begin one to three weeks following infection and include bladder infection with frequent, burning urination; abdominal pain; nausea; fever; and painful intercourse.

Diagnosis and treatment: Chlamydia is caused by a bacterium that is identified by a laboratory evaluation of tissue secretions taken with special swabs of the genital area or by a urine test.

Because women so rarely develop symptoms, Planned Parenthood suggests that a bladder infection in a male partner should be taken as a clue to chlamydia infection in the woman. Chlamydia can be treated successfully with oral antibiotics for both partners.

Complications: Complications of chlamydia include chronic urinary tract infection, inflammation, and damage; pelvic inflammatory disease (PID); ectopic pregnancy; male or female sterility; and arthritis.

Protection: Condoms generally provide good protection against chlamydia.

Cytomegalovirus (CMV)

This viral disease is the most common infection in America that is spread from a woman to her developing fetus.

Prevalence: Once associated mainly with immune-compromised conditions such as AIDS, cytomegalovirus(CMV) is now spreading among adults and children. About 60 to 70 percent of all people have been previously infected with the virus, often without knowing it.

Transmission: CMV is present in all bodily fluids, including saliva, urine, and breast milk, of infected people. The virus can penetrate most mucous membranes to enter the body, including membranes of the eyes, nose, and mouth, which is why it spreads so easily among children. Among adults, it is usually spread through sexual activity, including intimate kissing and touching that does not involve intercourse. CMV can be spread by a person with no symptoms. The virus can be transmitted to the fetus through the placenta or through the vagina at birth, or to a nursing infant through breast milk. The risk of harm to the fetus is greatest if the woman becomes infected during the first trimester.

Symptoms: Adults rarely develop symptoms with the initial infection. However, when CMV is transmitted to a fetus, it can cause severe illness and birth defects, including blindness and mental retardation, and death. When the virus is reactivated in an adult, symptoms include swollen glands, fatigue, fever, weakness, stomach or intestinal upset, and vision problems.

Diagnosis and treatment: A blood test can identify CMV. CMV has no cure, and the virus remains in the body for life. However, its symptoms can be controlled by using intravenous medications.

Complications: Long-term conditions resulting from the virus include blindness, brain damage, and nervous system damage.

Protection: Use condoms for vaginal, oral, and anal intercourse, but be aware that condoms alone are not enough. Also avoid all contact between body areas of mucous membrane tissue and any bodily fluids. That means avoiding oral kissing with inner lip and/or tongue contact; contact between the tongue and the eyes; genital kissing or licking; as well as intimate touching, which can spread the virus via the hands.

Gonorrhea (the "clap")

This common bacterial infection may go unnoticed by many women because most women have no symptoms.

Prevalence: About 1 million new cases are reported each year in the United States.

Transmission: Gonorrhea can be transmitted by vaginal, oral, and anal intercourse. The gonorrhea bacterium can also be harbored in the throat, making oral sex play risky. Gonorrhea can be spread by a person with no symptoms.

Symptoms: Eighty percent of women have no symptoms, whereas only 10 percent of men are without symptoms of infection. When symptoms develop, they usually do so within ten days of infection and include frequent, burning urination in men and women; in women, pelvic pain, fever, greenish-yellow vaginal discharge, and sometimes arthritis symptoms.

Diagnosis and treatment: Sometimes confused with chlamydia, gonorrhea is caused by a bacterium that is identified by laboratory analysis of fluid samples from the cervix, throat, urethra, or rectum. It may be treated with oral antibiotics for both partners, but most experts recommend an antibiotic injection to cover some more resistant strains of the bacteria and to destroy the organism throughout the body.

Complications: These include pelvic inflammatory disease (PID), ectopic pregnancy and the sterility that may result from the scarring of the tubes, arthritis, heart damage, and nervous system disorders.

Protection: Condoms usually provide good protection against gonorrhea, except when the bacterium is present in the throat, where deep kissing could possibly spread it to a partner.

Hepatitis B virus (HBV)

This virus is the only STD against which you can be vaccinated.

Prevalence: About 225,000 new cases are reported annually in the United States.

Transmission: Hepatitis B virus (HBV) is very contagious and is present in blood, semen, saliva, feces, and urine. The virus can penetrate most mucous membranes to enter the body, including membranes of the mouth, so it can be spread through intimate kissing and touching, in addition to being spread through vaginal, oral, and anal intercourse. It is also commonly spread through needle sharing or use of unclean needles for IV drugs, as well as by accidental sticks from contaminated needles (a risk for health care professionals). During pregnancy, an infected woman can transmit the virus to the fetus. The risk is especially high if the woman is infected during her last trimester (80 to 90 percent).

Symptoms: Note that people are contagious before symptoms occur. Early symptoms may develop within four weeks of infection and include fatigue, headache, fever, hives, nausea and vomiting, and low abdominal tenderness; later symptoms may reveal liver and kidney damage and include very dark urine, clay-colored stool, and yellowing of the skin and the whites of the eyes (jaundice).

Diagnosis and treatment: A blood test can identify the virus or the antibodies that develop after you have been exposed to it. Presently, no cure and no treatment are available for HBV, which can remain in the body for life. Ninety percent of infections clear on their own, without treatment, in four to eight weeks and those infected are no longer contagious after that time. The remaining 10 percent of people do not recover completely and remain contagious for life (this is termed being a carrier).

Complications: Complications of HBV include permanent severe liver and kidney damage, and, occasionally, death.

Protection: HBV is the only STD that can be prevented entirely by vaccination. It is now recommended that infants and children be vaccinated, as well as sexually active teens and adults, illegal drug users, and health care workers.

Herpes simplex viruses 1 and 2 (HSV)

Although herpes-1 is most often associated with cold sores and fever blisters, like herpes-2, it may be sexually transmitted.

Prevalence: The prevalence of herpes is on the rise. Approximately 500,000 new cases are reported in the United States each year.

Transmission: The active infection, which usually appears as an open sore caused by both HSV-1 and HSV-2, is very contagious. The viruses are also present in blood, semen, and saliva. In the past, a distinction was made between the type 1 and the type 2 virus because type 1 was thought to occur predominantly around the mouth and type 2 in the genital area. It is now known that both types can occur in or infect any area of the body. In addition, both forms of the virus can penetrate mucous membranes of the mouth, anus, vagina, penis, and the eyes, so both can be spread through intimate kissing and other touching, in addition to vaginal, oral, and anal intercourse. Some carriers of HSV continue to be contagious even between recurrences of symptoms.

Symptoms: HSV symptoms appear between 2 and 20 days after infection and include a rash with blistering, itching, painful sores in the oral and/or genital areas or elsewhere; burning with urination; swollen glands; fever; headache; and fatigue.

Diagnosis and treatment: The virus is identified by laboratory analysis of fluid swabbed from one of the sores, so seeing your health practitioner is important before the sores scab over and heal. No cure is presently available for HSV 1 or 2, and the virus remains in the body for life. However, symptoms can be controlled somewhat by medications, and a person with frequent outbreaks can take medication long term to suppress how often this occurs.

Complications: The open sores caused by herpes are most dangerous because they provide ready doors for other STDs to enter the body, particularly, HIV.

Protection: Condoms offer some protection for vaginal, oral, and anal intercourse when the virus is not active and no sores are present, but condoms alone do not provide complete protection even between recurrences. This is because they cannot cover all body surfaces at risk, and they do, on occasion, break. Avoid all contact between body areas of mucous membrane tissue and any bodily fluids. That means avoiding oral kissing with inner lip and/or tongue contact; contact between the tongue and the eyes; genital kissing or licking; as well as intimate touching, which can spread the virus via the hands.

Human immunodeficiency virus (HIV) and acquired immune deficiency syndrome (AIDS)

Human immunodeficiency virus (HIV) is the virus that ultimately causes acquired immune deficiency syndrome (AIDS) — and AIDS is the final, deadly stage of HIV infection. In the United States, HIV infection dates back to about 1978, though its recognition as the cause of AIDS became widespread only in the mid-1980s. HIV is a virus that attaches itself to *T lymphocytes,* an important type of immune cell in the bloodstream. Like all viruses, HIV eventually destroys the cells it occupies, in this case leaving the body's immune system crippled and ultimately unable to fight infection and disease. HIV remains the most dangerous STD because, as yet, no one has ever recovered from AIDS.

Prevalence: The good news is that after nearly two decades of devastation, both new cases of HIV infection and AIDS deaths are finally starting to decline. Nonetheless, AIDS is now the leading cause of death among men and women between the ages of 25 and 44 in the United States. Well over 1 million Americans are infected with HIV and, worldwide, 1 million children and nearly 10 million adults are infected — roughly half of whom are women.

Transmission: HIV is present in blood, semen, and breast milk. It is also present (but at lower levels) in saliva, sweat, and tears. Like other STD viruses, it can enter the body through the mucous membranes lining the vagina, rectum, urethra, and mouth, as well as through any breaks in the skin, such as abrasions, cuts, and sores. Fortunately, because HIV is only present in trace concentrations in saliva, sweat, and tears, it is not readily spread by kissing alone, as are CMV, hepatitis B, and herpes. And HIV cannot be spread by being coughed or sneezed on, holding hands, hugging, sweating, or crying with someone, or by using the same makeup or telephone as an HIV-infected person.

HIV is spread by vaginal, anal, and oral intercourse, as well as by nonsexual routes, including needle sharing, accidental puncture by an infected needle, and receiving blood transfusions, organ transplants, or artificial insemination from an infected person. Oral sex is a potential route of transmission and is particularly risky if you have recently had dental work or have any open sores or bleeding of the gums or mouth, which provide a direct route into the bloodstream.

Studies have shown that the vast majority of people who know they are HIV-infected do *not* inform their sexual partners of their HIV status. And people with HIV infection are contagious even during the early stages of infection when very few signs of infection are present. This is another reason it is so critical to assume that any new sexual partner is infected and protect yourself accordingly.

Symptoms: HIV infection has several stages, the last stage being AIDS, but HIV typically lives in the body for an average of ten years before the final, deadly complications of AIDS develop. The first stage is during the six months immediately following infection, when the immune system is developing antibodies against the virus. Individuals *may not test positive* for HIV in the first six months; however, they are very contagious during this period. Symptoms at this time last just a few weeks and include slight fever, headaches, fatigue, muscle aches, and swollen glands.

Next, there is usually a long "latent" stage, lasting 10 years on average, and up to 15 years in some cases. No symptoms are present during this stage, but silent damage to various body tissues is taking place nonetheless. In the third stage of infection, the first symptoms appear that could clue a person (or her health care provider) to the immune system damage being caused by HIV. They include swollen glands in the neck, armpits and groin, sometimes called *persistent, generalized lymphadenopathy;* fatigue; persistent fevers and night sweats; light-headedness; headaches; and a dry cough. This leads to a stage that some practitioners call *AIDS-related complex,* whose symptoms include persistent, generalized infections, such as severe viral or yeast infections; other STDs; purplish growths on the skin; or PID.

AIDS, the final stage of HIV infection, is defined by the following symptoms: rapid weight loss (10 percent or more of body weight) due to chronic diarrhea and loss of appetite, called *HIV-wasting syndrome;* brain dysfunction, due to HIV infection of the brain; pneumonias or other severe infections caused by particular organisms, called *opportunistic infections;* tuberculosis; and cancer, especially cervical cancer in women.

Diagnosis and treatment: The presence of HIV in the body is identified by a blood test (a urine test is being developed) for the presence of antibodies to the virus. The body needs six months to develop antibodies against HIV, so a blood test in the first six months after exposure may be falsely negative. AIDS, as the final complication or stage of HIV infection, is identified by the presence of the specific severe conditions and opportunistic infections known to be associated with AIDS, which take advantage of the person's weak immune system and lack of defenses.

So far, like all other viruses, the HIV infection has no cure. However, a growing number of drug treatments (similar to cancer drugs) are being developed that slow the progress of HIV infection, delaying end-stage AIDS conditions and prolonging the meaningful lives of people with HIV. Alternative or complementary medical therapies are not curative but can help relieve some of the pain and discomforts of AIDS.

Protection: Male or female condoms provide very good protection against HIV during vaginal, oral, or anal intercourse. However, if you have another STD that causes sores or other open lesions on the skin (no matter how small) — or if you have cuts or skin sores from any other cause — you are at much higher risk for transmission and must avoid any skin contact with your partner's semen or genital secretions. And if the infected partner has recently had a baby or is currently breast-feeding, any leakage of breast milk must also be avoided.

Human papilloma virus (HPV or genital warts)

This viral family is also associated with cervical cancer.

Prevalence: More than 60 varieties of human papilloma virus (HPV) exist, only a few of which cause infections in the genital region. That said, about 1 million new cases of HPV appear in the United States annually.

Transmission: HPV is transmitted by vaginal, oral, or anal intercourse and intimate skin-to-skin contact and can be spread by a person with no symptoms.

Symptoms: Most genital HPV infections exhibit no symptoms, but if symptoms do appear, they develop within two to three weeks of infection and include soft, itchy wartlike growths on the genitals or in the urethra or anus and, rarely, in the mouth or throat. The warts may grow more rapidly in pregnancy and when another STD is present.

Diagnosis and treatment: The virus can be identified by microscopic examination of tissue scrapings (such as a Pap test of the cervix) or by use of a magnifier (called a *colposcope*) at the time of your physical examination by your practitioner. Warts are treated surgically, by removal with laser or freezing techniques, but often recur because the virus itself may remain in the body even when the warts are removed.

Complications: Untreated warts can occasionally grow to block the openings of the bladder, anus, vagina, or throat, but the greatest danger with HPV is that it can develop into cancer of the cervix, vulva, anus, or for men, of the penis. Recent research has linked HPV to the rising prevalence of anal and cervical cancers.

Protection: Female condoms, which cover the external vulva as well as the vaginal or anal surfaces, provide the best protection, but the virus itself may shed beyond the area covered by the condom. If you are diagnosed with an abnormal Pap smear due to HPV or genital warts, make sure your partner sees a urologist or dermatologist. Treating your partner lowers the risk that you will be reinfected.

Syphilis

This complex disease was once very prevalent.

Prevalence: Syphilis is on the decline, probably due to more widespread screening (premarital and pregnancy blood tests) and condom use. Approximately 225,000 new cases are reported in the United States each year.

Transmission: Fluid from the open sores caused by early syphilis is very contagious, but the bacterium can also be spread by direct contact with the mucous membranes of an infected person. Syphilis can be spread by a person with no symptoms.

Symptoms: Symptoms in the early phase usually occur between three weeks and three months from the time of infection. Primary phase symptoms include sores on the genitals, in the vagina and on the cervix, or on the lips, in the mouth or anus, along with swollen glands in the same area. Secondary phase symptoms include body rashes, especially on the palms of the hands and soles of the feet; mild fever; fatigue; sore throat; hair loss; weight loss; continued swollen glands; headache; and muscle pains. Untreated syphilis can then go into a long "latent" phase with no symptoms, but the infectious organism remains in the body, often causing late phase, permanent complications.

Diagnosis and treatment: Syphilis is caused by a type of bacterium known as a *spirochete* and can be diagnosed by blood test or microscopic examination of spinal fluid or fluid from the sore. It can be treated successfully with antibiotics for both partners, but damage caused by failing to treat the disease early cannot be reversed.

Complications: One-third of those with untreated syphilis suffer permanent damage to the heart, brain, nervous system (*neurosyphilis*), and to other organs. Death may result.

Protection: Condoms provide good protection during vaginal, oral, or anal intercourse, especially female condoms if genital lesions are present. Because syphilis can also be spread by direct contact between mucous membranes, you should also avoid deep kissing and other, unprotected oral-sex play.

Trichomoniasis ("Trich")

This parasitic infection is a common cause of vaginal infections (vaginitis).

Prevalence: Up to 3 million new cases are reported in the United States each year.

Transmission: Trich is transmitted through vaginal intercourse and can be spread by a person with no obvious symptoms.

Symptoms: Men often have no symptoms. In women, symptoms appear 4 to 20 days after infection and include frothy, musty-smelling greenish discharge, sometimes with blood-tinged spotting; itching in and around the vagina; swelling of the glands in the groin; and sometimes bladder infection, with frequent, possibly painful urination. Trich often occurs with other STDs and may disguise their symptoms, making diagnosis more difficult.

Diagnosis and treatment: Trich is caused by a parasite that can be identified by microscopic examination of vaginal discharge and can be treated successfully with antibiotics for both partners. A follow-up exam is important, however. It checks for other, hidden STDs.

Complications: Untreated trich is uncomfortable to live with but is not associated with high rates of pelvic inflammatory disease or other complications.

Protection: Condoms provide good protection.

Chapter 23
Sexuality and Sexual Dysfunction

Sexuality isn't just about having sex. It's also about your sexual attitudes and practices, your thoughts and feelings about being female, and your relationships with others. Many things affect your sexuality, including your age, health, emotions, and values, how you were brought up, your religious beliefs, and culture.

Your sexual needs and desires can change dramatically over your lifetime. Your sexuality may be affected by biological events, such as pregnancy or menopause, as well as life events, such as pursuing a career or becoming a widow.

This chapter takes a closer look at sexuality and some of the events common to many women that may affect it. It explores some of the common sexual dysfunctions that women experience, as well as some practical ways to improve your sexual pleasure.

Your Sexuality

Your body goes through a lot of changes over the course of your lifetime. So do your attitudes and lifestyle. All these changes affect your sexuality (and your sex life itself).

Although sexuality begins at birth, most women don't think of their sexuality or begin to have an active sex life until they reach adolescence or adulthood. Every woman's experience is individual, but many women find that events such as finding a partner, breaking up, having a baby, losing a partner, and going through menopause affect their sex lives — for better or worse. Certainly, the decision to have a baby affects sexuality. Giving up birth control can give you a sense of sexual freedom and spontaneity that you may not have enjoyed previously.

But some women feel that sex becomes mechanical when they must have intercourse on certain dates, whether the desire is present or not. And after a woman does become pregnant, she may be concerned that intercourse can harm her unborn child by causing a miscarriage or premature labor.

Pregnancy itself causes changes in a woman's body that can affect her sex life, due in large part to the dramatic increase of hormones. Your interest in sex may vary depending on the stage of your pregnancy, and your sexual techniques may change of necessity, depending on the size and shape of your body. (If your belly is large, for example, you may need to be creative and experiment with positions.)

The actual birth of a baby also brings about changes that profoundly can affect your sex life. For starters, the doctor generally prohibits sex for about six weeks. As the hormone surge from pregnancy comes to a screeching stop, so does sexual desire. And if you breast-feed, high levels of *prolactin* (a hormone that helps to start and maintain the making of breast milk) keep levels of estrogen and testosterone low, which causes vaginal dryness and reduced sexual desire. And we haven't even mentioned the affects of sleepless nights and colicky babies.

What is an orgasm anyway?

Technically, an orgasm is a series of contractions of the pelvic muscles. In women, these contractions can be felt throughout the body. The majority of women can achieve orgasm only by stimulating their *clitoris* (a highly sensitive organ about the size of a pea located just above the opening of the urethra). This stimulation produces contractions around the entrance of the vagina that are called *vulvar orgasms*. This type of orgasm tends to be briefer and more intense than other types of orgasms. For others, vaginal stimulation produces a *uterine orgasm*.

After childbirth, however, a woman has increased blood flow to her pelvis, which can actually increase the intensity of her orgasms.

Women reach their sexual peak at around age 40 and have more orgasms than when they were younger.

By the time they hit their 50s, most women are going through menopause, which causes a sharp reduction in hormone levels. Some of the resulting changes (discussed in Chapter 20) can make intercourse uncomfortable or even painful.

Some women experience a change in arousal and orgasm. In other women, menopausal symptoms may temporarily affect desire. This does not mean, however, that menopause has to curtail your sex life or decrease your sexuality.

It's a myth that older adults are sexless. Most people have a hard time picturing their parents having sex, let alone their grandparents still being sexually active. But sexuality continues into old age. Even older women can do "it." As long as you have a receptive partner, fairly good health, and a positive attitude, there's no reason you cannot enjoy sexual activity or intimacy.

What may change, however, is how you expresses your sexuality. You may prefer to receive gratification through intimacy, touch, hugs, and kisses. If intercourse is no longer an option because of illness or lack of a partner, masturbation may be an alternative.

Sexual Dysfunction: When Things Don't Go Well Between the Sheets

What do you do if you suspect you have a sexual problem? Start by making an appointment with your gynecologist or doctor. If you're like most women, you're probably reluctant or embarrassed to talk with her about any type of sexual problem. Instead, you suffer in silence — perhaps needlessly. Many sexual problems have simple solutions and are easily treated. But don't assume that your doctor will ask you whether you're having problems with your sex life. Be assertive and speak up. Your doctor has probably cared for other women with sexual dysfunction; you won't be the first or the last.

Your doctor can determine whether a medical cause is present that she can treat or a medication that you can stop or change. If your doctor can find no physical cause for your problem, she may recommend a sex therapist, marriage counselor, or psychotherapist.

Work out that orgasm muscle!

Working out and strengthening your pubococcygeus, or PC, muscle can enhance your sexual pleasure. This muscle contracts and relaxes during orgasm, but it's not a muscle you see women working out in the gym. Exercising this muscle can help you have a longer, howling, sweat-dripping, heart-pounding orgasm. Although we can't give you any guarantees, you can generally increase the intensity of your orgasm — or maybe even experience orgasm if you've never had one before — just by strengthening this one small muscle with Kegel exercises.

To exercise your PC muscle, you first need to find it. You actually use it many times a day to stop the flow of urine. So, the next time you go to the bathroom, contract this muscle while you're urinating. You'll know you're contracting the right muscle because the stream of urine will stop. This is the feeling you should have when you exercise your PC muscle.

Test your PC muscle's strength by inserting two fingers into your vagina while lying down. Spread out your fingers and squeeze your PC muscle to try to bring your fingers together. Don't worry if your PC muscle is too weak to do this. If you practice your Kegel exercises faithfully, you should notice a significant improvement within several weeks.

To perform Kegel exercises, contract your PC muscle, hold it, and release it. Repeat this maneuver ten times. As your PC muscle becomes stronger, increase the number of repetitions to as many as 150 per day. Gradually increase to ten seconds of holding and ten seconds of releasing. You can work this muscle several times a day. Instead of stewing about the long grocery line, work on your orgasm. No one will ever know what you're doing — unless, of course, you have a sly grin on your face.

Causes of sexual dysfunction

Numerous factors can cause or contribute to sexual problems. Psychosocial factors, such as stress (see Chapter 1 for more information), fatigue, and emotions such as anger, can obviously affect your level of desire. A lack of privacy or religious beliefs may also have an effect, as may sexual inexperience and abuse (either sexual or physical). As discussed in the previous section, hormones, can have a profound effect on your sex life. Chronic illnesses, such as arthritis, cancer, diabetes, and cardiovascular disease, can affect sexual response both physically and psychologically. Mental illnesses, including depression (see Chapter 14), are also a common cause of sexual dysfunction. Medications that can cause sexual problems include alcohol, antidepressants, antihistamines, antihypertensives, antipsychotics, oral contraceptives, sleeping pills, and tranquilizers.

Types of sexual dysfunction

Four basic types of sexual dysfunction can keep a woman from enjoying a satisfying sexual relationship. They are

- Lack of desire
- The inability to have an orgasm *(anorgasmia)*
- Painful intercourse *(dyspareunia)*
- Spasm of the vaginal muscles *(vaginismus)*

Lack of desire

If you suffer from a loss of desire, or libido, you may still be able to have an orgasm even though you have little or no interest in sexual activities. If your partner initiates sex, you are often able to respond. Bear in mind, however, that if your sex drive isn't the same as your partner's, that doesn't mean you have a lack of desire. No two people have the same sex drive.

If you think that you have a lack of sexual desire and would like to have a more satisfying sex life, make an appointment with your doctor or gynecologist. There may be a treatable cause. For instance, a woman may experience a drop in sexual desire if she's had both her ovaries removed. Emotionally, many women feel that they have lost their femininity or sexuality after their ovaries are removed. Replacing hormones such as estrogen, progesterone, and testosterone can be helpful in improving desire. Not as much is known about how a hysterectomy affects sexual activity. If your doctor can't find a medical problem, she may recommend counseling or therapy. Often, a decrease in sexual desire is related to a problem in the relationship.

Anorgasmia

Anorgasmia occurs when a woman is unable to have an orgasm. Many women experience this problem at some time in their lives. A woman with primary anorgasmia has never experienced an orgasm, while a woman with secondary anorgasmia is able to have orgasms but isn't able to achieve orgasm with her present partner.

Some factors that can interfere with the ability to have an orgasm include sexual abuse, problems with a partner (such as poor hygiene) or the relationship (you just don't like him), an inexperienced or inattentive partner, and feelings of fear, anger, or guilt. An ability to masturbate to orgasm can help distinguish anorgasmia resulting from a psychological cause and anorgasmia from a physiological cause.

Dyspareunia

Feeling pain or discomfort with intercourse from time to time is not uncommon, but persistent painful intercourse *(dyspareunia)* isn't normal and should be checked out by your doctor. The cause can be as simple as vaginal dryness from not enough foreplay. Breast-feeding, menopause, removal of the ovaries, and certain medications, including antihistamines or even birth control pills can also cause vaginal dryness.

If your partner uses a latex condom, you may have an allergy to latex. Try switching brands. Other causes of pain that require treatment may include endometriosis, urinary tract or vaginal infections, sexually transmitted diseases, and sexual abuse.

A water-soluble lubricant such as K-Y Jelly can resolve the dryness. So can stopping an offending medication. By the way, more foreplay can also help. And it's fun! Some menopausal woman benefit from estrogen replacement therapy.

Vaginismus

A woman with *vaginismus* suffers from spasms of the muscles around the opening of the vagina, which can cause pain and be severe enough to prevent penetration. Vaginismus may be triggered by some of the same painful conditions that cause dyspareania, including endometriosis and urinary tract or vaginal infections. Or it may be triggered by fear or anxiety about sex, as well as by previous sexual trauma.

A woman may be treated with psychotherapy and the use of vaginal dilators (narrow tubes that stretch, or dilate, the vagina) to help the muscles learn to relax.

Enhancing your pleasure

What else can you do to improve your sex life? Here are some simple suggestions that can help you experience more pleasure:

✔ Practice safe sex (see Chapter 22) with a partner you care about.

✔ Communicate with your partner and your gynecologist.

✔ Show affection, hold hands. Know that experiencing sexual pleasure is okay.

✔ Reduce stress, learn to relax, take vacations, enjoy your work, and feel good about yourself.

✔ Eat healthily, limit how much alcohol you drink, exercise regularly, and get enough sleep.

✔ Practice your Kegel exercises.

✔ Only perform sexual activities that you feel good about, and don't compare your sexual response with that of other women.

Part V
Pregnancy

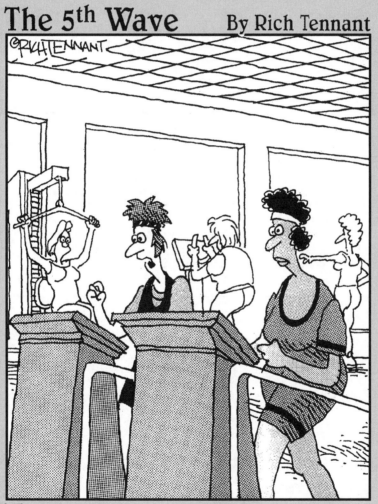

The 5th Wave   By Rich Tennant

"I exercised so much during my first pregnancy that the baby was born with athlete's foot."

In this part . . .

Despite advances in science and science fiction, pregnancy remains uniquely a women's domain — and it's one that can change your life. Knowing what to expect from your body — and your health care practitioner — before and during pregnancy, as well as during labor and after, can help you make this change with as little difficulty as possible.

Chapter 24

Choosing Your Childbirth

· ·

In This Chapter

▶ Choosing a health care practitioner for your pregnancy and birth

▶ Selecting a birth setting

▶ Understanding childbirth methods and options

· ·

*I*f you're thinking of having a baby or you just found out that you're pregnant, you have a number of very important decisions to make — from what to call your bundle of joy to how she'll come into the world.

You can't count on the stork to make these decisions. You have to make them yourself. Fortunately, you have several options available. This chapter looks at the various types of birth practitioners, birth settings, and childbirth methods, giving you the information you need to have the pregnancy and childbirth of your choice.

Choosing Your Practitioner

Choosing a health care practitioner to monitor your pregnancy and birth is one of the first and most important tasks you face after you discover that you're pregnant. After all, you're going to consult with this person for 40-plus weeks and you're entrusting him or her not only with your own health but also that of your unborn child.

You need to select your practitioner early because prenatal care cannot wait. (For more on prenatal care, see Chapter 25.) You can always switch to someone else later if you discover that you are uncomfortable with your choice. (See Chapter 27 for a list of questions to ask a prospective practitioner.)

A generation ago, the choice of a practitioner was not much of an issue. Most practitioners were pretty much the same — they treated their pregnant patients like military inductees who were expected to take orders and ask no questions. Today, the variety of birth attendants is substantial, and you can find one who is ideal for you.

Think about what you want out of childbirth, and look for a practitioner who is experienced and qualified and who shares your philosophy. You're likely to choose an obstetrician, a family practitioner, or a nurse-midwife.

The road most traveled: The obstetrician

Approximately four out of five babies born in the United States are delivered by an obstetrician-gynecologist. The majority of women choose an ob/gyn as their birth practitioner because they want a doctor on hand in case of a medical emergency during delivery. Obstetrical training focuses in large part on handling complications, and obstetricians are more likely to use interventions such as episiotomies and cesarean sections than other practitioners. (Chapter 26 discusses interventions.)

Ob/gyns are licensed physicians — M.D.'s or D.O.'s — who have completed an approved four-year program of specialty training (called a *residency*) in obstetrics and gynecology after medical school.

Many ob/gyns are board certified, which means that they have completed this postgraduate training and have passed an examination administered by a *specialty board,* a national board of professionals in that specialty field. Board certification is generally considered a minimum standard of excellence. Although certification does not guarantee competence, it is a good sign that a doctor is up-to-date on the procedures, theories, and success-failure rates in her specialty. It also ensures that the doctor has specialty training: A licensed physician may practice any specialty and call himself a specialist in a particular field, regardless of training or certification. You can find out if the obstetrician you are considering is board certified by contacting the American Board of Medical Specialties at 800-776-CERT or, if the obstetrician is a doctor of osteopathy, by calling the American Osteopathic Board of Obstetrics and Gynecology at 312-947-4630.

If your pregnancy is high risk, an obstetrician is the way to go. You may even be referred to a *perinatologist*, an obstetrician who specializes in maternal and fetal medicine.

The family way: The family practitioner

The family practitioner, chosen as birth practitioner by 10 to 12 percent of pregnant women, provides one-stop medical care for the entire family. A board-certified family practitioner must have three years of specialty training in primary care, including at least three months in obstetrics and gynecology. Many women prefer the continuity offered by a physician who can care for them before, during, and after pregnancy and who will act as their child's pediatrician.

While board certification does guarantee that a family practitioner has received some training in obstetrics, not every family practitioner has obstetrical experience. If you're considering asking your family practitioner to deliver your child, make sure that you ask her how many babies she has delivered and what percentage of her practice is obstetrics. Although most family practitioners do not perform delivery interventions, determining their philosophy in this area is important before making your selection. If a problem requiring intervention arises during your pregnancy or labor, a family practitioner may consult an obstetrician.

To find out if a family practitioner is board certified, contact the American Board of Medical Specialties or, if the doctor is an osteopathic doctor, contact the American Osteopathic Board of General Practice at 847-640-8477.

The historic choice: The midwife

Historically, most births were attended by women. Today, certified nurse-midwives are selected as birth practitioners by about 5 percent of pregnant women. The main attraction is the nurse-midwife's focus on you as the patient. She takes extra time to talk about your concerns, and she leans toward a "natural" childbirth with limited interventions. She also heavily stresses childbirth education.

A *certified nurse-midwife* is a registered nurse who has completed at least one year of obstetric training and passed a national certification examination. Nurse-midwives limit their practice to handling low-risk pregnancies, but they are trained to recognize signs of trouble, either during pregnancy or delivery. They won't hesitate to call in a doctor or specialist if necessary.

Nurse-midwives practice in a variety of settings — county hospitals, private hospitals, neighborhood health centers, and birthing centers. Some obstetricians have seen the value of nurse-midwives and added them to their staffs.

To find a certified nurse-midwife in your area, contact the American College of Nurse-Midwives, 818 Connecticut Ave., N.W., Suite 900, Washington, DC 90006; 202-728-9860.

Choosing a practice

Your potential birth attendant's type of practice may also influence your decision. Physicians in a solo practice provide their patients with the advantage of continuity. If you choose a doctor in solo practice, you will see the same doctor at each visit and during your delivery. However, if your doctor is unavailable at the time of birth, you could be stuck with a doctor whom you've never met.

If your physician is part of a group practice, however, you won't necessarily see him at each visit. Instead, you may meet each member of the group throughout your pregnancy. At delivery time, you'll probably have at least met the person who will get you through the grand finale.

Practices based in birth centers offer care for low-risk pregnancies, largely because the primary birth attendants are nurse-midwives.

Setting Your Site

As you're selecting your birth practitioner, you should also be considering where you want to deliver your child. The two often go hand in hand. (Most doctors will not deliver a child in your home, for example.) Also be sure to ask your insurance company what birthing locations it will cover — unless you're willing to foot the bill yourself.

Your birth setting choices generally include a hospital, a birth center, and your home. (You may give birth elsewhere, but it will likely be due to your baby's insistence, rather than your choice.)

Technological reassurance

For mothers who feel safer bringing their child into the world in a place filled with modern medical technology, a hospital is the obvious choice. Most babies today are born in hospitals.

If you live in an area where you have more than one hospital from which to choose, shop around for one that meets your standards. Many hospitals are getting the message that the medicalized deliveries of the 1950s and 1960s have become passé and are offering more family-oriented births. Among the latest additions to hospitals are *birthing rooms* — rooms in which you labor, deliver, and recover. The rooms are a bit more homey than the traditional hospital room, with windows, pictures on the wall, and comfortable chairs and beds. They are fully equipped for normal deliveries, but if you require a cesarean section, you'll be whisked away to a standard delivery room.

You'll also want to ask the representatives of the hospitals you're considering a number of questions, including questions about their cesarean-section rates, their use of interventions such as inducement and episiotomies, and the birth positions they encourage. You also should inquire about the childbirth preparation methods the staff is familiar with and those that the hospital offers (see "Childbirth Methods and Options" later in this chapter). Be sure to ask who may be in the delivery room — this is particularly important if you want someone (or several people) in addition to the father. Ask whether the baby may room with you or whether he must spend his nights in the nursery.

Almost as homey as home

For moms-to-be searching for a delivery that's a bit more laid-back, a birth center is a possible choice. Staffed predominantly by midwives, birth centers offer a middle ground between giving birth in a hospital and giving birth at home. The atmosphere tends to be relaxed. Very little medical intervention is planned, and the entire family is invited to participate.

Another benefit is that delivery in a birth center can be as much as 35 percent cheaper than delivery in a hospital. Not all insurance companies cover such deliveries, however.

Only women with low-risk pregnancies are permitted to give birth in a birth center. If complications develop during your pregnancy, you'll be referred to a physician and will have to plan on a hospital delivery. If the trouble arises during delivery, you'll likely be rushed to a hospital, where a doctor will attend your birth. You may want to consider a birth center's proximity to a hospital when making your choice.

Studies have shown birth centers to be a safe, cost-effective alternative to hospitals. About one in six women must be transferred to a hospital during delivery. Generally, first-time moms are the ones who must be moved — often because of stalled labor. The cesarean-section rate for birth centers is a very low 4.4 percent.

Some questions you may want ask of representatives of a birth center are

✔ Is the center freestanding or is it affiliated with a hospital?

✔ Does the center provide prenatal and postpartum care and education?

✔ Is the center accredited by a national organization?

✔ Are the primary caregivers certified nurse-midwives?

✔ Does the center have a physician backup?

✔ What preparations are made for emergencies?

✔ What hospital is the backup hospital?

No place like home

Fear or dislike of hospitals and the quest for the perfect birth experience are among the factors that drive women to give birth at home. Those who make this choice are likely to face harsh criticism from family and physicians who've been indoctrinated with the idea that doing so is unsafe. Proponents, however, argue that there is no safer place for a normal birth.

If home is your choice, the selection of your birth attendant is likely the most critical decision you will make. You must find someone qualified, with whom you feel comfortable, and who is willing to deliver your child in your home.

Childbirth preparation and education classes also are vital. You truly will have control over your birth and will not be able to rely on a medical staff to make decisions in the middle of your delivery. You must be acutely aware of every aspect of the birthing process, and you must be prepared to deal with it. For this reason, home births are not always the best option for first-time moms. Having your support person and family familiar with the particulars of the event is also key.

You must have a plan for emergency transportation to the hospital in the event of a difficult delivery or a problem with the baby. And you must prepare your home for caring for the newborn in those first few hours of life.

Childbirth Methods and Options

The days when all women in labor were anesthetized and gave birth strapped on their backs to a table with their legs raised in stirrups are gone. Today, women have a whole host of options for childbirth, including delivery methods, birthing positions, and breathing and relaxation techniques. Doctors and hospitals are considerably more flexible than in the past, but you still must make your preferences known in advance of your due date.

Education is everything

Before you consider one of several childbirth methods, it helps to attend a class in which you can learn the ins and outs of labor and the usefulness of different birthing methods. Childbirth preparation courses are just that — preparation for what is likely to be the most interesting day of your life. You — and your partner — can use them to learn what to expect, decide on a childbirth method, or learn such a method. You can take a course at any time during your pregnancy. The length, duration, and material covered varies depending on the course. Some hospitals and childbirth centers offer the choice of a series of classes for first-time moms, a "crash course" for those who already have an idea of what to expect, or a short refresher course if that's all you need.

The Methods

A host of childbirth methods are available. Among the most common are

- **Bradley:** Partner-coached childbirth is the focus of this method. It uses the six conditions found in the animal world that a woman requires to give birth naturally — darkness and solitude, quiet, physical comfort, physical relaxation, controlled breathing, and closed eyes. The method, which starts lessons early in pregnancy, also emphasizes nutrition and exercise to ease the discomforts of pregnancy and to prepare for childbirth.

- **Dick-Read:** This method is premised on the idea that women fear childbirth. The fear creates tension, which produces pain in a vicious tension-pain cycle. With Dick-Read, women use knowledge, breathing, and relaxation techniques to eliminate fear and thus make pain more tolerable. The method also uses visualization techniques and involves men in the delivery.

- **Lamaze:** By learning exercises and breathing techniques, women who practice the Lamaze method learn to block pain. Also known as *psychoprophylaxis* because it prevents pain psychologically, the Lamaze method works on the theory of conditioned reflexes: Contractions serve as a stimulus to relax certain muscles through controlled breathing, which blocks pain. Pain sensations are also blocked by concentrating on distracting stimuli, such as staring at a focal point.

- **LeBoyer:** Known as the birth-without-violence method, LeBoyer advocates delivery in a dark, quiet room without medical interventions such as forceps. LeBoyer recommends soft music and lights and delivery into a warm tub as the body of the baby emerges. Newborns in this technique also are placed immediately on their mothers' abdomens for a massage.

Sit, stand, or flop on your back?

A laboring woman can work through delivery in any number of positions, given her flexibility and that of her birth attendant. The old method of lying flat on your back (known as the *lithotomy position*) is giving way to sitting and squatting, simply because birth attendants have recognized the advantages of gravity. In addition, research has found that an upright position reduces the length of labor and reduces maternal trauma (such as vaginal tears) during delivery. Surveys indicate that most women prefer to stand, sit, or walk during labor.

Most delivery rooms these days are equipped with a birthing bed, which is a wide comfortable piece of furniture that tilts the woman into a semi-squatting position. The bottom of the bed pulls away to allow the birth attendant access to the baby.

Birthing chairs are somewhat less common. They support a woman in a full sitting position and provide even more gravity.

The birth cushion aids women who deliver in a squatting position. It is a U-shaped cushion that supports a woman's thighs and has handles to help her push out the baby.

Women have also delivered in a kneeling position or on their sides. In some instances, birthing under water has been known to hasten a stalled labor.

If you are interested in giving birth in an alternative position, discuss it with your practitioner as soon as possible. Some positions, such as squatting, may require special preparation to enhance flexibility.

Why take a class?

Still not sure whether you're ready to sign up for a childbirth preparation class? Here are some reasons that may help you make up your mind:

- ✔ The class begins with a description of what to expect before labor begins and how things change through the various stages of labor.

- ✔ The class gives you an opportunity to learn methods for dealing with the pain of labor.

- ✔ The class gives you the chance to ask questions of professionals on a regular basis.

- ✔ The class gives you an opportunity to spend time with other expectant couples and to share your experiences.

- ✔ The class provides a wealth of information for dads who may have little idea of what's been happening during the pregnancy and no clue about the ordeal and wonder of delivery.

- ✔ Increased knowledge means increased confidence in the delivery room, which can result in less stress and, consequently, a more comfortable labor, both mentally and physically.

Chapter 25

A Healthy Pregnancy

. . . .

. . . .

*F*or many women, getting pregnant is something they do first and think through later. But if you know what to do and what to expect, you can give yourself and your baby the best chances for health and well-being during pregnancy — and after. This chapter tells you how to prepare for pregnancy, what will happen to your body (and your baby) during pregnancy, and how to keep yourself and your baby healthy to reduce the risk of complications. This chapter also discusses common complications and how they're handled.

Starting Out Right

Start with an annual gynecologic and complete physical exam. This way, you and your health care provider can get a good baseline picture of your reproductive and general health. Be sure to get a breast exam — your breast tissue will change as a result of the high hormonal levels of pregnancy. Your physical should also include a heart, lung, and blood pressure check, thyroid check, urine check, lifestyle review, and blood work — you need to know early on what problems, if any, you may face during pregnancy.

This is also the ideal time to discuss with your practitioner the kinds of risk factors that could affect the health of your baby once you become pregnant. The three major types of fetal risk factors you will need to address are

- Risks involving your general health such as a pre-existing chronic illness that could affect the safety and well-being of your pregnancy
- Risks involving your genetic makeup and your partner's, any portion of which your offspring can inherit
- Risks involving external or environmental hazards that you may be exposed to

To evaluate these risk factors your practitioner needs to

- Take a personal medical history from each of you or update it if you have given one before.
- Take a family history from each of you, including all known illnesses, surgeries, causes of death, inherited disorders, children born with birth defects, mental retardation, or disabilities.
- Order blood studies to provide information about any need for early preventive health measures that you or your baby may need, and to settle some other questions about fetal risk factors.

Two to three months before you start trying to conceive, you should discontinue your method of birth control and begin to follow the lifestyle recomendations in "Taking Steps to a Healthy Pregnancy."

Just before trying to conceive, stop taking all over-the-counter medicines, as well as medicinal herbal supplements, unless you have discussed their use with your practitioner. Acetaminophen (Tylenol) is considered safe. Herbal medicines, although "natural," contain active ingredients that can have powerful effects on your developing baby.

Stages of Uncomplicated Pregnancy

Health providers refer to pregnancy in terms of *trimesters,* or thirds, each one lasting three months. Here are some highlights of what your baby and your body will be up to for these nine months.

Blood tests

In addition to the standard blood tests that measure your overall health status, you may also want to consider the following:

✔ **A rubella (German measles) screen:** If you are not immune to this disease, exposure to the virus during the first trimester of pregnancy can cause fetal deafness, cataracts, heart defects, and/or mental retardation in your unborn baby. If you are not yet pregnant, you can receive a vaccine and wait three months before conceiving.

✔ **A toxoplasmosis screen:** Toxoplasmosis is an infection caused by a parasite that lives in raw meat and in some mammals, such as cats. If you are apt to have any contact with cat feces during your pregnancy, you may want to find out whether or not you are already immune to this viral illness — which can cause blindness, mental retardation, and *neural tube defects* (a type of birth defect in the fetus of a newly infected mother).

✔ **An HIV screen:** Human immunodeficiency virus (HIV), the virus that causes AIDS, is generally passed from mother to baby during pregnancy, and, possibly, through breast-feeding after birth. You should receive an HIV screening if you, or any of your past or present sexual partners are health care workers who may have been exposed to the virus through occupational duties, are gay or bisexual, share needles with anyone, have ever had another sexually transmitted disease, or have received a blood transfusion or blood product before 1985.

✔ **A varicella (chicken pox) screen:** If you do not know whether you have had chicken pox, you should have a test to see if you are immune. If you are not, you can be vaccinated against the disease, which may be serious in pregnant women and can sometimes affect your unborn baby as well.

Your baby's first trimester

During the first month, your baby's basic organ systems begin forming, and the heart starts to beat. Arm and leg buds appear, and by the third month, arms and legs, hands and feet, and fingers and toes are fully formed. The basic structure for all major organs and organ systems has been established by the end of the second month. The fetus has a complete skeleton made of cartilage, is able to move, and the first set of tooth buds appear. During the third month, real bone begins to replace cartilage, the sex organs are formed, and your baby's gender may be possible to distinguish by ultrasound. He or she begins to look very human, and sucking, swallowing, and breathing movements appear. The heart forms its four chambers and pumps blood through the major vessels. The placenta, umbilical cord, and amniotic sac with its fluid become fully formed.

Your first trimester

Even while your baby is undergoing some of his most important physical development, you may be feeling your worst. Though not all women experience problems such as nausea in the first trimester, most women have some degree of difficulty with queasiness and other discomforts, which usually sets in six to nine weeks after their last menstrual period.

Your uterus grows larger and becomes soft. Your blood volume increases rapidly. Common but minor discomforts include sleepiness, needing to urinate more frequently, intestinal gas and/or bloating, food aversions and cravings, and breast changes such as darkening of the *areolas* (the pigmented circle surrounding the nipple), fullness, or tingling. More troublesome discomforts include nausea and vomiting (which can occur at any time of the day, not just in the morning), heartburn, constipation, and fatigue.

Your baby's second trimester

During the second trimester, your baby grows (on average) in length from 3 or 4 inches to over a foot, and in weight from just an ounce to $1^1/_2$ pounds. He grows hair on his head and nails on his fingers and toes. By the end of the sixth month, he has his finger- and toe-prints; he can hear; and his eyelids separate so that the eyes can open. His skin is paper thin, with no fat stores beneath to help him regulate hunger and warmth. But the various organ systems are now beginning to function as they will have to do after birth: If your baby were born at the end of the second trimester, he would have a chance of survival in most major medical centers.

Your second trimester

The fourth, fifth, and sixth months generally give some relief from the annoyances and miseries of the preceding three, without the awkwardness and fatigue of the three that will follow. Your appearance will start to take on the "look" of pregnancy, and your energy will probably pick up.

By about the middle of this trimester, the top *(fundus)* of your uterus will expand upward to the level of your navel. Also, around the 20th week, you will begin feeling your baby's activity regularly. Over the next month, these movements will develop into vigorous activity. Your breasts may continue to enlarge, the nipples and areolas to darken, and a lightly pigmented line from your navel to your pubic bone may appear on your abdomen. Some women also develop pigmented patches elsewhere. You may also develop mild swelling *(edema)* in your feet and ankles by month five or six.

Among the discomforts that may continue are heartburn and constipation. You may become faint or dizzy when you sit up or move rapidly. You may also begin noticing new veins in your legs, varicose veins, or nasal or ear stuffiness. Low backaches and strains can begin to cause problems, especially by the sixth month. Other common problems include headaches, hemorrhoids, nosebleeds, leg cramps, and discomfort in the lower abdomen caused by the stretching of a major uterine support ligament.

Your baby's third trimester

This period is when your baby's real preparation for life outside the womb begins. Fat stores are deposited under his skin, and he gains an average of about $1/2$ pound per week during this trimester. His brain grows rapidly throughout this trimester, he gains an additional 6 inches in length, and his bones gain more and more calcium to strengthen them for weight-bearing movement outside the womb. His own blood supply grows, and all organ systems fine-tune themselves for independent function. His lungs remain immature by the end of the eighth month, but if he were born early now, most other organ systems would be quite functional.

Your third trimester

The third trimester is when your body and mind make final preparations for labor, birth, and life with a newborn.

Emotionally, you may notice yourself beginning to wonder and worry more about getting through childbirth. Physically, your body is hard at work with preparations, such as blood volume expansion (to replace blood lost during childbirth), uterine muscle development, and preparations for milk production. By the eighth month, your fundus will reach the level of your *diaphragm* (a muscle that lies between your lungs and stomach), and you may begin to feel short of breath — especially following exertion. *Braxton-Hicks uterine contractions* (which often begin occurring in the second trimester) occur now with increasing frequency. Although these muscle contractions are sometimes referred to as "false" labor pains, they serve a purpose by allowing the uterus to exercise itself — rehearsing for "real" labor by building up its tone, strength, and endurance. Also in the eighth month, you may begin noticing occasional breast leakage of a clear to yellowish fluid, *colostrum,* which will be your baby's first "milk." By the middle of this trimester, you will probably begin to feel weary of your weight and bulk. Your energy level may begin to wane.

Sometime in the ninth month, your baby will probably start to descend in your pelvis, relieving your short-windedness and cramped stomach, but causing you to urinate more often from the pressure on your bladder.

Discomforts that may continue from earlier months include heartburn, leg cramps, hemorrhoids, and fatigue. You may also experience insomnia (see Chapter 13), trouble getting comfortable in bed, and stretch marks.

Taking Steps to a Healthy Pregnancy

In most cases, healthy eating, gentle, regular exercise, and a few careful, informed lifestyle choices can, together, do far more to boost the likelihood of having a healthy pregnancy and a healthy newborn than any number of medical treatments and procedures could hope to do. The initiative rests mostly with you to see that your daily routines contribute to your well-being and that of your baby, rather than detracting from them.

Careful examination of your lifestyle is a first, and most crucial, step in protecting your baby's health and your own. You can start with these tips:

✔ **Quit smoking:** Women who smoke have more difficulty becoming pregnant, have a higher incidence of miscarriage and stillbirth, and give birth to more low-birthweight babies than women who do not smoke. Smoking also raises your risk of complications, Sudden infant death syndrome (SIDS) is ten times more common among babies of smoking mothers than babies of nonsmokers. Secondhand smoke is also implicated with some of these conditions.

✔ **Reduce or eliminate alcohol intake (not to mention the use of any "recreational" drugs):** Moderate to heavy alcohol use leads to *fetal alcohol syndrome,* a group of birth defects that can include heart defects, facial deformity, growth retardation, and mental retardation.

✔ **Reduce or eliminate caffeine intake:** Caffeine has been linked with a higher rate of miscarriage and, in large quantities, could be a factor in some birth defects.

✔ **Exercise regularly:** Your daily activities tend to stress the same muscle and nerve groups over and over, but they don't stretch or strengthen other, less-used but complementary muscles that can help support your body when you go into labor. Your goals are qualities, such as flexibility, coordination, concentration, and endurance. The American College of Obstetricians and Gynecologists recommends regular, low-impact exercise, done three times a week or more. A good routine is 5 to 10 minutes of warm-up, 15 to 30 minutes of exercise, and 5 to 10 minutes of cooldown.

The two most highly recommended types of exercise are walking and lap swimming. High-impact sports, such as skiing, and competitive contact sports are risky and not recommended. Diving, surfing, and scuba diving are also not recommended. Most other kinds of sports are safe if you were accustomed to them before pregnancy.

Why bother with exercise?

More than one study has shown that women who exercise regularly throughout pregnancy and are in good cardiovascular health

✔ Give birth to healthier babies

✔ Experience less pain and difficulty during labor

✔ Have fewer back pain problems

✔ Return to their prepregnancy weight faster

✔ **Drink at least 6 to 8 glasses of water (about 2 quarts) a day:** Sufficient water helps prevent constipation, fatigue, headaches, painful uterine contractions, and urinary tract infections.

✔ **Aim for a healthy weight:** If you are significantly underweight before pregnancy, you run a higher risk of premature labor, of having a low-birthweight baby, and of early infant death. You may even have difficulty getting pregnant. Although it once appeared that babies of overweight women were somewhat protected from these complications, research has shown that very overweight women also run a risk for preterm delivery. The major risks for overweight moms in pregnancy are those to the mom herself; namely, an increased chance of developing gestational diabetes, blood clots, high blood pressure, and greater risk of surgical complications if cesarean section is necessary.

Although the exact cause of these complications is not understood, it appears that reaching and maintaining a healthy body weight before pregnancy creates a healthier environment for your baby during pregnancy. Discuss the appropriate weight gain for you with your health care professional.

✔ **Eat a well-balanced diet, high in nutrients, but low in fat:** The nutrient building materials most crucial to your baby's healthy development are protein, certain fatty acids, and a wide range of vitamins and minerals, along with sufficient energy to fuel the construction work. Many women take a daily multivitamin supplement, and some choose to take a prescription, high-dose, prenatal vitamin and mineral supplement. Table 25-1 lists vitamin and mineral needs during pregnancy. The National Research Council lists the following requirements for 18 of the most widely researched vitamin and mineral elements.

How much weight to gain ...?

According to the Institute of Medicine guidelines, *Nutrition During Pregnancy,* the following ranges of weight gain are appropriate for women during pregnancy:

Prepregnancy Category	*Recommended Gain (lbs.)*
Underweight	28 – 40 pounds
Optimal healthy weight	25 – 35 pounds
Overweight	15 – 25 pounds
Obese	15 pounds, not much more

Table 25-1   Vitamin and Mineral Needs During Pregnancy

Vitamin or Mineral	*Amount*
Protein (grams)	60
Vitamin A (micrograms)	800
Vitamin D (micrograms)	10
Vitamin E (milligrams)	10
Vitamin K (micrograms)	65
Vitamin C (milligrams)	70
Thiamin (milligrams)	1.5
Riboflavin (milligrams)	1.6
Niacin (milligrams)	17
Vitamin B_6 (milligrams)	2.2
Folic Acid (micrograms)	400
Vitamin B_{12} (micrograms)	2.2
Calcium (milligrams)	1200
Phosphorus (milligrams)	1200
Magnesium (milligrams)	320
Iron (milligrams)	30
Zinc (milligrams)	15
Iodine (micrograms)	175

Your Prenatal Care

Whether you select an obstetrician, midwife, or family practitioner for your obstetrical care, many aspects of your care during pregnancy will be the same. Examine your own expectations, philosophy, and beliefs about health care and pregnancy before your first appointment. That way, the caregiver you choose can more adequately address your needs and priorities throughout pregnancy and the birth of your baby.

Your first visit

Your first appointment will probably be the longest, lasting from 30 to 90 minutes. At this time, your caregiver should take a complete personal medical history from you as well as a complete family history, including as much about your partner's family as you can provide. If you haven't had a prepregnancy physical exam, have a physical now. You can arrange routine blood work, and any blood screens, including screening for genetic problems that you need based on your personal and family histories on this visit.

Emotional health during pregnancy

Pregnancy is hard physical work, and it is emotionally demanding. Every pregnant woman experiences uncertainties about her future with her baby, in varying degrees, so you are clearly not alone. You may also have money issues, big brothers or sisters to prepare, or step-family issues to address. You probably have job decisions ahead, a sense of loss of the life you had before this pregnancy, and your sex life can become anything from a creative challenge to a chore. To make the future more approachable and the present less anxious, keep the lines of communication open between you and your partner, you and your kids, and you and your doctor; try planning a new budget, and then try living with it for a month; explore possible ways of reducing the stress in your life, and take prenatal classes to meet other women in the same situation.

Also be aware that if you have previously experienced either depression or other major disturbances of your emotional well-being, you are at significantly higher risk for developing the same or a related problem either during pregnancy or in the first postpartum year. Even if you have never suffered a mood or anxiety disorder in the past, having a first episode during the childbearing year is possible.

Mood and anxiety disorders are the most common pregnancy complication that American women experience. Estimates range from 10 to 12 percent for the prevalence of depression alone in the childbearing year, and up to 25 to 33 percent for the whole spectrum of mood and anxiety disturbances (for more information about mood and anxiety disorders, see Chapter 14). Do not try to handle these problems on your own. These are often biological, not just psychological, illnesses, and your pregnancy adds an additional biological component to your condition. If you're in pain, ask someone you trust to help you find a competent and compassionate professional to help you.

The long haul

After the first visit, most practitioners will want to see you on approximately the following schedule:

- ✔ Once every three to six weeks through 28 weeks of gestation
- ✔ Once every two to three weeks from 29 to 36 weeks of gestation
- ✔ Once every week from 36 weeks of gestation until the birth of your baby

If you or your baby have any risk factors, have developed complications, or you are carrying multiple babies, your practitioner will want to see you more often.

Between your second appointment and your eighth month, your visits will follow a similar routine. Your practitioner will do the following:

- ✔ Check your weight and test your urine for sugar and protein (these simple urine checks screen for early signs of gestational diabetes and preeclampsia. For more information, see "Complications of Pregnancy").
- ✔ Review the time period since your last visit, determine your baby's weeks of gestation, see how you are feeling, and address any problems or questions you may have.
- ✔ Review your chart and weight gain, check for needed tests, or offer optional ones.
- ✔ Measure your blood pressure and, possibly, check your pulse.
- ✔ Beginning at about 12 weeks, listen through your abdomen for your baby's heart rate.
- ✔ Beginning at about 20 weeks, measure your fundal height, from the top of your pubic bone to the top of your uterus, to assess your baby's growth rate.

Most practitioners perform a routine, in-office blood screen for anemia at one or two points in the pregnancy. Most also routinely screen for gestational diabetes at 24 to 28 weeks (see "Complications of Pregnancy").

In most cases, you do not need to have internal examinations throughout your pregnancy. Your practitioner will want to perform an internal exam as you get closer to your due date, however.

Prenatal Risks and Testing

Pregnancy has its risks, though most mothers and babies come through it well. If you are a typical woman going through pregnancy, your risk of having a child born with a major structural (physical) disability, from any cause, is roughly 4 percent. The risk of having a baby with a milder, correctable structural defect is about 10 to 11 percent.

But finding out ahead of time about these problems is not easy — not even with the most advanced prenatal tests. Further complicating matters, the vast majority of birth defects are not structural at all but involve problems with bodily parts that appear normal but do not work properly. These functional defects account for as much as 85 percent of all birth defects and many of these escape detection until well after birth.

The kinds of risks involved are as varied as people are. Generally, however, the kinds of risks that concern most people fall within one of four groups:

✔ Genetic defects, which cause a wide variety of fundamental disabilities for a fetus, many severe

✔ Environmental hazards, called *teratogens,* which harm an otherwise healthy fetus at some point during or throughout pregnancy

✔ Chronic maternal illnesses, which affect a fetus indirectly through their effects on the mother's ability to support the demands of pregnancy

✔ Complications of pregnancy, in which a healthy mother and baby are endangered by a problem related to the pregnancy itself

Some of the risks and complications that mothers and babies experience are not understood well enough to place them in any one of these groups. For example, miscarriage — which many specialists believe occurs much more often than was once thought — could result from genetic abnormalities or from the effect of an environmental hazard at a critical period or from the indirect effect of a maternal illness. Similarly, well over half of all birth defects have no single, identifiable cause. Here we focus on risks that are reasonably well understood and on ways of managing or minimizing them.

Genetic defects

A *genetic defect* is a disability or group of disabilities caused by an error in the genetic blueprint present within the person's cells — an error that originates before birth. The two basic types of genetic defects you may need to be concerned with are as follows:

✔ **Chromosomal defects:** Errors involving an entire chromosome among the 23 pairs that are formed at the time of conception (see "Genetics: Understanding the basics of reproducing yourself")

✔ **Single-gene defects:** Hereditary defects involving just one, or a few, genes among the thousands passed on from parent to child and contained in each chromosome

Although these problems may concern anyone, some people are at higher risk than others. You should seriously consider genetic counseling and testing if you or your partner

- ✔ Are over age 35
- ✔ Know or suspect you suffer from a genetic disorder or carry a gene for a genetic disorder
- ✔ Have had a previous child with a genetic disorder, birth defect, or mental retardation
- ✔ Know or suspect a member of your family suffers from a genetic disorder or carries a gene for a genetic disorder
- ✔ Have been exposed to any harmful, environmental substances that could increase that chance of a genetic defect occurring in your egg or sperm cells or in the developing fetus

An experienced genetics counselor is the best-qualified person to discuss these problems with you, answer your questions, and help you proceed. Almost all teaching university medical centers have genetics departments, where you can receive counseling and testing. (The sidebar "Genetics: Understanding the basics of reproducing yourself" offers some basic information to get you started.)

Chromosomal defects

Chromosomal abnormalities may originate inside the woman's egg, within her partner's sperm, or when the chromosomes of each combine to form the 23 chromosomal pairs inside the fertilized egg. Many major birth defects and syndromes result from abnormalities involving a chromosome. The most familiar — and most common — of these chromosomal defects is known as *Down syndrome.*

Because Down syndrome is so familiar, many people think it is the only important genetic defect for which to be tested. But there are many different major chromosome-defective syndromes that produce serious disabilities. Some of these syndromes cause disabilities that are so serious that an affected newborn often lives only a few days to a few weeks after birth; others are relatively mild.

Fetal chromosomal abnormalities become more common as you (and your partner) grow older, though it is generally only maternal age that is used in age breakdowns of risk. Presently, chromosomal defects are not treatable or reversible. If you are 35 or older, your doctor may suggest *amniocentesis,* an examination of the amniotic fluid, or chorionic villi sampling (CVS) to test for chromosomal or other genetic abnormalities.

Genetics: Understanding the basics of reproducing yourself

Growing up, people learn that they are "half" their mother and "half" their father, but how does this really work inside a fertilized egg?

Unlike all other cells in our bodies, each of which has 23 pairs of chromosomes, our reproductive cells alone (a woman's *ova*, or eggs, and a man's sperm) each carry half that number — 23 lone, unpaired chromosomes, all looking for a date on a Saturday night.

When an ovum and sperm cell unite, they each contribute their 23 lone chromosomes to create 23 pairs. But unlike the 23 chromosome pairs inside every other cell of the newly conceiving mother's body, each of the 23 pairs inside her fertilized egg contains just half her own body's genetic material, or genes; the other half of each pair is supplied entirely from the genetic material of her partner — genes that his sperm released when it penetrated her egg. And because each pair of chromosomes within the fertilized egg is a balanced mix, every one of the cells that normally develops into a fetus, from this first cell, contain a precise mix of half mom's genes, the other half dad's.

Of these 23 pairs of chromosomes inside the fertilized egg, 22 pairs (known as *autosomes*) appear roughly the same in both males and females and guide every aspect of the developing fetus's characteristics, except his or her gender and sexual characteristics. The twenty-third pair (known as the *sex chromosomes*) alone determines gender. These chromosomes are commonly referred to as the x-x pair in girls, and the x-y pair in boys because of their appearance.

This difference comes about because the woman's sex chromosomes are both "x." The lone (unpaired) chromosome that she contributes within the egg can only be an "x." By contrast, the sperm produced by a man's body can contain either a lone "x" or a lone "y," depending on which half of the sex-chromosome pair ended up in any one particular sperm cell. Consequently, the man's genetic contribution to the fertilized egg determines the gender of the resulting fetus.

Hereditary defects

Other genetically determined birth defects result from a defect of one (or two or several) gene contained within one of the chromosomes. The occurrence of hereditary defects are unaffected by your age but instead have a predictable, mathematical probability of causing a defect in your offspring. These defects do not occur within just the egg or sperm cell, but are present in the genetic blueprint within every cell of the affected parent, and are passed on from parent to child.

So, identifying whether your baby may be at risk for one of these defects can start by having a blood screening done on yourself and/or your partner. Depending on the disorder, one or both of you need to test positive for your baby to have a risk of inheriting that disorder. If one of you does test positive, you are identified as a carrier of the particular disorder. *Carriers* are people who carry a defective gene within one of their chromosomes, even though the gene does not cause the abnormality to be expressed (or manifested) in those individuals themselves.

If you or your partner has a hereditary disorder or is a carrier, finding out whether your baby has inherited the disorder requires prenatal genetic testing. In some disorders, both partners have to be carriers of the same defect in order for the illness to be expressed in one of their offspring (*autosomal recessive conditions*). In others, even when only one partner carries the defect, the condition has a 50:50 chance of affecting a child (*autosomal dominant conditions*). Many other conditions have more complex patterns of inheritance. And in the case of a great many single-gene defects, multiple other factors also come into the picture. In these cases, prenatal genetic testing may not always be able to answer whether your baby will develop the disorder in question.

All in all, several thousand hereditary and multifactorial genetic conditions have been identified, with the number increasing steadily. Just how common or how serious any particular condition is varies widely. A genetics counselor is most able to help you in this area. Currently, no method is available for correcting genetic defects before conception. However, methods are available for extremely early embryo testing so that you will know at an early stage whether your embryo is likely to have inherited a defect.

Prenatal testing

Four prenatal tests are currently in wide use throughout the United States to screen for fetal abnormalities. The first three tests are used specifically to screen for genetic defects:

- **Triple screen:** The least invasive of these tests is also known as the "alpha plus" or "multiple marker." This test, which is performed on the mother between the 16th and 21st weeks of pregnancy, screens the levels of three substances in the blood; obstetricians widely encourage this test as a relatively simple tool for learning whether a fetus may be at higher risk for either a chromosomal abnormality or a neural tube defect. The three substances measured are present in particular concentrations in the mother's blood when a fetus is healthy. If the test shows that any of these substances are present at higher or lower concentrations than expected, this may indicate a genetic (such as Down syndrome) or neural tube (such as spina bifida) abnormality. But each of these three substances changes in concentration from week to week during pregnancy, and gestational age is difficult to determine. In addition, the triple-screen blood test cannot screen for specific genetic or chromosomal abnormalities. It only provides an indication of a higher likelihood that some type of abnormality exists, when one or more of the three levels is outside the expected range.

✔ **Amniocentesis:** Amnio is usually performed between 14 and 16 weeks after your last menstrual period in order to make possible earlier decisions about pregnancy termination. An amnio is performed under ultrasound guidance and involves the insertion of a needle through the mother's abdominal wall, uterine wall, and into the amniotic sac of the fetus, in order to remove a small sample of amniotic fluid containing the fetus' cells. These cells are then studied to detect any chromosomal or hereditary genetic defects. In addition, an amnio can usually detect neural tube defects, as well as some other nongenetic birth defects. But amniocentesis is invasive and carries some risks. Midtrimester amniocentesis (at 15 to 16 weeks) usually is said to have about a 1 in 200 (0.5 percent) risk of serious complications, such as infection, maternal bleeding, miscarriage, fetal injury, or, rarely, fetal death.

✔ **Chorionic villi sampling:** CVS is performed earlier in pregnancy than amniocentesis — generally between the 9th and 11th weeks of pregnancy. CVS, like amnio, is performed with the guidance of ultrasound imaging. A catheter is inserted, either through the vagina and cervix or through the abdominal wall by using a needle, into the chorionic villus tissue, which lies between the amniotic sac and the uterine wall and later develops into the placenta. A small sample of cells are removed, and then studied to learn about the genetic attributes of the growing fetus. CVS can identify chromosomal and hereditary defects; however, it cannot detect neural tube defects. CVS has only been performed in the United States since 1983. But so far, statistics indicate the risk of miscarriage following the procedure runs about 1 percent. Other potential risks include uterine cramping, spotting, and amniotic fluid leakage into the vagina.

Amniocentesis or CVS cannot usually detect environmentally induced birth defects. The impact of many defects, which are not structural, but functional, can only be identified after birth when a baby's or child's functional development can be observed and charted. An ultrasound can sometimes identify when a teratogen does produce a structural defect, though.

✔ **Ultrasound:** Also called sonogram, this test is most common and familiar of the prenatal tests. It cannot actually identify genetic defects specifically, although it does allow your doctor to observe for evidence of structural (physical) abnormalities.

Ultrasound imaging is produced by bouncing sound waves off the physical structures of your baby's body within your uterus. A transducer, which is moved back and forth across the outside of your abdomen, emits these ultra high-frequency sound waves. A computer then analyzes the returning echoes of sound, constructing a picture (sonogram) of the physical structures that are present. Ultrasound imaging has no known risks or complications.

Although you need to know that each of these tests is available to you, genetics testing is a very personal decision. Ideally, it should be undertaken only after thorough discussion with your partner, as well as detailed discussion with your doctor or a genetics counselor about the specific purpose of any proposed test, its risks, benefits, the actions you may or may not want to take based on the test's results, and possible medical consequences of the procedure for you and your baby.

Environmental hazards

Even under the best conditions, living cells occasionally make errors when they copy their genetic blueprint for passing on to new cells. But these errors, which cause genes to mutate, can occur more frequently when conditions are not the best — when the cells are stressed by hazardous environmental agents, referred to by medical specialists as *teratogens*. A wide variety of teratogens can be harmful to a developing fetus, some are more dangerous than others, and many are particularly damaging during specific periods in your unborn baby's development. Major teratogens for a developing fetus include the following:

- Alcohol you consume during pregnancy, as well as "recreational" drugs you use

- Cigarettes or secondhand smoke

- Infections that you contract or that are active during your pregnancy

- Hazardous chemicals, fumes, industrial pollutants, and radiation (x-rays), as well as radioactive substances you may be exposed to

- Dietary chemical exposures, including herbicide and pesticide residues in plant food sources, trace steroids or antibiotics in animal food sources, and trace metals found in some seafood, caffeine, and, possibly, some chemical food additives.

- Some prescription and over-the-counter medicines when taken during pregnancy

You can maximize the odds of a good outcome by reducing your exposure to harmful substances in the environment, following nutritional advice, and taking care of yourself, although "following the rules" does not necessarily guarantee a healthy baby.

It may be helpful to know that, in some cases, environmental factors act cumulatively, so the less total exposure, the lower the risk. But in other cases, the crucial question is when the exposure took place. Some environmental hazards are devastating to a particular system only during a specific critical period. You should know that the first trimester does not hold all the major critical periods for your baby's development as many people believe. Exposure to environmental hazards in the middle or last trimester can be equally damaging to an organ's ability to work the way it should as exposure in the first trimester can be to the proper formation of that organ.

Pregnancy safety hotlines exist in most major cities, where you can call to find out the risks to your baby from exposure to almost any drug, chemical substance, virus, or other agent for which established outcomes are known.

Chronic illnesses and you

Similar to environmental hazards, chronic illness in pregnancy can stress your developing baby either through the indirect effects of the illness or through the impact of drugs or other treatments you must take to manage the illness. Maternal conditions such as diabetes mellitus, epilepsy, high blood pressure, or thyroid disease can lead to fetal problems ranging from heart defects or cleft palate, to poor placental function and fetal growth restriction, to skeletal problems or mental retardation. Asthma, depression, and heart conditions are not associated with known birth defects, but they often involve the use of medication that could pose risks.

Here are some steps that can help keep you and your baby on course:

- ✔ If you are not yet pregnant, consider carefully the risks involved and ask your doctor about managing your condition through pregnancy.

- ✔ Learn all you can about your illness in pregnancy so that you can best know what to expect and plan for it.

- ✔ Consult your nearest teratology hotline for information on the effects of your condition — and of any medications you may need to take — on your baby's prenatal development.

- ✔ Don't deny or minimize your illness; failing to take prescribed medication or treatments because you're concerned about possible teratogenic effects only creates a different risk for your baby — a mother whose health is unstable and cannot take the best possible care of her baby.

- ✔ Pay attention to your body's changes with pregnancy and its effect on your condition; write notes on a calendar to keep track of the changes.

- ✔ Record any medication adjustments or results of medical testing you undergo.

- ✔ Identify your red flags — the early signs and symptoms that warn you of a temporary worsening of your condition — and respond to them.

- ✔ Get your doctors talking to each other when needed so that you're not always having to serve as the messenger between specialists.

Your doctors, as well as any teaching university medical center library or teratology information service, can help you find information about the effects of specific illnesses and their treatments on pregnancy outcomes and longer term child development.

Complications of Pregnancy

Some medical problems can result directly from the continuing progress of your pregnancy, due to physical factors or limitations about your health that never presented a problem until you became pregnant. Other complications are unique to pregnancy and pose no risk apart from it.

Rh incompatibilities

Rh is a type of protein, called an *antigen,* that is on the surface of red blood cells. If a woman's blood does *not* have the Rh antigen (making her blood Rh-negative) and she becomes pregnant with a fetus who carries this antigen from its father (an Rh-positive fetus), problems can arise. When the mother's blood travels to her fetus, the mother's immune system makes antibodies to attack the "foreign," Rh-positive blood, which can result in red blood cell destruction for the fetus, leading to anemia, toxic levels of red blood cell breakdown products, and, in rare cases, even fetal death.

For this reason, pregnant women who are Rh-negative are routinely given a medicine called Rhogam, which fools the immune system and prevents it from making antibodies to destroy Rh-positive blood, at the beginning of the third trimester (28 weeks) and again within 72 hours of birth. If Rhogam is not given and the baby is Rh-positive, the baby must be given a blood transfusion possibly even before birth to replace destroyed red blood cells with Rh-negative blood, which will not be attacked by the mother's antibodies. An Rh screen can be performed with the battery of bloodwork done during the pregnancy to determine whether you may have a problem.

Preeclampsia and eclampsia

Eclampsia and its precursor, *preeclampsia,* are serious complications of pregnancy marked in the early phase by rising maternal blood pressure, headaches, fluid retention, protein in the urine, visual disturbances, and abdominal pain. These symptoms of preeclampsia can ultimately progress into full-blown eclampsia (also called *toxemia*), involving convulsions during or after labor or birth, possible stroke or kidney failure, coma, and, sometimes, death. Eclampsia is also associated with premature separation of the placenta from the walls of the uterus (called *abruptio placentae*), as well as other complications that can cause fetal death.

About 6 percent of pregnant women develop the symptoms of preeclampsia, usually during the third trimester of pregnancy. You are at particular risk if

 ✔ You are a pregnant teenager or are over 40.

> ✔ You have an underlying, chronic medical condition, such as high blood pressure, kidney disease, diabetes mellitus, or another autoimmune disorder, such as lupus or rheumatoid arthritis.
>
> ✔ You have a multiple pregnancy.
>
> ✔ You are experiencing your first pregnancy.

The mechanisms that cause preeclampsia are still not understood, yet, partly due to improving prenatal care, only 0.1 percent of all pregnant women actually go on to develop eclampsia. Because the cause is unknown, the only real treatment is effecting the birth of the baby.

Gestational diabetes

Gestational diabetes, or diabetes of pregnancy, is a condition of abnormally high blood sugar (glucose) levels, which appear for the first time when you are pregnant. (For more information on diabetes, see Chapter 17.)

High maternal blood glucose levels lead to abnormally large growth of the fetus, making vaginal birth more difficult. There is evidence that women who are diabetic before pregnancy not only give birth to larger babies, but are at increased risk for problems such as birth defects, excess amniotic fluid, miscarriage, premature labor, stillbirth, and fetal problems such as imma-ture lung development. The women are also at increased risk of developing diabetes later in life. Gestational diabetes can usually be controlled with diet, but insulin may be required.

Premature labor, placenta previa, and abruptio placentae

Premature labor is any labor that begins before the completion of 37 weeks of gestation. Poor nutrition, heavy smoking, use of recreational drugs or other teratogens, a history of surgery on your cervix or uterus, and mater-nal illness can all predispose your baby to premature birth. Pregnant teens and women carrying multiple fetuses are also vulnerable to premature labor.

Occasionally, premature labor contractions are preceded by vaginal bleed-ing, with or without pain. This can signal one of two serious complications: *placenta previa*, in which the placenta lies low in the uterus and covers (or partly covers) the cervix; or *abruptio placentae*, the premature separation of the placenta from the uterine wall. Both conditions, which can also occur at term, are more common in older women who have had other pregnancies, and abruptio placentae is significantly more common in women with high blood pressure who smoke or use cocaine or who develop eclampsia in their third trimester.

Both conditions can usually be diagnosed with ultrasound if time allows. Sometimes placenta previa resolves on its own. If at the time of delivery, the placenta still covers and blocks the cervix entirely, a cesarean section (c-section) birth is generally necessary (see Chapter 26 for more information about c-sections). Detachment of the placenta may occur if labor starts and the cervix begins to open, cutting off circulation (and oxygen) to the fetus. Abruptio placentae, unless very minor and nonprogressive, often requires rapid delivery or c-section birth to protect the mother from excessive blood loss and the baby from loss of oxygen and nutrients.

Other Risks and Pregnancy Loss

Three other major complications are distinct in that they nearly always lead to loss of a pregnancy and can have other serious health consequences for you, as well. They are

- **Ectopic pregnancy:** Chapter 18 discusses this condition.

- **Molar pregnancy:** A molar pregnancy occurs when the tissues that would normally surround a fertilized egg grows out of control into a clump of tumor cells, instead of develop into the placenta. Without a placenta, the embryo cannot survive, but the clump of tumor cells often continues to grow rapidly. The most important issue is making sure that the entire growth of tumor cells is discharged from the uterus. If any question remains as to whether the entire mole has been expelled from the uterus, a D&C (dilation and curettage) or vacuum aspiration (suction evacuation) procedure of the uterus is done.

- **Miscarriage:** *Miscarriage,* referred to medically as *spontaneous abortion,* is technically defined as any loss of a pregnancy that occurs before the completion of 20 weeks of gestation. The word is commonly used, however, to refer to any pregnancy loss, even in the third trimester. Most specialists now estimate that between 20 and 25 percent of all pregnancies end in miscarriage. In the majority of miscarriages that occur in the first eight weeks of pregnancy, a serious genetic problem exists with the embryo.

A miscarriage that does not expel all the tissues of the fetus and placenta (called an *incomplete abortion*) or one that is accompanied by no bleeding or discharge (called a *missed abortion*) will need to be followed by surgical removal of these tissues.

If you lose a baby to miscarriage, you will need time to heal emotionally, as well as physically. Most doctors recommend waiting at least three menstrual cycles before stopping birth control and trying to become pregnant again.

Chapter 26
Labor and Delivery

● ●

In This Chapter

▶ Determining whether you're in labor

▶ Understanding childbirth interventions

▶ Delivering by cesarean section

▶ Recovering from childbirth

● ●

For roughly nine months you've carried around extra weight and endured a backache, swollen feet, and pressure on your stomach and bladder. Yet the one thought that your mind has likely focused on is your impending labor and delivery. This chapter discusses what your body will go through — both on its own and at the hands of health care professionals — during the three stages of labor and in the weeks following your baby's birth.

Going into Labor?

Contrary to the portrayal of labor in movies, determining when labor begins is not always easy. Some early indicators that labor is imminent are

✔ The gradual descent of the baby into the pelvis (at least for first-time moms)

✔ Increased vaginal discharge

✔ Loss of the mucus plug that acts as a natural barrier at the level of the cervix

✔ Pink or bloody discharge known as "show"

✔ Contractions more intense and frequent than the "practice" contractions of the eighth and ninth month known as Braxton-Hicks

The most obvious sign that there's no going back is the breaking of water. The amniotic membranes that protect the fetus generally burst once labor begins (although in 20 percent of pregnant women they burst before labor begins). If your water breaks, you should phone your birth practitioner immediately, even if you don't feel any contractions. And be sure to note the color of the liquid; your practitioner is likely to ask because a brownish color could indicate fetal distress.

Your practitioner should tell you ahead of time how far apart your contractions should be before you call him. Usually doctors won't send you to the hospital until your contractions are three to five minutes apart for at least one hour unless you have had several babies already or have a history of fast labor. But don't hesitate to call if you're concerned or have questions.

The Stages of Labor

The first stage of labor generally lasts 12 hours for first-time moms, from the moment of the first timeable contraction to full dilation of the *cervix* (the lowermost portion of the uterus). The cervix, which normally has only a very small opening at its center, must dilate, or open, to a width of about 10 centimeters (about 4 inches) to let the baby pass through. (See Figure 26-1.)

Pushing and delivery of the baby are the highlights of the second stage, which averages two hours for the first baby (generally less with subsequent babies), from full dilation to delivery. As you push, your baby makes his or her way down the birth canal, generally head first.

The third stage of labor involves the passage of the *placenta,* or afterbirth, which helped nourish your baby during his or her nine months of development. The placenta is expelled with a few final contractions, though they are far less severe than those required for your baby's exit. This stage lasts about five minutes.

Medical Interventions

If you've opted to give birth in a hospital with a doctor as your birth attendant, you will have a number of choices, called medical interventions, to speed your baby's delivery or ease your labor. Some women are comforted by the use of medical technology and encourage it. Others prefer a more "natural" childbirth with little outside assistance.

Considering all these possibilities and discussing them thoroughly with your doctor long before your labor begins is important. Your doctor needs to know your preferences. Some women even prepare a birth plan, detailing

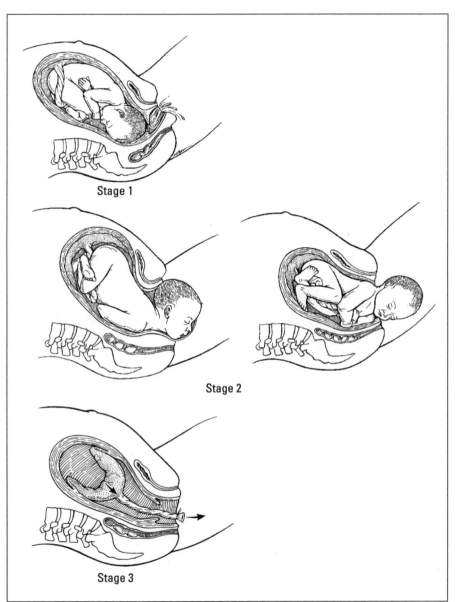

Stage 1

Stage 2

Stage 3

Figure 26-1:
The stages
of labor.

what procedures they will and will not condone. Although you may feel confident that you've negotiated every aspect of your labor and delivery with your doctor, be prepared to have your plan thrown out the window in the event of an emergency, or if you discover labor's unpredictability.

The following sections present the most common childbirth interventions.

Inducement

Doctors *induce* or *augment* labor in approximately one in three deliveries, when, for any number of reasons, it is decided to help out Mother Nature. Inducing labor means starting the process when you're not yet in labor. Augmenting means making labor contractions that have already begun stronger and more efficient.

The hormone *oxytocin* (Pitocin) is the primary medication used to induce or augment labor. It is administered intravenously, and the dose is controlled until contractions are regular.

A less-controlled method of inducing labor is to break a woman's water, or amniotic membranes. This procedure is known as *amniotomy*. Once the water is broken, labor usually starts within 12 hours. The membrane is broken with a surgical instrument.

Fetal monitoring

Once reserved for high-risk pregnancies, the use of an electronic fetal monitor is now quite common. This monitor measures uterine contractions and fetal heart rate to track how the fetus is handling labor. External monitors are strapped to the woman's abdomen. Some monitors are portable and allow a woman to walk during labor. Others may be removed between readings to allow the woman some freedom. Internal monitors, which are attached to the part of the baby that is exiting first, are considered more accurate, but they eliminate some of a woman's mobility during labor.

Although some hospitals electronically monitor all births, others monitor only those women with high-risk pregnancies, women who are having a difficult labor, or fetuses who appear to be in distress.

Epidurals and other drugs

Your mother or grandmother may tell you that she was unconscious during the delivery of her children. For generations, physicians typically anesthetized laboring women to eliminate their pain. In the 1950s and 1960s, however, women began to take charge and demand to fully participate in childbirth. Today, the choices for pain relief are quite varied, and women are the primary decision makers when it comes to accepting a drug.

Women who just can't tolerate the agony of labor or whose long labor is causing stress (which affects contractions and may limit the ability to push) may benefit from pain medication. Various narcotics are available. However, you should be aware of the potential side effects of pain medications before labor begins so that you can make an informed decision when the time comes.

In other cases, local or regional anesthesia is used. Both types of anesthesia involve the injection of a numbing medication. Local anesthesia is used to numb a specific area (such as the *perineum* — the area between the vagina and anus), while regional anesthesia is used to numb a larger area — generally the lower half of the body.

The most widely used form of regional anesthesia is the lumbar epidural, which has gained in popularity because of the ease of administration and the relative safety for both mother and child. Administered through a needle in the back, the epidural blocks pain from the point of insertion down through the woman's legs, while leaving her mentally alert.

Episiotomy

A laboring mother may gladly accept pain medication, but she is less likely to ask for an *episiotomy,* an incision made in the perineal tissue toward the anus in order to enlarge the vagina. Episiotomies are performed more frequently in first births to make extra room for the baby's head.

Forceps delivery

Occasionally a baby becomes stuck in the birth canal, resulting in fetal and maternal distress and a prolonged labor that pushing alone cannot rectify. In these instances, when the baby is near the vaginal opening, *forceps* — metal instruments resembling spoons — are inserted and placed around the baby's head to guide him through the birth canal. Infants who are stuck very high in the birth canal are brought into the world by cesarean delivery.

Complications of a forceps delivery are lacerations and bleeding in the mother and bruising or, very rarely, skull fracture for the baby. The mother will also need an episiotomy and likely will require pain medication.

Vacuum extraction

An alternative to forceps is the vacuum extractor. In this procedure, a suction cup is placed on the baby's head and a vacuum is created to ease the baby through the birth canal. Complications are similar to those with forceps deliveries.

Cesarean Section

A very common medical intervention, and one that you may be concerned about, is the cesarean-section delivery. Because approximately one in five babies delivered in the United States is delivered via cesarean section (c-section), it is a process you should understand, be prepared for, and discuss with your doctor. If you seek to deliver your baby vaginally, look for a doctor and hospital with low rates of cesareans who are willing to try alternatives.

A *c-section* is a surgical procedure in which the woman's abdomen is cut open for removal of the baby. In most cases, it is as safe as a vaginal delivery for the baby. The controversy centers on the necessity of c-sections and their safety for the mother.

When is a c-section necessary?

A c-section is not always called for in the following instances, but your chances of having one are more likely if any of them apply to you:

- You've had a previous c-section, and the reason for that c-section (an abnormally small pelvis, for example) still exists.

  Although experts once believed that any woman who has had one c-section must always deliver that way, newer studies show that women can deliver vaginally in subsequent pregnancies about 80 percent of the time.

- Your baby's presentation is *breech* (bottom or feet first) or *transverse* (lying across the pelvic opening, neither head nor feet first) instead of the normal head-first presentation.

- Your labor does not progress despite augmentation procedures.

- You're expecting more than one baby.

- You have a serious condition, such as *placenta previa* (when the placenta blocks the opening of the cervix), *abruptio placentae* (separation of the placenta from the uterine wall), or active herpes.

- Your baby's head is too big to pass through your pelvis.

- The fetus is in distress as evidenced by an abnormal heart rate on the monitor or on an ultrasound.

What you should ask your doctor

If you are concerned about the possibility of undergoing a cesarean section, express your concerns to your doctor. And make sure that you know her stance on the issue. Here are some questions to ask:

✔ **What is your c-section rate?** Seek out a doctor with a rate less than the 21 percent national average.

✔ **In the event my labor stalls, what alternatives are you willing to try before calling for surgery?** A doctor should consider allowing you to try different birthing positions, get some rest, or even give labor a nudge with some oxytocin.

✔ **What is your experience with vaginal breech deliveries, vaginal births after** previous cesareans, large babies, and any other "abnormal" factors?

✔ **If the baby is breech, would you try turning it before labor begins so as to avoid a c-section?**

✔ **What kind of pain medications and anesthesia do you use?** Will I be awake to watch the birth?

✔ **May my husband or coach be present for the delivery whether I am awake or not?**

✔ **Will I be able to hold and nurse my baby right after surgery?**

✔ **What length of recovery do you expect for an uncomplicated c-section?**

Postpartum

Once you force that wrinkled little baby into the world, you'll breathe a sigh of relief. But don't think you're going to jump up, put on a pair of your prepregnancy jeans and run out to the mall. Your body has had 40 weeks of pregnancy and several hours or days of labor trauma to contend with. Recovery takes as long as six weeks, and you may still have physical issues to resolve as much as a year from now.

Viewing the new you

When you were pregnant, you may have had a glow about you. Now, you may have bloodshot eyes and small broken veins in your face from pushing. Sitting or walking straight may be tough because of sore muscles and even sorer incisions. And where once you had a full, round belly, a gelatinous blob now taunts you.

Your hair may begin to fall out — in clumps — to make up for the shining, full head of hair you had throughout pregnancy. Don't worry. It will grow back.

Moving forward: Your body's still working

The blood and tissue that nourished and housed your baby doesn't just disappear overnight. You will bleed for several days as your body rids itself of what is no longer necessary. The heavy, bright red discharge will subside and gradually turn brownish, but it will taper for up to six weeks.

You may notice some periodlike cramping, particularly when you nurse if you're breast-feeding. These are small contractions that help eliminate some of the discharge and quickly shrink the uterus back to its normal size.

Your doctor will give you a list of activities that you must put on hold until your postpartum checkup in four to six weeks. Sex is out. So are dieting and rigorous exercise. Walking, however, is acceptable and even encouraged.

Recovering from a c-section

Except for not having a rather sore vaginal area, many of the recovery symptoms for cesarean delivery are the same as those for a vaginal delivery. You'll have that periodlike cramping, bloody discharge, and hormonal changes. However, you'll also be recovering from a surgery, which means dealing with care of an incision, additional pain, and more physical limitations.

After your anesthesia wears off, you may want to accept the offer of pain medication.

You'll also be instructed to regularly hold a pillow to your belly and cough up mucus to prevent pneumonia from developing in your lungs. The pillow helps brace the incision so that coughing is less painful. You'll be encouraged to walk around to maintain good circulation.

You'll be instructed not to lift anything heavy, meaning over 25 pounds, for the first four to six weeks.

Crying, crying, crying

You probably expect some high-pitched wails from your newborn, but many new mothers find themselves sobbing uncontrollably at the drop of a hat. You may find it's not all that different than the hormonal roller coaster you rode in on nine months ago. Don't panic. Your levels of progesterone and estrogen, no longer needed to support your pregnancy, have plummeted, wreaking havoc with your emotions.

That said, keep a handle on your emotional state. Your hormonal episodes may easily turn into a mild form of depression known as the *baby blues*. This type of depression is quite common — it's estimated that between 50 to 75 percent of postpartum moms feel mildly depressed. Postpartum depression may begin in the first week, though it occasionally can turn up months later. Mild temporary depression generally doesn't require treatment and will simply go away on its own. The symptoms of postpartum depression include anxiety or panic attacks, extreme mood swings, feelings of inadequacy, feelings of anger toward the baby or partner, insomnia or excessive fatigue, lack of interest in the baby, lack of interest in sex, uncontrollable crying, and withdrawal from partner and friends.

If your depression persists for more than two weeks and you're having trouble sleeping (without help from your newborn), are not interested in food, seek medical help. If you are feeling aggressive toward your baby or feel suicidal, seek help immediately. Counseling is in order for women suffering from severe postpartum depression.

Breast-feeding

You have many options in raising your child, and one of the first is whether to breast-feed. In fact, this is one decision you should make before your baby is born.

Benefits and disadvantages of breast-feeding

The American Academy of Pediatrics now recommends breast-feeding infants for the first year of life. In making this recommendation, the Academy cites studies showing breast-fed babies are healthier and breast-feeding mothers recover more quickly from delivery and are less likely to develop breast cancer.

Breast milk contains 100 ingredients not found in cow's milk that cannot be completely duplicated in commercial formulas. Breast milk is also more digestible, meaning less infant constipation. And breast milk contains *antibodies,* immune system components that protect babies against a wide range of disease-causing bacteria and viruses — protection that recent research indicates may extend into childhood and even adulthood.

Experts say that almost all new moms can breast-feed. A breast-feeding woman should eat an extra 500 calories per day — while maintaining a healthy diet — to maintain proper milk production. She also should consume at least eight 8-ounce glasses of water each day.

If you breast-feed, your baby needs no water, formula, or solid food for the first four to six months: Breast milk is enough. It's also recommended that you not give your baby a bottle until she is four weeks old. The change in nipple can confuse her. (Make sure the hospital staff knows that you don't want your baby getting a bottle in the nursery.)

The only real disadvantage to breast-feeding is the extra work it places on the mother because all feedings are her responsibility. And because babies digest human milk more quickly than they do formula, breast-fed babies require more frequent feedings. As a result, breast-feeding mothers can become exhausted and stressed out. They can also experience sore breasts, clothing soiled by leaking milk, and infection of the breast (for more information on breast infection, see Chapter 19).

One way to diminish the stress and allow others in the family to take part in feeding is to allow dad to burp and comfort the baby after each feeding. Another solution is to express milk from the breast with a small pump, allowing others to take over some feedings.

Contrary to popular belief, breast-feeding is not a perfect form of contraception. Although a woman may not ovulate as soon after delivery if she is nursing, she still may ovulate before ever having any menstrual bleeding. Given this uncertainty, another form of birth control is recommended.

How is it done?

According to lactation experts, breast-feeding for the first time within an hour of delivery is crucial to the learning process. At this point, the baby is getting only *colostrum*, a clear, yellowish liquid that's packed with nutrients and antibodies.

Before you breast-feed, wash your hands because you may need to stick a finger in your child's mouth to break the suction around your nipple.

Get into a comfortable position. Use several pillows to support your arm and the baby. You can hold the baby in three basic holds, though you may discover more as you and your baby adapt to the process.

- ✔ **Front hold:** Cradle your baby's head in the crook of your arm, then roll her toward you so that she's lying on her side, her belly to your chest.

- ✔ **Football hold:** Tuck your baby's head under your arm so that her legs are behind you and her head is at your breast; support her head on your lap.

- ✔ **Lying down:** Both you and your baby should lie on your sides, her tummy facing your chest. Offer her the breast closest to the mattress.

Tickle the baby's lips. Instinctively, the baby will open her mouth. Then guide your nipple and some of the areola (the pigmented area around the nipple) into her mouth (see Figure 26-2). Milk comes from the ducts surrounding the nipple, so just sucking on the nipple does no good.

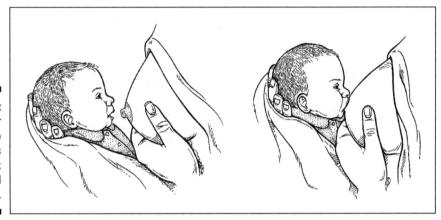

Figure 26-2:
Guide your nipple to your baby's mouth; she will latch on.

After your baby latches on, your nipple is pressed against the roof of her mouth and her tongue is under the nipple. Her bottom lip is rolled out.

To disengage your sucking baby, place a finger in the corner of her mouth to break the suction.

It's generally recommended that you use both breasts at each feeding, burping your baby when you switch and when you're finished. Your baby will often nurse from 15 to 40 minutes at a time and will let you know when she's had enough. You're likely to nurse as many as 10 to 12 times per day.

If your breasts get too full (you'll know this because they will feel like they are about to burst), try the following:

✔ Breast-feed every two to three hours around the clock.

✔ Take a hot shower or place warm washcloths on your breasts before feeding.

✔ Express some milk with a pump or by hand if they still are full at the end of a feeding.

The pumping option

If you're returning to work or you just need some time to yourself, you can collect breast milk and store it for use by someone else while you're away. You can pump your breasts by hand, but if collecting breast milk is going to be a regular occurrence, you may consider a pump. Several electric and battery-operated pumps also are on the market. For information on pumping methods, contact the local chapter of the La Leche League.

Breast milk is safe at room temperature for a few hours; however, immediate refrigeration is recommended. You can store fresh milk in the refrigerator up to 72 hours. You may store frozen milk in the back of the freezer portion of a refrigerator-freezer for up to six months or in a -20 degree Celsius deep freezer for up to 12 months. Once defrosted, store the milk in the refrigerator and make sure that it is consumed within 24 hours.

Freeze breast milk in 2- to 4-ounce portions — they thaw more quickly. To defrost milk, place it in the refrigerator overnight or under warm running water. NEVER microwave breast milk; it can change the milk's composition and may burn your baby.

The Formula Option

Some women can't nurse their babies because of a physical ailment or prior breast surgery or because of a problem with the baby. Others try but run into pain and infections that make breast-feeding stressful. Still others simply prefer to bottle feed.

If you plan to feed your baby formula, ask your practitioner to recommend the formula that is best for your baby. Most formulas are made from cow's milk, which may not be suitable for all infants. Infants who have difficulty digesting cow's milk-based formulas or who are allergic to them may benefit from soy-based formulas.

Formula comes in three forms: prepared formula that is ready for use, liquid concentrate that must be diluted with water, and powdered formula that must be mixed with water. If you use either the liquid or powdered formula, be sure to follow the mixing instructions to ensure that your baby is getting the right amounts of the nutrients he or she needs.

Part VI
The Part of Tens

"Sandy says she's *going* to work on her cat-cow. Sounds more like a science experiment than a yoga posture to me."

In this part . . .

If you're expecting David Letterman-style humor, you've come to the wrong place. We take our top ten list seriously — and more practically give you ten questions to ask a prospective childbirth practitioner, ten ways to make a gynecologic exam more comfortable, and ten medical Web sites that are useful for women.

Chapter 27

Ten Questions to Ask a Prospective Childbirth Practitioner

- -

In This Chapter

▶ Checking qualifications

▶ Costing out maternity care

▶ Finding a practitioner who meets your needs

▶ Determining a practitioner's M.O.

- -

*I*f you're expecting, or hope to be, choosing a childbirth practitioner is among the first of many important decisions that await you. As Chapter 24 discusses, choosing a practitioner who is in tune with your individual wants and needs is important. Here are ten questions that can help you narrow your search.

What Are Your Credentials?

Your search for a childbirth practitioner, like your search for any other health care practitioner, should begin with a basic background check. If you're looking for a physician — perhaps an obstetrician or a family practitioner — you want know whether she holds a medical degree, is board certified, or has undergone any specialized or postgraduate study. You also want to know how long the practitioner has been in practice and whether she has staff privileges at the hospital or birth center of your choice. If you're looking for a nurse-midwife, you want to know whether she's been certified by the American College of Nurse-Midwives and whether she is licensed to practice in your state. You also want to know whether she practices at the hospital or birth center of your choice.

How Much Does Maternity Care and Delivery Cost?

Costs for normal maternity care and delivery vary significantly from practitioner to practitioner and region to region. No matter where you live, having a baby is a big investment. And although you don't want to put a price on your child's head, cost is an issue you may want to consider when choosing a birth practitioner. Ask those you are considering what they charge for normal prenatal care and delivery and what that fee covers. Make sure that any fee includes office visits and routine lab work. Ask how the fee must be paid. Is a fee schedule or payment plan available? And find out whether your insurance is accepted and what it covers.

How Frequent and How Long Are Appointments?

You want to know how frequently your practitioner expects to see you and also how long visits will last. Make sure to ask how long the typical wait is. Like other doctors, some childbirth practitioners overbook, or schedule too many appointments in too short a time frame. The results of this practice may include hurried consultations and long waits. If you want to make the most of your visits and your time is valuable to you, you will want to know whether overbooking is the case with the practitioners you are considering.

What Prenatal Tests and Procedures Do You Recommend?

As Chapter 25 details, you can choose from quite a few prenatal tests and procedures, and you may wish to undergo some and not others. Knowing your prospective birth practitioner's take on these can help you narrow your decision.

Do You Encourage Breast-Feeding?

If you intend to breast-feed your child, you'll want to know whether your childbirth practitioner supports the practice. Although most doctors aren't experts in breast-feeding, particularly not in the area of "how-to" advice, if you plan to breast-feed, their support can be helpful — particularly if you want to breast-feed immediately after birth. (For more discussion of breast-feeding, check out Chapter 26.)

What Method of Childbirth Preparation Do You Prefer and Why?

If you've not yet decided what type of childbirth preparation method is right for you, discussing the options available to you with your prospective practitioner may help you make that decision. If you have already made up your mind on this important issue, you'll want to know whether your prospective practitioner supports your decision. (Check out Chapter 24 for more information about childbirth preparation methods.)

What Is Your Cesarean Section Rate?

If you want to avoid a cesarean section, look for a practitioner with a range of 7.6 to 12 percent. Ask what criteria she follows in deciding whether to deliver by cesarean. Does she hold the now-outdated belief that after a woman has delivered by cesarean, all her future deliveries must also be by cesarean?

How Often Do You Use Intervention Methods During Labor?

If you prefer a childbirth with as few interventions as possible, you want to know in what percentage of births your prospective practitioner induces labor, performs episiotomies, or uses forceps or vacuum extraction. (Chapter 26 contains more details about childbirth interventions.)

Do You Routinely Use Drugs to Manage Pain During Labor?

Whether you want a drug-free delivery or the assurance of pain relief, you want to ask your prospective childbirth practitioner this question. You also want to know what medications — analgesic or anesthetic — she generally uses. (Chapter 26 outlines the different options for medication.)

Do You Encourage Trying Different Birthing Positions?

If you're flexible in this area, you want a practitioner who is flexible, too. You want a practitioner who will let you give birth in the position that is most comfortable for you — not in the position that is most convenient for him. And walking and squatting have been known to shorten labor in some women, so a practitioner who encourages you to try a different position may be less likely to use childbirth interventions. (For more information on birthing positions, see Chapter 24.)

Chapter 28

Ten Ways to Make a Gynecologic Exam More Comfortable

In This Chapter

▶ Finding a doctor you trust
▶ Understanding what's going on
▶ Doing what you can for yourself

*N*o wonder no woman looks forward to having a gynecologic exam. You're in a very vulnerable position. You can't see what's happening. You may be nervous. You may feel sensations that are unfamiliar to you. And when your practitioner performs a Pap test or breast exam, you are forced to confront the reality of life-threatening diseases such as breast cancer and cervical cancer.

But those screening procedures may save your life. Regular gynecologic exams may detect sexually transmitted diseases and other problems early on, before they lead to sterility and other complications. In short, regular gynecologic exams are an important part of ensuring your fertility, reducing your chances of complications during pregnancy and childbirth, and increasing your chance of catching female cancers early. So, the discomfort is not without reward.

That said, this chapter discusses ways to make the exam more comfortable.

Choose Your Practitioner Carefully

You already know how important it is to choose a health care practitioner who is qualified, available, and who meets your needs as a health care consumer. You want to find a practitioner with whom you feel comfortable. The comfort factor is even more important when it comes to choosing the practitioner who will perform your gynecologic exam. After all, this person sees and hears what few others will. Can you trust this person with the more intimate aspects of your anatomy and life? If you're not comfortable with your practitioner, your exam may be off to an uncomfortable start.

Consider Your Practitioner's Gender

Gender may come into play in your choice of a health care practitioner to perform a gynecologic exam. Although you can find qualified practitioners of both genders, some women are uncomfortable having a man perform their gynecologic exam and may find talking about the intimate aspects of their life easier with a female rather than a male practitioner. Gender is purely a matter of personal preference, but it can influence your level of comfort during the exam. If you're uncomfortable with the idea of a male practitioner, choose a woman. If you're comfortable with either gender, choose the practitioner you are most comfortable with who has the qualifications to treat any specific condition you may have. *Remember:* You can always request the presence of a female nurse during the exam if that makes you feel more comfortable.

Know What to Expect

Knowing what will happen during your exam can be of great comfort — especially if this visit is your first-ever gynecologic exam, your first exam with a new practitioner, or an exam in which you will experience a procedure for the first time. (If you've never had a gynecologic exam, see Chapter 2 for an explanation of what happens during one.) If this visit is your first exam with a new practitioner, ask her or her staff in advance what procedures she follows. If you're undergoing a new procedure, read about it or ask about it when you schedule the exam. *Remember:* You can't see much of what is going on during the exam. Knowing what is going to occur and how it will feel may ease your mind.

Consider Taking Someone with You

If this visit is your first gynecologic exam or you have had a bad experience in the past, you may feel more comfortable if you have your mother, partner, or a close friend with you to offer moral support during the exam. Be aware, however, that having another person with you may in some way compromise your ability to ask questions or speak freely with your practitioner about your symptoms or experiences.

Empty Your Bladder

A gynecologic exam can put pressure on your bladder, making you feel the need to urinate. To prevent this discomfort, visit the restroom before you visit the examining room. First, however, inquire whether your doctor may want a urine sample to analyze in case of a bladder infection. If you are having symptoms such as pain with urination or going to the bathroom frequently, let the doctor or nurse know before you empty your bladder.

Ask Questions

If you have any questions — about the procedures to be performed, about why certain procedures are being performed, or about your reproductive health in general — ask before the exam begins. The exam will be a much more positive experience for you if you have an open conversation with your practitioner and leave with your questions answered.

Ask Your Practitioner to Give You a Play-by-Play

Because most of your reproductive system is internal, you'll be unable to see what's happening during much of the exam. And even if you know what to expect, you may not know what is happening at any given point unless you are told. Ask your practitioner to let you know what she's doing as it is happening.

Ask Your Practitioner to Take Comfort Measures

Your practitioner can do a lot of little things to make you more comfortable during the exam. For example, she can put cloth covers over the metal stirrups to keep your feet warm or warm the speculum (an instrument shaped like a duckbill with a handle) before she inserts it into your vagina. And if you have a smaller vagina, she may be able to use a smaller speculum. If you're concerned about the size of the instrument, ask your practitioner to show it to you. Ask her whether it's the smallest available, and ask her to agree to withdraw it if you experience any pain.

Try to Relax

Some women experience pressure in the bladder or rectum when the speculum is in place. If you relax your muscles, you can relieve this pressure and make your rectal exam less uncomfortable. Take deep slow breaths and relax your muscles, particularly those in your hips, between your legs and your abdomen. And try to think of something pleasant, such as lying on the beach or sitting on a mountain top.

Remember That You Are in Charge

Although you may feel as though you are in a vulnerable position during a gynecologic exam, you are still in control. Let your practitioner know whether anything is too uncomfortable or painful. Ask any questions you have. Remove the drape sheet, if you wish, to see your practitioner's face. And remember that you can stop the examination if you feel it is necessary.

Also warn your practitioner in advance if you have had any past experiences that may make this exam especially uncomfortable such as a history of sexual abuse. Most doctors will be far more patient with you if you warn them in advance.

Chapter 29

Ten Best Medical Web Sites to Visit

*T*hese days, you don't have to leave your house to amass quite a bit of health information. If you have a computer and access to the Internet, a world of information is at your fingertips — from basic information about individual conditions to detailed articles from medical journals.

This chapter gives you ten of the best health and medical Web sites for women.

Health Finder

www.healthfinder.gov

Maintained by the Department of Health and Human Services, this Web site provides a wealth of information on health care resources, including several pages devoted exclusively to women. These include pages on hot topics, support groups, and the women's communities page, which provides resources for women in various roles and lifestyles, including mothers and retirees.

PubMed

www.ncbi.nlm.nih.gov/PubMed

Sponsored by the National Library of Medicine, this site provides free access to the 9 million citations in the library's MEDLINE database, which references articles published in nearly 4,000 medical journals.

Physician Select

www.ama-assn.org/aps/amahg.htm

Maintained by the American Medical Association, Physician Select provides the name, address, education, specialty, and board certification of most U.S. doctors.

The National Institutes of Health

www.nih.gov/health

This site, sponsored by the National Institutes of Health, serves as a gateway to a variety of governmental health information resources.

The National Women's Health Information Center

www.4woman.org

A service of the U.S. Public Health Service's Office on Women's Health, this site provides a gateway to a vast array of federal and other women's health information resources. The center also maintains a toll-free information referral line (800-994-WOMAN; TDD: 800-220-5446) from 9 a.m. to 5 p.m. EST Monday through Friday for people without Internet access.

The Women's Health Initiative

www.nhlbi.nih.gov/nhlbi/whi1/

This site provides information about the Women's Health Initiative, a large, ongoing study focusing on the major causes of death, disability, and frailty in postmenopausal women. This 15-year research program is sponsored by the National Institutes of Health and the National Heart, Lung, and Blood Institute.

American Medical Women's Association Health Topics

www.amwa-doc.org

This site, sponsored by an organization of doctors dedicated to women's health, provides information about a variety of different medical issues of interest to women, including thyroid conditions, the effects of smoking, and keeping your skin, hair, and nails healthy.

The American Heart Association's Women's Web Site

www.women.americanheart.org

This site provides detailed information on heart disease and stroke, including statistics and risks unique to women. In addition, the site provides tips for keeping your heart healthy.

The Women's Cancer Network Site

www.wcn.org/

Sponsored by the Society of Gynecologic Oncologists, this site provides information about gynecologic cancer, as well as referrals to gynecologic specialists. The site offers the latest news about cancer research and includes a survey that helps you assess your personal risk level for various cancers.

CancerNET

www.cancernet.nci.nih.gov/

This site, sponsored by the National Cancer Institute, provides fact sheets, news, information on cancer prevention, screening, treatment, and ongoing clinical trials, as well as a bibliographic database.

Index

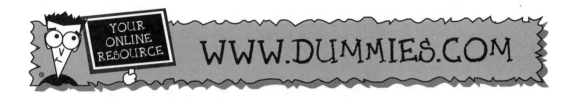

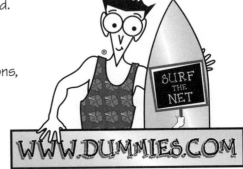

IDG BOOKS WORLDWIDE BOOK REGISTRATION

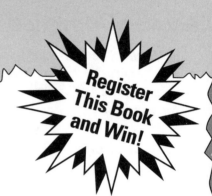

Register This Book and Win!

We want to hear from you!

Visit **http://my2cents.dummies.com** to register this book and tell us how you liked it!

✔ Get entered in our monthly prize giveaway.

✔ Give us feedback about this book — tell us what you like best, what you like least, or maybe what you'd like to ask the author and us to change!

✔ Let us know any other *...For Dummies*® topics that interest you.

Your feedback helps us determine what books to publish, tells us what coverage to add as we revise our books, and lets us know whether we're meeting your needs as a *...For Dummies* reader. You're our most valuable resource, and what you have to say is important to us!

Not on the Web yet? It's easy to get started with *Dummies 101*®: *The Internet For Windows*® *98* or *The Internet For Dummies*®, 5th Edition, at local retailers everywhere.

Or let us know what you think by sending us a letter at the following address:

...For Dummies Book Registration
Dummies Press
7260 Shadeland Station, Suite 100
Indianapolis, IN 46256-3945
Fax 317-596-5498

™

BESTSELLING
BOOK SERIES